ADVANCES IN SURGICAL PATHOLOGY:
LUNG CANCER

ADVANCES IN SURGICAL PATHOLOGY SERIES

Series Editors: Philip T. Cagle, MD, and Timothy Craig Allen, MD, JD

Advances in Surgical Pathology: Lung Cancer
Philip T. Cagle and Timothy Craig Allen, *2010*

Advances in Surgical Pathology: Gastric Cancer
Dongfeng Tan and Gregory Y. Lauwers, *2010*

Advances in Surgical Pathology: Endometrial Cancer
Anna Sienko, *2011*

Advances in Surgical Pathology: Malignant Mesothelioma
Richard Attanoos, *2012*

Advances in Surgical Pathology: Prostate Cancer
Jae Y. Ro, Steven S. Shen and Alberto G. Ayala, *2012*

ADVANCES IN SURGICAL PATHOLOGY:
LUNG CANCER

SERIES EDITORS

Philip T. Cagle, MD
Professor of Pathology
Weill Medical College of Cornell
    University
New York, New York
Director, Pulmonary Pathology
The Methodist Hospital
Houston, Texas

Timothy Craig Allen, MD, JD
Professor of Pathology
Chairman, Department of Pathology
The University of Texas Health Science
    Center at Tyler
Tyler, Texas

BOOK AUTHORS

Philip T. Cagle, MD
Professor of Pathology
Weill Medical College of Cornell University
New York, New York
Director, Pulmonary Pathology
The Methodist Hospital
Houston, Texas

Timothy Craig Allen, MD, JD
Professor of Pathology
Chairman, Department of Pathology
The University of Texas Health Science
    Center at Tyler
Tyler, Texas

Sanja Dacic, MD, PhD
Associate Professor of Pathology
Department of Pathology
University of Pittsburgh Medical Center
Pittsburgh, Pennsylvania

Keith M. Kerr, MD
Consultant Pathologist,
Aberdeen Royal Infirmary & Aberdeen
    University Medical School
Foresterhill, Aberdeen
Scotland, United Kingdom

Mary Beth Beasley, MD
Associate Professor of Pathology
Mt. Sinai Medical Center
New York, New York

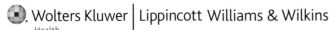
Wolters Kluwer | Lippincott Williams & Wilkins
Health

Philadelphia · Baltimore · New York · London
Buenos Aires · Hong Kong · Sydney · Tokyo

Senior Executive Editor: Jonathan W. Pine, Jr.
Product Manager: Marian Bellus
Vendor manager: Bridgett Dougherty
Senior Manufacturing Manager: Benjamin Rivera
Senior Marketing Manager: Angela Panetta
Creative Director: Doug Smock
Production Service: SPi Technologies

Library of Congress Cataloging-in-Publication Data
  Advances in surgical pathology. Lung cancer / Philip T. Cagle . . . [et al.].
      p. ; cm.—(Advances in surgical pathology series)
  Other title: Lung cancer
  Includes bibliographical references and index.
  ISBN 978-1-60547-591-2 (alk. paper)
 1. Lungs—Cancer—Pathophysiology.
 I. Cagle, Philip T. II. Title: Lung cancer. III. Series: Advances in surgical pathology series.
  [DNLM: 1. Lung Neoplasms—pathology—Atlases. WF 17 A244 2011]
  RC280.L8A38 2011
  616.99'424—dc22

2010025180

Care has been taken to confirm the accuracy of the information presented and to describe generally accepted practices. However, the authors, editors, and publisher are not responsible for errors or omissions or for any consequences from application of the information in this book and make no warranty, expressed or implied, with respect to the currency, completeness, or accuracy of the contents of the publication. Application of this information in a particular situation remains the professional responsibility of the practitioner; the clinical treatments described and recommended may not be considered absolute and universal recommendations.

The authors, editors, and publisher have exerted every effort to ensure that drug selection and dosage set forth in this text are in accordance with the current recommendations and practice at the time of publication. However, in view of ongoing research, changes in government regulations, and the constant flow of information relating to drug therapy and drug reactions, the reader is urged to check the package insert for each drug for any change in indications and dosage and for added warnings and precautions. This is particularly important when the recommended agent is a new or infrequently employed drug.

Some drugs and medical devices presented in this publication have Food and Drug Administration (FDA) clearance for limited use in restricted research settings. It is the responsibility of the health care provider to ascertain the FDA status of each drug or device planned for use in his or her clinical practice.

Visit Lippincott Williams & Wilkins on the Internet at: LWW.COM. Lippincott Williams & Wilkins customer service representatives are available from 8:30 am to 6 pm, EST.

9 8 7 6 5 4 3 2 1

To my wife, Kirsten
Philip T. Cagle, MD

To my children, Caitlin and Erin, and my wife, Fran
Timothy Craig Allen, MD, JD

To Andrew and Sasha, my boys
Sanja Dacic, MD, PhD

To my wife, Gillian
Keith M. Kerr, MD

To my family
Mary Beth Beasley, MD

Series Overview

Expectations for the pathologist practicing today exceed those for pathologists in practice only a few years ago. In addition to the rapid growth of knowledge and new technologies in the field of pathology, recent years have seen the emergence of many trends that significantly impact the traditional practice of pathology including the subspecialized multidisciplinary approach to patient care, personalized therapeutics including targeted molecular therapies and imaging techniques such as endoscopic microscopy, molecular radiology, and imaging multimodality theranostics that compete with conventional light microscopy. In order to remain a viable member of the patient care team, the pathologist must keep up with growing knowledge in traditional subjects as well as in new areas of expertise such as molecular testing. Additionally, the pathologist is subject to an increasing number of credentialing requirements and, for those now completing training, self-assessment modules for maintenance of certification, which require the pathologist to be examined on the recent advances in pathology in order to sustain their qualifications to practice.

Each volume in the new series "Advances in Surgical Pathology" focuses on a specific subject in pathology that has undergone recent advancement in terms of knowledge, technical procedures, application, and/or integration as part of current trends in pathology and medicine. Each book includes an accompanying Solution site with a fully searchable online version of the text and image bank. This series of books not only updates the pathologist on recently acquired knowledge but also emphasizes the new uses of that knowledge within the context of the changing landscape of pathology practice in the 21st century. Rather than information in a vacuum, the pathologist is educated on how to apply the new knowledge as part of a subspecialized multidisciplinary team and for purposes of personalized patient therapy.

Each volume in the series is divided into the following sections: (1) Overview—updates the pathologist on the general topic, including epidemiology, bringing the pathologist generally up-to-date on a topic as a basis for the more specialized sections that follow. (2) Histopathology—reviews histopathology and specific recent changes that warrant more description and more illustration, for example, recently described entities and recent revisions in classifications. This also emphasizes histopathology figures to illustrate recently described entities and to demonstrate the basis for classification changes so that the pathologist is able to understand and recognize these changes. (3) Imaging—reviews the impact of imaging techniques on histopathologic diagnosis and on the practice of pathology. An example of the former is the use of increasingly sensitive high-resolution CT scan in the diagnosis of interstitial lung diseases. An example of the latter is the use of multimodality theranostics rather than traditional histopathology for the diagnosis and treatment of lung cancer. Figures linking the radiologic images to the histopathology are emphasized. (4) Molecular pathology—a review and update on specific molecular pathology as it applies to specific diseases for the practicing pathologist in regard to molecular diagnostics and molecular therapeutics. An example of the former is the identification of a specific fusion gene to diagnose synovial sarcoma. An example of the latter is the identification of specific EGFR mutations in pulmonary adenocarcinoma and its relationship to treatment with EGFR antagonists. (5) For those volumes dealing with cancers (Lung Cancer, Breast Cancer, Prostate Cancer, Colon Cancer, etc.), additional sections include Preneoplastic and Preinvasive Lesions, which emphasize histopathologic figures and Staging, particularly emphasizing the new staging systems and illustrating specific problems in staging.

These books will assist the pathologist in daily practice in the modern setting and provide a basis for interacting with other physicians in patient care. They will also provide the timely updates in knowledge that are necessary for daily practice, for current credentialing, and for maintenance of certification. As such, this series is invaluable at all levels of experience to pathologists in practice who need to keep up with advances for their daily performance and their periodic credentialing and to pathologists-in-training who will apply this knowledge to their boards and their future practice. In the latter case, this series will serve as a useful library for pathology training programs.

Preface

Our knowledge and concepts about lung cancer have been undergoing a major revolution over the past few years. Among the areas that have been impacted are development of molecular targeted therapies including implications for the role of cell type diagnosis by the pathologist, significant proposed revisions to cell type and subtype classification (especially regarding adenocarcinomas), advances in imaging including multimodality theranostics, revisions to staging, progress in molecular diagnostics, and advancement of our understanding of premalignant and preinvasive lesions.

For those readers who need to update on the pathology of lung cancer and associated disciplines, whether for routine practice, for participation in multidisciplinary tumor boards, or for examinations, including boards and maintenance of certification, the editors of this book have provided a succinct, comprehensible overview of lung cancer emphasizing updated information from the ongoing revolution in this field. Copious high-resolution color images are used to illustrate in detail the various pathologic features covered in the discussion. Our intent is for this book to be a pragmatic tool for study and for practice.

The editors wish to acknowledge the contributions made by many of our colleagues to this ongoing transformation of the pathology of lung cancer. While we cannot begin to list everyone who has contributed to these recent advances, two individuals stand out as leaders in proposing the revisions to both the staging and the classification of lung cancer. In particular, Dr. William D. Travis of Memorial Sloan Kettering Cancer Center and Dr. Elisabeth Brambilla of Centre Hospitalier Universitaire Albert Michallon provided the pathology leadership for the various individuals and societies (International Association for the Study of Lung Cancer, American Thoracic Society, and European Respiratory Society) for the proposed new classification of pulmonary adenocarcinoma and related recommendations. Dr. Travis and Dr. Brambilla have long been at the forefront of lung cancer pathology and led the 1999 and 2004 World Health Organization classifications of lung tumors. The editors wish to especially acknowledge their contributions to this field.

The reader should note that the proposals for changes to the classification of lung cancer, particularly pulmonary adenocarcinoma, are not yet finalized, some recommendations will probably continue to be debated and it remains for the World Health Organization to adopt a new classification in the future.

Philip T. Cagle, MD
Timothy Craig Allen, MD, JD
Sanja Dacic, MD, PhD
Keith M. Kerr, MD
Mary Beth Beasley, MD

Contents

SECTION III. Imaging

SECTION IV. Molecular Pathology

SECTION V. Staging

SECTION VI. Preneoplastic and Preinvasive Lesions

ADVANCES IN SURGICAL PATHOLOGY:
LUNG CANCER

Overview of Lung Cancer

Epidemiology and Demographics of Lung Cancer

1

▶ Philip T. Cagle

Lung cancer remains the leading cause of cancer deaths in the United States,[1] Europe,[2] and worldwide.[3] In 2002, worldwide an estimated 1.35 million people were diagnosed with lung cancer and 1.18 million died of the cancer, the largest number for any type of cancer.[3,4] In the United States, there were an estimated 159,390 deaths from lung cancer in 2009 (88,900 deaths in men and 70,490 in women), surpassing the next three most common causes of cancer deaths (colon, breast, and prostate cancers) combined.[1] Five-year survival among lung cancer patients is poor and, worldwide, varies between 6% and 14% for men and 7% and 18% for women.[4]

Tobacco smoking causes more than 90% of lung cancers in men and 75% to 85% of lung cancers in women in the United States and Europe.[5] Worldwide, tobacco smoking causes an estimated 85% of lung cancer in men and 47% of lung cancer in women.[3] In the United States and other developed countries, changes in smoking habits have resulted in a slight decrease in lung cancer among men in recent years and a stabilization of the incidence in women. However, the rates continue to rise in less developed countries,[1–4] and the estimated numbers of lung cancer cases worldwide have increased by 51% since 1985, although in men this seems to be largely the result of population increase and aging.[3]

Only about 10% of tobacco smokers ever develop lung cancer. Host factors, including difference in enzymes that metabolize carcinogens in tobacco smoke and differences in enzymes that repair DNA, impact the development of lung cancer as do the length and amount of exposure to tobacco smoke.[5–7] Generally, there is a latency period of 20 to 40 years, or more, after the first exposure to tobacco smoke before a smoker is diagnosed with lung cancer. Although the risk of death from lung cancer decreases after smoking cessation compared to those who continue to smoke, the risk does not return to the level of a never smoker. Compared to never smokers, the risk of lung cancer in a former smoker may remain elevated 25 years or more after smoking cessation, although it is much less than that in those smokers who do not quit.[5,8–12]

Although tobacco smoke is overwhelmingly the major risk factor for lung cancer, the number of lung cancers occurring among never smokers is not insignificant.[13–20] Worldwide, about 15% of men with lung cancer and 53% of women with lung cancer are never smokers.[3] In the United States, death rates from lung cancer among never smokers are comparable to death rates from leukemia and endometrial cancer in women and death rates from cancers of the esophagus, kidney, and liver in men.[13,17,19] The death rate from lung cancer among Chinese women who have never smoked is particularly high.[3,19] Therefore, women of Asian descent with lung cancer are often never smokers and their lung cancers are often adenocarcinoma histology.[3,19] Risk factors for lung cancer in never smokers include environmental tobacco smoke (secondhand smoke), exposure to cooking fumes (particularly in Chinese women), inherited genetic susceptibility, occupational and environmental exposures (radon, asbestos, arsenic, etc.), hormonal factors, preexisting lung disease, outdoor pollution, dietary factors, human immunodeficiency virus, human papillomavirus, and ionizing radiation.[14,19]

References

1. Jemal A, Siegel R, Ward E, et al. Cancer statistics. *CA Cancer J Clin.* 2009;59:225–249.
2. Ferlay J, Autier P, Boniol M, et al. Estimates of the cancer incidence and mortality in Europe in 2006. *Ann Oncol.* 2007;18:581–592.
3. Parkin DM, Bray F, Ferlay J, et al. Global cancer statistics, 2002. *CA Cancer J Clin.* 2005;55:74–108.
4. Youlden DR, Cramb SM, Baade PD. The International Epidemiology of Lung Cancer: geographical distribution and secular trends. *J Thorac Oncol.* 2008;3(8):819–831.
5. Cagle PT. Carcinoma of the lung. In: Churg AM, Myers JL, Tazelaar HD, Wright JL, eds. *Pathology of the Lung.* 3rd ed. New York, NY: Thieme Medical Publishers; 2005:413–479.
6. Cagle PT, Jagirdar J, Popper H. Molecular pathology and genetics of lung cancer. In: Tomashefski J, editor-in-chief, Cagle PT, Farver C, Fraire A, eds. *Dail and Hammar's Pulmonary Pathology.* New York, NY: Springer; 2008.
7. Cagle PT, Allen TC. Genetic susceptibility to lung cancer. In: Zander D, Popper HH, Jaigrdar J, Haque A, Cagle PT, Barrios R, eds. *Molecular Pathology of Lung Diseases.* New York, NY: Springer-Verlag; 2008.
8. Alberg AJ, Semet JM. Epidemiology of lung cancer. *Chest* 2003;123(suppl):21S–49S.
9. Wynder EL, Stellman SD. Impact of long-term filter cigarette usage on lung and larynx cancer risk: a case-control study. *J Natl Cancer Inst.* 1979:62:471–477.
10. Pathak DR, Samet JM, Humble CG, et al. Determinants of lung cancer risk in cigarette smokers in New Mexico. *J Natl Cancer Inst.* 1986;76:597–604.
11. US Department of Health and Human Services: *The health benefits of smoking cessation.* US Department of Health and Human Services, Public Health Service, Centers for Disease Control, Center for Chronic Disease Prevention and Health Promotion, Office on Smoking and Health. DHHS Publication No. (CDC) 89-8416, 1990.
12. Hrubec Z, McLaughlin JK. Former cigarette smoking and mortality among US veterans: a 26-year follow-up, 1954–1980. In: Burns DM, Garfinkel L, Samet JM, eds. *Changes in Cigarette-related Disease Risks and Their Implications for Prevention and Control.* Bethesda, MD: US Government Printing Office; 1997:501–530.
13. Thun MJ, Henley SJ, Calle EE. Tobacco use and cancer: an epidemiologic perspective for geneticists. *Oncogene.* 2002;21:7307–7325.
14. Subramanian J, Govindan R. Lung cancer in never smokers: a review. *J Clin Oncol.* 2007;25(5): 561–570.
15. Subramanian J, Velcheti V, Gao F, et al. Presentation and stage-specific outcomes of lifelong never-smokers with non-small cell lung cancer (NSCLC). *J Thorac Oncol.* 2007;2(9):827–830.
16. Subramanian J, Govindan R. Molecular genetics of lung cancer in people who have never smoked. *Lancet Oncol.* 2008;9(7):676–682.
17. Ries L, Melbert D, Krapcho M, et al. SEER cancer statistics review, 1975–2004. Bethesda, MD: National Cancer Institute; 2008.
18. Rudin CM, Avila-Tang E, Harris CC, et al. Lung cancer in never smokers: molecular profiles and therapeutic implications. *Clin Cancer Res.* 2009;15(18):5646–5661.
19. Samet JM, Avila-Tang E, Boffetta P, et al. Lung cancer in never smokers: clinical epidemiology and environmental risk factors. *Clin Cancer Res.* 2009;15(18):5626–5645.
20. Morgensztern D, Waqar S, Subramanian J, et al. Improving survival for stage IV non-small cell lung cancer: a surveillance, epidemiology, and end results survey from 1990 to 2005. *J Thorac Oncol.* 2009; [Epub ahead of print].

Clinicopathologic Overview of Lung Cancer

2

▶ Philip T. Cagle

TRADITIONAL HISTOLOGIC CELL TYPES

Histologic classification and tumor stage are critical to the diagnosis and treatment of lung cancer and pathologists have a vital role in determining both.[1–6] Although sarcomas, lymphomas, and other nonepithelial malignancies may very rarely arise as primary tumors in the lung, the term "lung cancer" almost always refers to primary carcinoma of the lung and that is how the term is used in this book. Traditionally, lung cancers have been divided into two major categories based on histologic features and cell type that also imply other characteristic features including response to conventional therapy: non–small cell lung carcinoma (NSCLC) and small cell lung carcinoma (SCLC). NSCLCs include three major cell types (adenocarcinoma, squamous cell carcinoma, and large cell carcinoma) that may be additionally divided into subtypes and variants (see Chapters 3–8). In addition to SCLCs, there are other less common forms of neuroendocrine carcinomas of the lung (see Chapters 9–12). There are also several rare forms of primary lung carcinoma (see Chapters 13–16). Further details on all of the cell types and subtypes of lung cancer, including proposed revisions to classification, are found in the subsequent chapters of this book. In the past, the term "bronchogenic carcinoma" was used interchangeably with lung cancer or lung carcinoma, but, in recognition of the peripheral nature of many lung cancers and the changing concepts of lung cancer origins, we will not use this term.[1–6]

In recent years, there has been a significant increase in information about lung cancer, with new insights in histologic classification, pathological-clinical correlations, imaging, molecular pathology and therapy protocols, including molecular targeted therapy, and multimodality theranostics.[7–12] Correlation of certain molecular mutations with histologic cell type has been noted (see Chapter 21). As a result, the International Association for the Study of Lung Cancer, American Thoracic Society, and European Respiratory Society, with the pathology component under the leadership of Dr. William Travis,[8] are in the process of proposing revisions to the traditional classification, diagnosis, and staging of lung cancer and handling of specimens. Of particular importance to pathologists, significant revisions to the histologic classification of pulmonary adenocarcinomas have been proposed (see Chapters 3–5).[8]

HISTOLOGIC SUBTYPES IN DIAGNOSIS AND TREATMENT

Therapy of lung cancer is based on cell type and stage. Early-stage NSCLCs are treated with surgery, and SCLCs, the vast majority of which are in advanced stage at presentation, are treated with chemotherapy and radiation therapy. Most NSCLCs are also advanced at the time of presentation and are diagnosed on small biopsy or cytology specimens, rather than resection specimens. Double-agent platinum-based chemotherapy (e.g., carboplatin/paclitaxel) is the usual first-line therapy for NSCLC patients with good performance status. Administration of two platinum-based chemotherapy agents extends survival, enhances quality of life, and decreases disease symptoms.

Adding a third cytotoxic agent does not add any clinical benefit, although it may increase toxicity. On the other hand, adding new molecular targeted therapies such as bevacizumab to platinum-based agents may improve survival compared with platinum-based therapy alone. Docetaxel, pemetrexed, and erlotinib may be used in lung cancer patients who have progressed on first-line therapy.[9–11]

Oncologists are increasingly in need of a specific cell type diagnosis for new lung cancer therapies, and simply diagnosing "non–small cell carcinoma" is no longer as adequate as it once was. Whenever possible, the diagnosis of "non–small cell carcinoma" should not be used, but rather a specific cell type (e.g., squamous cell carcinoma or adenocarcinoma) should be diagnosed, using special stains, immunohistochemistry, or molecular techniques. The latter has significant implications for patient therapy, since advanced stage adenocarcinomas, but not squamous cell carcinomas, may respond to pemetrexed therapy. In addition, patients with adenocarcinomas may respond to bevacizumab therapy, but patients with squamous cell carcinoma who receive bevacizumab therapy are at risk of developing severe, even life-threatening, hemorrhage. In addition, other potential targets of molecular targeted therapy tend to have histologic associations, for example, K-ras mutations in mucinous adenocarcinomas and epidermal growth factor receptor mutations in nonmucinous bronchioloalveolar carcinomas in specific populations (see Chapter 22).[9–11]

However, the term "non–small cell carcinoma" will not disappear completely in the foreseeable future. Most lung cancers are diagnosed by small biopsies or cytology specimens, not surgical resection specimens. If the sampled area is poorly differentiated, a diagnosis of "non–small cell carcinoma" may occasionally be unavoidable, although use of ancillary studies and suggestion of the favored cell type should be provided if possible.[8]

Use of the term "large cell carcinoma" has been gradually disappearing from pathologic diagnoses over the last several years and is being replaced by more specific cell types (e.g., large cell neuroendocrine carcinoma). For those lung cancers that are not SCLCs and cannot be further classified as a more specific cell type, the term "non–small cell carcinoma, not otherwise specified" remains useful.[8]

LUNG CANCER SCREENING

As noted in Chapter 1, lung cancer remains the leading cause of cancer deaths in the United States, in Europe, and in the world as a whole. In the 1970s, lung cancer screening with chest x-ray and sputum cytology was not found to be effective in reducing the number of advanced lung cancers or in reducing lung cancer mortality. In recent years, there has been renewed interest in lung cancer screening using high-resolution computed tomography. Results have not yielded a decreased incidence of advanced lung cancers, and information about survival is not yet available. New concepts about the natural history of lung cancer are being proposed on the basis of these screening studies.[12–16]

References

1. Travis WD, Brambilla E, Muller-Hermelink HK, et al. eds. *World Health Organisation Classification of Tumours. Pathology and Genetics of Tumours of the Lung, Pleura, Thymus and Heart.* Lyon: IARC Press; 2004:35–44.
2. Cagle PT. Carcinoma of the lung. In: Churg AM, Myers JL, Tazelaar HD, Wright JL, eds. *Pathology of the Lung.* 3rd ed. New York, NY: Thieme Medical Publishers; 2005:413–479.
3. Laga AC, Allen T, Ostrowski M, et al. Adenocarcinoma. In: Cagle PT, editor-in-chief. *The Color Atlas and Text of Pulmonary Pathology.* 2nd ed. New York, NY: Lippincott Williams & Wilkins; 2008:31–35.

4. Flieder DB, Hammar SP. Common non-small cell carcinomas and their variants. In: Tomashefski J, editor-in-chief, Cagle PT, Farver C, Fraire A, eds. *Dail and Hammar's Pulmonary Pathology*. Vol 2, 3rd ed. New York, NY: Springer; 2008:216–307.

5. Jones KD. Malignant epithelial neoplasms. In: Cagle PT, Allen TC, Beasley MB, eds. *Diagnostic Pulmonary Pathology*. 2nd ed. New York, NY: Informa; 2008:611–626.

6. Kwon KY, Kerr KM, Ro JY. Non-small cell carcinomas. In: Cagle PT, Allen TC, Kerr KM, editors-in-chief. *Transbronchial and Endobronchial Biopsies*. New York, NY: Lippincott Williams & Wilkins; 2009:7–19.

7. Kerr KM. Pulmonary adenocarcinomas: classification and reporting. *Histopathology*. 2009;54(1):12–27.

8. Travis WD, Brambilla E, Noguchi M, et al. The new IASLC/ATS/ERS international multidisciplinary lung adenocarcinoma classification. *J Thorac Oncol*. 2009;4(Suppl. 1):s86–s89.

9. Stinchcombe TE, Socinski MA. Current treatments for advanced stage non-small cell lung cancer. *Proc Am Thorac Soc*. 2009;6(2):233–241.

10. Selvaggi G, Scagliotti GV. Histologic subtype in NSCLC: does it matter? *Oncology (Williston Park)*. 2009;23(13):1133–1140.

11. Rossi A, Maione P, Bareschino MA, et al. The emerging role of histology in the choice of first-line treatment of advanced non-small cell lung cancer: implication in the clinical decision-making. *Curr Med Chem*. 2010; [Epub ahead of print].

12. Chirieac LR, Flieder DB. High-resolution computed tomography screening for lung cancer: unexpected findings and new controversies regarding adenocarcinogenesis. *Arch Pathol Lab Med*. 2010;134(1):41–48.

13. Bach PB, Jett JR, Pastorino U, et al. Computed tomography screening and lung cancer outcomes. *JAMA*. 2007;297(9):953–961.

14. Bach PB. Is our natural-history model of lung cancer wrong? *Lancet Oncol*. 2008 Jul;9(7):693–697.

15. Warner E, Jotkowitz A, Maimon N. Lung cancer screening—are we there yet? *Eur J Intern Med*. 2010;21(1):6–11.

16. Tanner NT, Silvestri GA. An up to date look at lung cancer screening. *Cell Adh Migr*. 2010 18;4(1); [Epub ahead of print].

Histopathology

Adenocarcinoma

3

▶ Philip T. Cagle
▶ Keith M. Kerr

Adenocarcinomas are defined as carcinomas with gland formation and/or mucin production. Adenocarcinomas are the most frequently occurring cell type of pulmonary carcinoma in the industrialized world, replacing squamous cell carcinomas over the past several decades in North America and Western Europe, possibly because of alterations in smoking exposure caused by modifications in cigarettes, including the use of filters (see Chapter 27). In the 1950s, adenocarcinomas accounted for as few as 5% of lung cancers, but currently adenocarcinomas account for 35% to 50% of lung cancers in most series.[1–10] Adenocarcinomas have long been the most frequent cell type in Asian countries. In the past, adenocarcinomas were more frequent in women than in men in North America and Europe, but the general increase in the frequency of adenocarcinoma has been associated with a major shift in cell types in men, so that today adenocarcinoma is the most frequent cell type in both sexes. Although most adenocarcinomas are caused by tobacco smoking, adenocarcinoma is the most frequent cell type in patients who have never smoked.[11–17]

In this chapter, we review the histopathology of pulmonary adenocarcinoma based on the current 2004 World Health Organization (WHO) classification. Revisions to the current classification are being proposed and these are discussed in Chapter 5. The 2004 WHO classification divides pulmonary adenocarcinomas into acinar, papillary, bronchioloalveolar, solid adenocarcinomas with mucin production, and mixed subtypes and includes several variants (fetal adenocarcinoma, mucinous or colloid carcinoma, mucinous cystadenocarcinoma, signet ring adenocarcinoma, and clear cell carcinoma).[18] Since bronchioloalveolar carcinoma is distinct from other forms of adenocarcinoma and by definition is carcinoma-in-situ, which introduces unique issues, it is discussed separately in Chapter 4.[19,20] As mentioned above, there are a number of concerns with the 2004 WHO classification and revisions are being proposed, including recognition that most adenocarcinomas have mixed histologic patterns and should be classified according to their predominant subtype,[21–27] replacing the term bronchioloalveolar carcinoma with adenocarcinoma-in-situ[10] and differentiating adenocarcinoma from squamous cell carcinoma whenever possible, minimizing the use of the term non–small cell carcinoma. These and other proposed revisions are discussed in Chapter 5.

ADENOCARCINOMA, GROSS FEATURES

Most pulmonary adenocarcinomas are peripheral in location, and most peripheral primary carcinomas of the lung are adenocarcinomas, although pulmonary adenocarcinomas may be central in location. Due to their peripheral location, adenocarcinomas may be discovered as an incidental mass, nodule, or "coin lesion" on imaging studies performed for other reasons and may not present with clinical symptoms (Fig. 3-1). Typically, they are gray-white, firm, lobulated masses, often with central scarring and anthracotic pigment (Fig. 3-2). In some cases, part or all of the peripheral margin of the tumor is ill-defined. Subpleural tumors may be associated with pleural puckering (Figs. 3-3 and 3-4). As noted, central desmoplastic reaction, or scar, is common and necrosis may be present, but cavitation is unusual. Not surprisingly, because of their location, adenocarcinomas are the most likely cell type to invade the pleura and extend onto the pleural surface.[18,21–24]

FIGURE 3-1 Chest x-ray shows peripheral mass in the right upper lung zone. This mass was diagnosed as a pulmonary adenocarcinoma. (Courtesy of Ronald E. Fisher, M.D., Ph.D.)

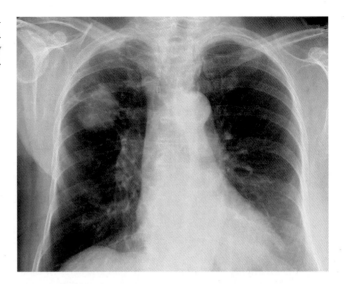

FIGURE 3-2 Lobectomy specimen containing a bisected subpleural adenocarcinoma. The cut surface of the tumor displays a lobulated firm mass with central scarring and anthracotic pigment.

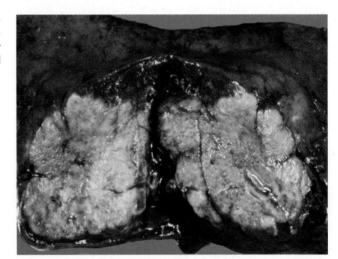

FIGURE 3-3 Pleural surface of lobectomy specimen shows "puckered" pleura with a central depression from a scar associated with a subpleural tumor mass.

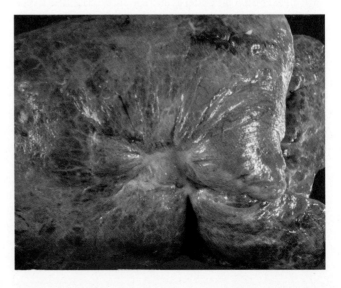

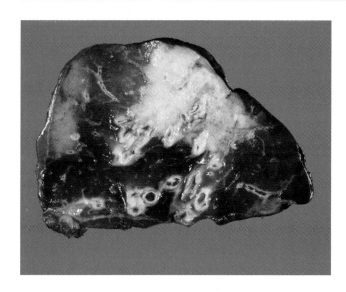

FIGURE 3-4 Cut surface of same specimen as in Figure 3-3 shows subpleural adenocarcinoma with scar causing puckering of overlying pleura.

The so-called "scar cancers" of the lung were once thought to be adenocarcinomas that arose from a preexisting scar, for example, from a focus of tuberculosis or healed pneumonia. It is now recognized that the vast majority of these tumors are adenocarcinomas with central desmoplastic reaction and the cancer has preceded the "scar" and not vice versa.[28–30] Rarely, carcinomas may grow predominantly on the pleural surface and encase the lung in a gross pattern similar to diffuse malignant mesothelioma and are referred to as "pseudomesotheliomatous carcinomas." The majority of carcinomas that grow in this "pseudomesotheliomatous" pattern arise as primary subpleural adenocarcinomas of the lung (Fig. 3-5).[31–33]

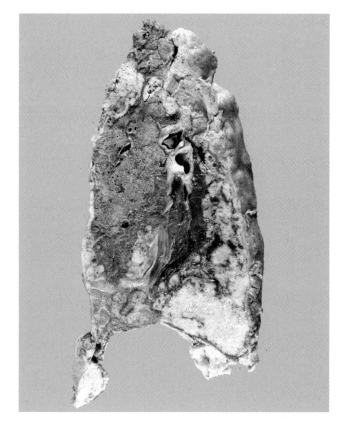

FIGURE 3-5 This subpleural adenocarcinoma has grown primarily in a "pseudomesotheliomatous" pattern over the visceral pleural surface.

ADENOCARCINOMA, HISTOLOGY

The current WHO classification of pulmonary adenocarcinomas includes several major subtypes: acinar, papillary, bronchioloalveolar, solid adenocarcinoma with mucin production, and mixed. If sampled adequately, virtually all pulmonary adenocarcinomas are of mixed subtype, although one subtype usually predominates.[18,21–27] It has been proposed that this long-standing observation should be addressed in a new classification system (see Chapter 5).[10]

The acinar pattern consists of formation of glands or tubules with malignant epithelial cells lining the central lumens of various shapes, sizes, and complexity (Figs. 3-6–3-8). The solid pattern consists of sheets or nests of large, polygonal cells with vesicular nuclei, prominent nucleoli, and comparatively abundant eosinophilic cytoplasm (Figs. 3-9 and 3-10). Intracytoplasmic mucin can be demonstrated with periodic acid Schiff with diastase, mucicarmine, and/or Alcian blue stains (Figs. 3-11 and 3-12). Current WHO criteria recommend at least five mucin positive cells in each of two high power fields for classification as a solid adenocarcinoma with mucin. Papillary adenocarcinomas consist of malignant epithelial cells lining the fibrovascular cores or papillae (Figs. 3-13 and 3-14). In contrast to the simple epithelial tufts seen in some bronchioloalveolar carcinomas, papillary adenocarcinomas have secondary and tertiary papillary structures that obliterate the underlying lung architecture. A distinctive type of pulmonary adenocarcinoma

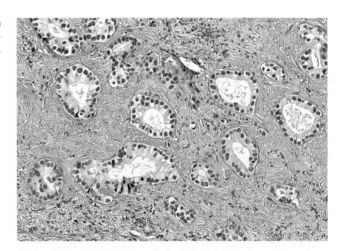

FIGURE 3-6 Medium power shows an acinar pattern of adenocarcinoma composed of glands of varying size and shape.

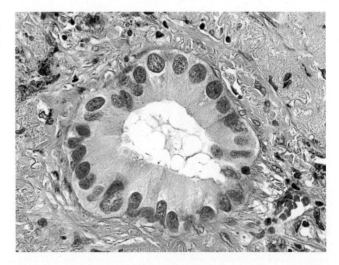

FIGURE 3-7 High power of acinar pattern shows a single gland with a roughly oval lumen lined by malignant columnar cells with basal nuclei.

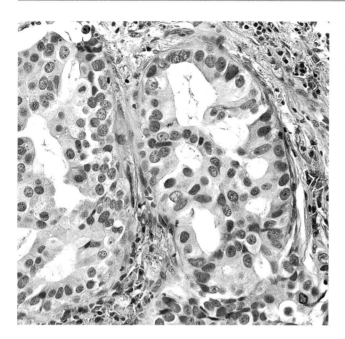

FIGURE 3-8 High power of acinar pattern shows glands with greater architectural complexity consisting of back-to-back glands or cribriforming.

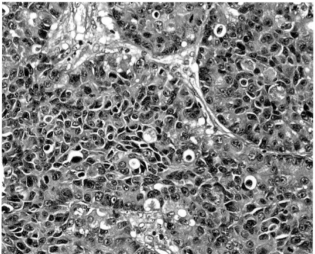

FIGURE 3-9 Low power shows solid pattern of adenocarcinoma with nests of polygonal cells.

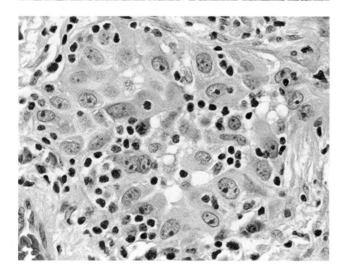

FIGURE 3-10 High power of solid pattern shows nest of polygonal cells with vesicular nuclei and prominent nucleoli.

FIGURE 3-11 Nest of polygonal cells with vesicular nuclei and prominent nucleoli displays intracytoplasmic mucin on Alcian blue stain in multiple cells, confirming that the tumor is an adenocarcinoma with solid pattern.

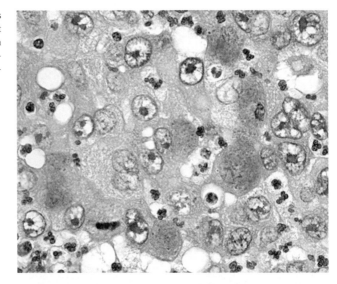

FIGURE 3-12 Mucicarmine stain verifies the presence of mucin, which stains red in the cytoplasm of multiple cancer cells in a solid pattern adenocarcinoma.

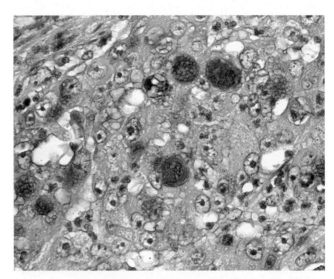

FIGURE 3-13 Medium power of papillary adenocarcinoma shows relatively complex branching fibrovascular cores lined by malignant columnar cells.

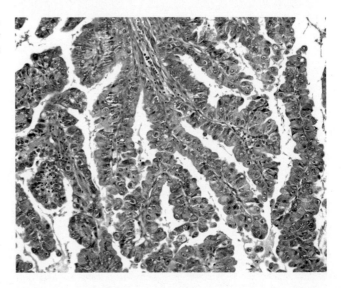

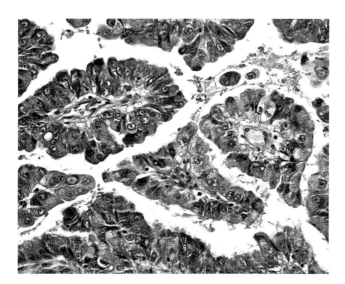

FIGURE 3-14 Malignant columnar cells line fibrous cores containing blood vessels in this high power of papillary adenocarcinoma.

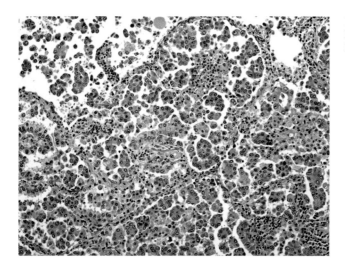

FIGURE 3-15 Low power of micropapillary pattern shows multiple simple papillary clusters of malignant cells.

is micropapillary adenocarcinoma. These tumors have simple papillary structures without fibrovascular cores and are associated with an unfavorable prognosis (Figs. 3-15 and 3-16).[18,21–25,34] It has been proposed that "micropapillary pattern, predominant" be recognized as a subtype under "invasive adenocarcinoma" distinct from "papillary pattern, predominant" (see Chapter 5).[10]

Bronchioloalveolar carcinomas are noninvasive carcinomas that grow in a lepidic fashion (Figs. 3-17 and 3-18), and it has recently been proposed that bronchioloalveolar carcinomas should be designated "adenocarcinoma-in-situ."[10] Bronchioloalveolar carcinomas are discussed separately in Chapter 4 and proposed revisions to their classification in Chapter 5.

There are also several variants of adenocarcinoma that are recognized in the 2004 WHO classification: fetal adenocarcinoma, mucinous or colloid carcinoma, mucinous cystadenocarcinoma, signet ring adenocarcinoma, and clear cell carcinoma.[18] Fetal adenocarcinomas have a histopathologic pattern that resembles fetal lung and consist of tubules lined by glycogen-containing columnar cells (Figs. 3-19–3-21). Fetal adenocarcinomas may be well-differentiated (formerly classified with pulmonary blastomas) or high-grade. Mucinous or colloid adenocarcinomas consist of strips of cytologically bland columnar tumor cells and individual tumor cells floating in pools of mucin (Figs. 3-22 and 3-23). Mucinous cystadenocarcinomas consist of mucin-filled cysts

FIGURE 3-16 Papillary clusters of adenocarcinoma cells lack fibrovascular cores or complex architecture in this high power of micropapillary pattern.

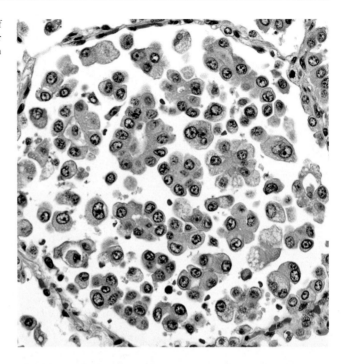

FIGURE 3-16 Papillary clusters of adenocarcinoma cells lack fibrovascular cores or complex architecture in this high power of micropapillary pattern.

FIGURE 3-17 Low power of a bronchioloalveolar adenocarcinoma, or adenocarcinoma-in-situ, shows a lepidic pattern in which intact alveolar septa are lined by single files of relatively uniform malignant cells without invasion of the underlying stroma.

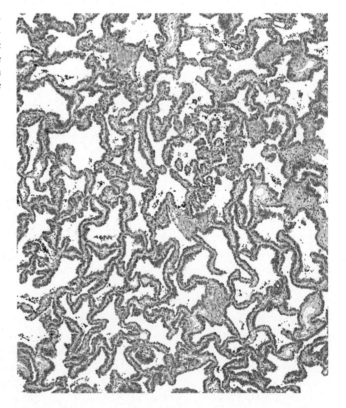

lined by columnar goblet cells containing apical mucin (Fig. 3-24). Signet ring adenocarcinoma consists of tumor cells that resemble signet rings, with large mucin vacuoles filling the cytoplasm and pushing the nuclei to one edge (Fig. 3-25). Clear cell adenocarcinomas consist of malignant cells with clear cytoplasm (Fig. 3-26).[18,21–25] It has been proposed that these latter two subtype

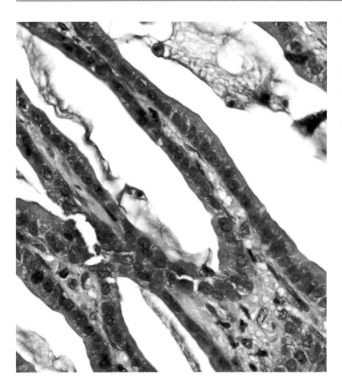

FIGURE 3-18 In this high power of a bronchioloalveolar adenocarcinoma, or adenocarcinoma-in-situ, relatively uniform malignant cells grow in a single row replacing the pneumocytes of the septal surfaces without invasion of the underlying alveolar septa, referred to as a lepidic pattern.

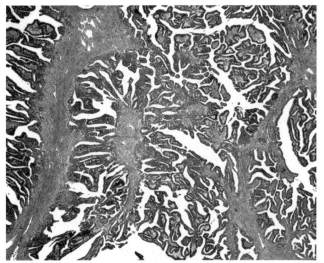

FIGURE 3-19 Low power of a fetal adenocarcinoma displays a complex branching pattern of tubules lined by columnar cells.

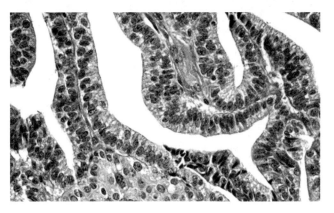

FIGURE 3-20 High power demonstrates the columnar cells with intracytoplasmic vacuoles and relatively uniform nuclei lining the tubules in a well-differentiated fetal adenocarcinoma.

FIGURE 3-21 High power of a fetal adenocarcinoma includes a morule consisting of an oval nest of polygonal cells with eosinophilic cytoplasm.

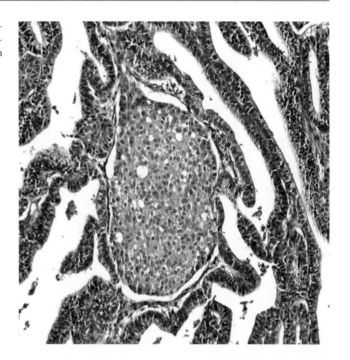

FIGURE 3-22 Low power of mucinous or colloid adenocarcinoma shows pools of mucin and strips of cytologically bland columnar tumor cells.

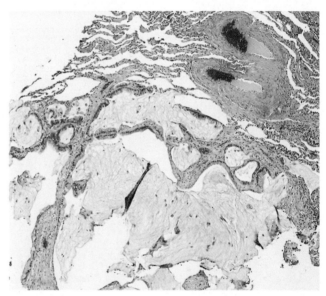

variants no longer be recognized as separate subtype variants, but rather as cytologic variants that may occur in several of the adenocarcinoma subtypes (see Chapter 5).

Adenocarcinoma may also occur in combination with other lung cancer histological subtypes.[18] When it occurs with small cell carcinoma, a diagnosis of combined small cell carcinoma should be given (Fig. 3-27). The combination with squamous cell carcinoma, adenosquamous carcinoma, has a separate category in the 2004 WHO classification, but is a very rare tumor. In the authors' experience, in surgically resected tumors, adenocarcinoma is more likely to be encountered in combination with large cell neuroendocrine carcinoma or sarcomatoid carcinoma.

As noted, most adenocarcinomas have mixtures of subtype patterns, for example, mixtures of acinar patterns and solid patterns.[18,21–25] Tumor-Node-Metastasis (TNM) stage is

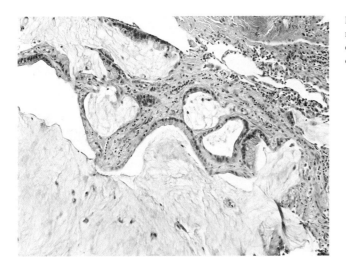

FIGURE 3-23 Medium power of mucinous or colloid adenocarcinoma has pool of mucin lined by cytologically bland columnar cells.

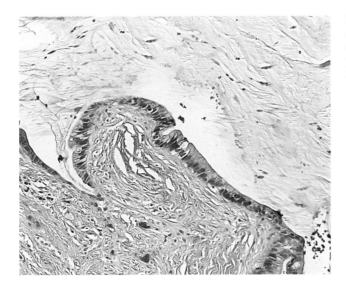

FIGURE 3-24 In this high power of cystadenocarcinoma, columnar goblet cells with moderate nuclear pleomorphism and containing apical mucin line a mucin-filled cyst.

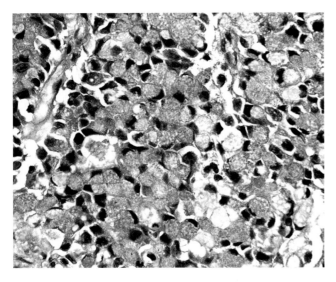

FIGURE 3-25 Signet ring cells with their nuclei pushed to one edge by large intracytoplasmic mucin vacuoles are present in this high power of a pulmonary adenocarcinoma.

FIGURE 3-26 High power of a pulmonary adenocarcinoma composed of cells
with clear cytoplasm.

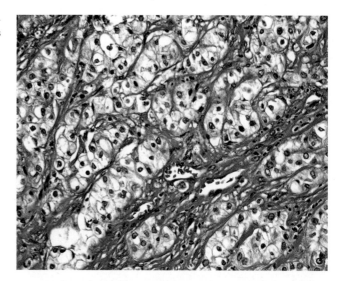

FIGURE 3-27 High power of combined
small cell carcinoma with an acinar pattern of adenocarcinoma in the lower left
portion of the image and small cell carcinoma with crush artifact and tumor
necrosis in the upper and right portions
of the image.

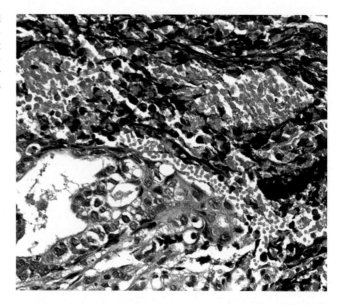

currently the most important predictor of prognosis for pulmonary adenocarcinoma, as it is
for other lung cancers, but the mixture of subtypes and grade or degree of differentiation also
have influence on prognosis. High grade is associated with greater cytologic pleomorphism
and higher mitotic rate. Prominent formation of glands tends to be generally associated with
better differentiated or low-grade tumors, and extensive solid pattern tends to be more often
associated with poorer differentiated or high-grade tumors.[21-25] As already noted, a micropapillary component is believed to be associated with a poorer prognosis. Adenocarcinomas often
have an in-situ bronchioloalveolar component growing in a noninvasive lepidic fashion at the
periphery of the tumor. Studies indicate that the greater the amount or percentage of bronchioloalveolar component of a mixed pattern adenocarcinoma, the better the prognosis.[35-38] Pulmonary adenocarcinomas that are predominantly bronchioloalveolar or lepidic pattern and
have foci of minimal invasion have a particularly excellent prognosis and the term "minimally
invasive adenocarcinoma" has been proposed for these tumors. The definition of "minimal
invasion" is currently being deliberated and invasion of 5 mm or less has been proposed.[39-41]
These issues are further discussed in Chapter 5.

ADENOCARCINOMA, IMMUNOHISTOCHEMISTRY

The most important reasons for performing immunostaining on a pulmonary adenocarcinoma are to confirm the primary site of a tumor (see Chapter 17) and, more recently, to confirm adenocarcinoma cell type as opposed to squamous cell carcinoma cell type before starting bevacizumab or pemetrexed therapy (see Chapter 22). Most pulmonary adenocarcinomas are immunopositive for a variety of cytokeratins including AE1/AE3, CK7 (Fig. 3-28), and CAM 5.2, but are usually immunonegative for CK5/6 (which is usually immunopositive in squamous cell carcinomas) and CK20 (except for mucinous bronchioloalveolar carcinoma discussed in Chapter 4, some mucinous adenocarcinomas and in the newly proposed category of enteric adenocarcinomas discussed in Chapter 5).[42–45] Thyroid transcription factor-1 (TTF-1) shows nuclear immunopositivity in 75% to 85% of pulmonary adenocarcinomas and is used routinely in many laboratories to support the pulmonary origin of an adenocarcinoma (Figs. 3-29 and 3-30). This biomarker is also

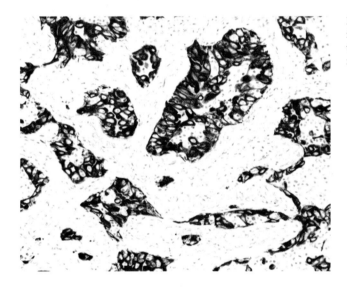

FIGURE 3-28 CK7 is immunopositive in the cytoplasm of the malignant cells of this predominantly solid pattern pulmonary adenocarcinoma.

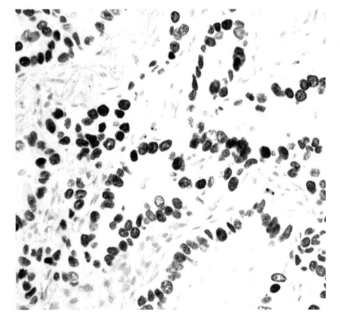

FIGURE 3-29 TTF-1 is immunopositive in the nuclei of the malignant cells of this predominantly acinar pattern adenocarcinoma.

FIGURE 3-30 TTF-1 is also immunopositive in the nuclei of nonneoplastic
normal and reactive type 2 pneumocytes
and this may serve as an internal positive
control for TTF-1 immunostaining.

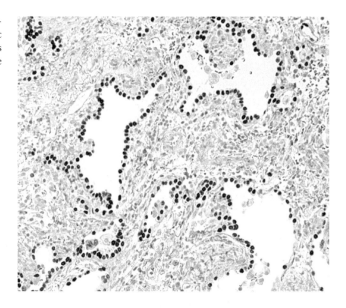

immunopositive in thyroid carcinomas, and thyroglobulin immunostain can be used to rule out a thyroid primary if the differential includes thyroid cancer.[43,44,46–49] Multiple other traditional carcinoma and adenocarcinoma markers are immunopositive in pulmonary adenocarcinoma including carcinoembryonic antigen, MOC-31, B72.3, and carcinoma antigen-125. Immunohistochemistry for surfactant proteins A and B are of limited value because they are less sensitive than TTF-1 and may be positive in adenocarcinomas metastatic to the lung.[20–25,43,44]

ADENOCARCINOMA, DIFFERENTIAL DIAGNOSIS

As mentioned in Chapters 5, 6, 7, and 22, differentiation of the solid pattern of adenocarcinoma from squamous cell carcinoma is particularly important in selecting patients for several chemotherapeutic agents; for example, bevacizumab therapy due to the potential for fatal hemorrhage in patients with squamous cell carcinoma. An immunohistochemistry panel consisting of p63 and CK5/6, which are frequently immunopositive in squamous cell carcinoma, and TTF-1, which is frequently immunopositive in adenocarcinoma, have been proposed for this differential diagnosis.[42–45] It is worth bearing in mind that large cell neuroendocrine carcinomas (see Chapter 8) often express TTF-1 and may have a cribriform or glandular architecture that can be mistaken for adenocarcinoma, especially of enteric type. The primary differential diagnoses for pulmonary adenocarcinoma are adenocarcinomas metastatic to the lung from other organs and other cancers of various types (carcinomas, melanoma, diffuse malignant mesothelioma, etc.), primary to the lung or metastatic to the lung from other sites. Metastatic tumors to the lung and their diagnosis, including immunostaining patterns, are discussed in detail in Chapter 17. Molecular profiling and micro-RNA profiling are under investigation as techniques to identify the primary site and cell type of cancers, including differentiating pulmonary adenocarcinomas from other cancers.[50–56] The molecular diagnostics of lung cancer is further discussed in Chapter 21.

ADENOCARCINOMA, HISTOGENESIS

Atypical adenomatous hyperplasia is believed to be the precursor lesion of peripheral pulmonary adenocarcinomas and progression from atypical adenomatous hyperplasia to adenocarcinoma-in-situ (bronchioloalveolar carcinoma) to invasive adenocarcinoma has been proposed.[57–66] Atypical adenomatous hyperplasia is discussed in detail in Chapter 27.

References

1. Vincent RG, Pickren JW, Lane WW, et al. The changing histopathology of lung cancer. A review of 1962 cases. *Cancer*. 1977;39:1647–1655, 1962.
2. Cox JD, Yesner RA. Adenocarcinoma of the lung: recent results from the Veterans Administration Lung Group. *Am Rev Resp Dis*. 1979;120:1025–1029.
3. Valaitis J, Warren S, Gamble D. Increasing incidence of adenocarcinoma of the lung. *Cancer*. 1981;47:1042–1046.
4. Percy C, Sobin S. Surveillance, epidemiology, and end results lung cancer data applied to the World Health Organization's classifications of lung tumors. *J Natl Cancer Inst*. 1983;70:663–666.
5. Dodds L, Davis S, Polissar L. A population-based study of lung cancer incidence trends by histologic type, 1974–81. *J Natl Cancer Inst*. 1986;76:21–29.
6. Wu AH, Henderson BE, Thomas DC, et al. Secular trends in histologic types of lung cancer. *J Natl Cancer Inst*. 1986;77:53–56.
7. Yoshimi I, Ohshima A, Ajiki W, et al. A comparison of trends in the incidence rate of lung cancer by histological type in the Osaka Cancer Registry, Japan and in the Surveillance, Epidemiology and End Results Program, USA. *Jpn J Clin Oncol*. 2003;33(2):98–104.
8. Devesa SS, Bray F, Vizcano AP, et al. International lung cancer trends by histologic type: male: female differences diminishing and adenocarcinoma rates rising. *Int J Cancer*. 2005;117:294–299.
9. Chen F, Cole P, Bina WF. Time trend and geographic patterns of lung adenocarcinoma in the United States. *Cancer Epidemiol Biomarkers Prev*. 2007;16:2724–2729.
10. Kerr KM. Pulmonary adenocarcinomas: classification and reporting. *Histopathology*. 2009;54(1): 12–27.
11. Subramanian J, Govindan R. Lung cancer in never smokers: a review. *J Clin Oncol*. 2007;25(5): 561–570.
12. Subramanian J, Velcheti V, Gao F, et al. Presentation and stage-specific outcomes of lifelong never-smokers with non-small cell lung cancer (NSCLC). *J Thorac Oncol*. 2007;2(9):827–830.
13. Subramanian J, Govindan R. Molecular genetics of lung cancer in people who have never smoked. *Lancet Oncol*. 2008;9(7):676–682.
14. Ries L, Melbert D, Krapcho M, et al. SEER cancer statistics review, 1975–2004. Bethesda, MD: National Cancer Institute; 2008.
15. Rudin CM, Avila-Tang E, Harris CC, et al. Lung cancer in never smokers: molecular profiles and therapeutic implications. *Clin Cancer Res*. 2009;15(18):5646–5661.
16. Samet JM, Avila-Tang E, Boffetta P, et al. Lung cancer in never smokers: clinical epidemiology and environmental risk factors. *Clin Cancer Res*. 2009;15(18):5626–5645.
17. Morgensztern D, Waqar S, Subramanian J, et al. Improving survival for stage IV non-small cell lung cancer: a surveillance, epidemiology, and end results survey from 1990 to 2005. *J Thorac Oncol*. 2009 Sep 11; [Epub ahead of print].
18. Colby TV, Noguchi M, Henschke C, et al. Adenocarcinoma. In: Travis WD, Brambilla E, Muller-Hermelink HK, Harris CC, eds. *World Health Organisation Classification of Tumours. Pathology and Genetics of Tumours of the Lung, Pleura, Thymus and Heart*. Lyon: IARC Press; 2004:35–44.
19. Christiani DC, Pao W, DeMartini JC, et al. BAC consensus conference, November 4–6, 2004: epidemiology, pathogenesis, and preclinical models. *J Thorac Oncol*. 2006;1(9 suppl):S2–S7.
20. Gordon IO, Sitterding S, Mackinnon AC, et al. Update in neoplastic lung diseases and mesothelioma. *Arch Pathol Lab Med*. 2009;133(7):1106–1115.
21. Cagle PT. Carcinoma of the lung. In: Churg AM, Myers JL, Tazelaar HD, Wright JL, eds. *Pathology of the Lung*. 3rd ed. New York, NY: Thieme Medical Publishers; 2005.
22. Laga AC, Allen T, Ostrowski M, et al. Adenocarcinoma. In: Cagle PT, editor-in-chief. *The Color Atlas and Text of Pulmonary Pathology*. 2nd ed. New York, NY: Lippincott Williams & Wilkins; 2008.
23. Flieder DB, Hammar SP. Common non-small cell carcinomas and their variants. In: Tomashefski J, editor-in-chief, Cagle PT, Farver C, Fraire A, eds. *Dail and Hammar's Pulmonary Pathology*. Vol 2, 3rd ed. New York, NY: Springer; 2008:216–307.
24. Jones KD. Malignant epithelial neoplasms. In: Cagle PT, Allen TC, Beasley MB, eds. *Diagnostic Pulmonary Pathology*. 2nd ed. New York, NY: Informa; 2008:611–626.

25. Kwon KY, Kerr KM, Ro JY. Non-small cell carcinomas. In: Cagle PT, Allen TC, Kerr KM, editors-in-chief. *Transbronchial and Endobronchial Biopsies.* New York, NY: Lippincott Williams & Wilkins; 2009:7–19.

26. Yesner R. Histopathology of lung cancer. *Semin Ultrasound CT MR.* 1988;9:4–26.

27. Roggli VL, Volmer RT, Greenberg SD, et al. Lung cancer heterogeneity: a blinded and randomized study of 100 consecutive cases. *Hum Pathol.* 1985;16:569–579.

28. Shimosato Y, Suzuki A, Hashimoto T, et al. Prognostic implications of fibrotic focus (scar) in small peripheral lung cancers. *Am J Surg Pathol.* 1980;4:365–373.

29. Madri JA, Carter D. Scar cancers of the lung: origin and significance. *Hum Pathol.* 15:625–631, 1984.

30. Cagle PT, Cohle SD, Greenberg SD. Natural history of pulmonary scar cancers: clinical and pathologic implications. *Cancer.* 1985;56:2031–2035.

31. Koss M, Travis W, Moran C, et al. Pseudomesotheliomatous adenocarcinoma: a reappraisal. *Semin Diagnosis Pathol.* 1992;9:117–123.

32. Attanoos RL, Gibbs AR. 'Pseudomesotheliomatous' carcinomas of the pleura: a 10-year analysis of cases from the Environmental Lung Disease Research Group, Cardiff. *Histopathology.* 2003;43(5):444–452.

33. Kobashi Y, Matsushima T, Irei T. Clinicopathological analysis of lung cancer resembling malignant pleural mesothelioma. *Respirology.* 2005;10(5):660–665.

34. Amin MB, Tamboli P, Merchant SH, et al. Micropapillary component in lung adenocarcinoma: a distinctive histologic feature with possible prognostic significance. *Am J Surg Pathol.* 2002; 26(3):358–364.

35. Castro CY, Coffey DM, Medeiros LJ, et al. Prognostic significance of percentage of bronchioloalveolar pattern in adenocarcinomas of the lung. *Ann Diagn Pathol.* 2001;5(5):274–284.

36. Lin DM, Ma Y, Zheng S, et al. Prognostic value of bronchioloalveolar carcinoma component in lung adenocarcinoma. *Histol Histopathol.* 2006;21(6):627–632.

37. Sakao Y, Miyamoto H, Sakuraba M, et al. Prognostic significance of a histologic subtype in small adenocarcinoma of the lung: the impact of nonbronchioloalveolar carcinoma components. *Ann Thorac Surg.* 2007;83(1):209–214.

38. Anami Y, Iijima T, Suzuki K, et al. Bronchioloalveolar carcinoma (lepidic growth) component is a more useful prognostic factor than lymph node metastasis. *J Thorac Oncol.* 2009;4(8):951–958.

39. Terasaki H, Niki T, Matsuno Y, et al. Lung adenocarcinoma with mixed bronchioloalveolar and invasive components: clinicopathological features, subclassification by extent of invasive foci, and immunohistochemical characterization. *Am J Surg Pathol.* 2003;27(7):937–951.

40. Yim J, Zhu LC, Chiriboga L, et al. Histologic features are important prognostic indicators in early stages lung adenocarcinomas. *Mod Pathol.* 2007;20(2):233–241.

41. Dacic S. Minimally invasive adenocarcinomas of the lung. *Adv Anat Pathol.* 2009 May;16(3):166–171.

42. Kargi A, Gurel D, Tuna B. The diagnostic value of TTF-1, CK 5/6, and p63 immunostaining in classification of lung carcinomas. *Appl Immunohistochem Mol Morphol.* 2007;15(4):415–420.

43. Jagirdar J. Application of immunohistochemistry to the diagnosis of primary and metastatic carcinoma to the lung. *Arch Pathol Lab Med.* 2008;132(3):384–396.

44. Beasley MB. Immunohistochemistry of pulmonary and pleural neoplasia. *Arch Pathol Lab Med.* 2008;132(7):1062–1072.

45. Khayyata S, Yun S, Pasha T, et al. Value of P63 and CK5/6 in distinguishing squamous cell carcinoma from adenocarcinoma in lung fine-needle aspiration specimens. *Diagn Cytopathol.* 2009;37(3): 178–183.

46. Loo PS, Thomas SC, Fyfe MN, et al. Immunohistochemical subtyping of undifferentiated non-small cell carcinomas in bronchial biopsy specimens. *J Thorac Oncol* 2010;5(4):442–447.

47. Ikeda K, Clark JC, Shaw-White JR, et al. Gene structure and expression of human thyroid transcription factor-1 in respiratory epithelial cells. *J Biol Chem.* 1995;270(14):8108–8114.

48. Bejarano PA, Baughman RP, Biddinger PW, et al. Surfactant proteins and thyroid transcription factor-1 in pulmonary and breast carcinomas. *Mod Pathol.* 1996;9(4):445–452.

49. Khoor A, Whitsett JA, Stahlman MT, et al. Utility of surfactant protein B precursor and thyroid transcription factor 1 in differentiating adenocarcinoma of the lung from malignant mesothelioma. *Hum Pathol.* 1999;30(6):695–700.

50. Tan D, Li Q, Deeb G, et al. Thyroid transcription factor-1 expression prevalence and its clinical implications in non-small cell lung cancer: a high-throughput tissue microarray and immunohistochemistry study. *Hum Pathol.* 2003;34(6):597–604.

51. Khan J, Wei JS, Ringner M, et al. Classification and diagnostic prediction of cancers using gene expression profiling and artificial neural networks. *Nat Med.* 2001;7:673–679.

52. Ramaswamy S, Tamayo P, Rifkin R, et al. Multiclass cancer diagnosis using tumor gene expression signatures. *Proc Natl Acad Sci USA*. 2001;98:15149–15154.

53. Ma XJ, Patel R, Wang X, et al. Molecular classification of human cancers using a 92-gene real-time quantitative polymerase chain reaction assay. *Arch Pathol Lab Med*. 2006;130:465–473.

54. Takeuchi T, Tomida S, Yatabe Y, et al. Expression profile-defined classification of lung adenocarcinoma shows close relationship with underlying major genetic changes and clinicopathologic behaviors. *J Clin Oncol*. 2006;24(11):1679–1688.

55. Yanaihara N, Caplen N, Bowman E, et al. Unique microRNA molecular profiles in lung cancer diagnosis and prognosis. *Cancer Cell*. 2006;9(3):189–198.

56. Jay C, Nemunaitis J, Chen P, et al. miRNA profiling for diagnosis and prognosis of human cancer. *DNA Cell Biol*. 2007;26(5):293–300.

57. Wang QZ, Xu W, Habib N, et al. Potential uses of microRNA in lung cancer diagnosis, prognosis, and therapy. *Curr Cancer Drug Targets*. 2009;9(4):572–594.

58. Miller RR, Nelems B, Evans KG, et al. Glandular neoplasia of the lung. A proposed analogy to colonic tumours. *Cancer*. 1988;61:1009–1014.

59. Miller RR. Bronchioloalveolar cell adenomas. *Am J Surg Pathol*. 1990;14:904–912.

60. Chapman AD, Kerr KM. The association between atypical adenomatous hyperplasia and primary lung cancer. *Br J Cancer*. 2000;83(5):632–636.

61. Mori M, Rao SK, Popper HH, et al. Atypical adenomatous hyperplasia of the lung: a probable forerunner in the development of adenocarcinoma of the lung. *Mod Pathol*. 2001;14(2):72–84.

62. Kerr KM. Pulmonary preinvasive neoplasia. *J Clin Pathol*. 2001;54(4):257–271.

63. Ullmann R, Bongiovanni M, Halbwedl I, et al. Is high-grade adenomatous hyperplasia an early bronchioloalveolar adenocarcinoma? *J Pathol*. 2003 Nov;201(3):371–376.

64. Kerr KM, Fraire AE, Pugatch B, et al. Atypical adenomatous hyperplasia. In: Travis WD, Brambilla E, Muller-Hermelink HK, et al., eds. *World Health Organisation Classification of Tumours. Pathology and Genetics of Tumours of the Lung, Pleura, Thymus and Heart*. Lyon: IARC press; 2004:73–75.

65. Kerr KM, Fraire AE. Pre-invasive disease. In: Tomashefski JF, editor-in-chief, Cagle PT, Farver CF, Fraire AE, eds. *Dail and Hammar's Pulmonary Pathology*. Vol II, 3rd ed. New York, NY: Springer; 2008:158–215.

66. Kerr KM. Preneoplastic and preinvasive lesions. In: Cagle PT, Allen TC, Beasley MB, eds. *Diagnostic Pulmonary Pathology*. 2nd ed. New York, NY: Informa; 2008:519–537.

4 Bronchioloalveolar Carcinoma/ Adenocarcinoma-in-Situ

▶ Philip T. Cagle
▶ Keith M. Kerr

First described by Averill Liebow in 1960,[1] bronchioloalveolar carcinomas (BACs) were thought to be derived from the peripheral pulmonary epithelium with tumor cells resembling Clara cells, goblet cells, or type II pneumocytes. The characteristic histologic feature was growth of the tumor cells along the surface of intact alveolar septa, referred to as lepidic growth. Prior to 1999, both adenocarcinomas with pure lepidic growth pattern and adenocarcinomas with a prominent BAC component mixed with invasive components were diagnosed as BACs and included in published studies as BACs. Currently, BAC is histologically defined as an adenocarcinoma-in-situ (AIS) that grows in a lepidic manner, replacing the original pulmonary epithelial lining, along intact alveolar septa *without invasion* into the underlying stroma, pleura, or lymphovascular spaces (Figs. 4-1–4-3).[2–15]

BACs are most frequently nonmucinous, but mucinous and mixed nonmucinous and mucinous types are described. Most of the preceding remarks apply to nonmucinous BAC rather than mucinous BAC. The nonmucinous and mucinous variants have critical differences in their histopathology, gross, radiology, molecular pathology, and clinical features and are, therefore, discussed separately.[2–15] Traditionally, the nonmucinous tumor cells are thought to resemble Clara cells or type II pneumocytes and mucinous tumor cells are thought to resemble goblet cells. Most of this chapter focuses on the nonmucinous type, which is more frequent than the mucinous type (>2/3 of BAC) and is generally considered to be the form that fits into the progression scheme from atypical adenomatous hyperplasia (AAH) to BAC (adenocarcinoma-in-situ) to invasive peripheral adenocarcinoma (see Chapter 27).[2–15] The frequency with which an individual pathologist may see one type rather than the other will, however, depend on the country in which he or she practices and the local protocols relating to lung cancer screening and thoracic surgical practice.

This current definition of BAC was first adopted in the 1999 World Health Organization classification,[2] was continued in the 2004 World Health Organization classification,[3] and is based largely on the study of small, peripheral adenocarcinomas by Noguchi et al.[16] Noguchi et al.'s original study[16] and subsequent studies[17–24] support the concept of progression from BAC or AIS to minimally invasive adenocarcinomas that have a prominent BAC component. Noguchi Type A tumors consist of pure BAC, Type B tumors consist of BAC with alveolar collapse and fibrosis, and Type C tumors consist of a predominantly BAC pattern with foci of invasion and associated fibroblastic proliferation. Noguchi Type A and B tumors have a 5-year survival rate of 100%, whereas Noguchi Type C tumors have a 5-year survival rate of 75%.[16] Some experts are proposing that the term bronchioloalveolar carcinoma be discarded and that pure localized BAC tumors (Noguchi Type A and B) be designated AIS. In this proposed classification, adenocarcinomas with minimal invasion would also be recognized (see Chapter 5).[14]

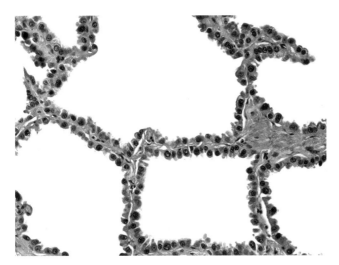

FIGURE 4-1 Medium power shows a BAC or an AIS growing in a lepidic pattern. Minimally thickened alveolar septa are lined by rows of single, relatively uniform cuboidal cells with round cytologically bland nuclei, adjacent one to another without gaps. The septal architecture is preserved and no invasion of the septa is present. Some cells have small apical snouts. A few cells have small intranuclear inclusions.

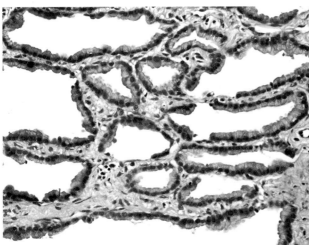

FIGURE 4-2 Medium power shows another example of BAC/AIS. The alveolar septal architecture is preserved, but the septa show mild fibrous thickening. Monotonous, cytologically bland, low columnar cells line the surfaces of the septa, replacing the pneumocytes, in a lepidic pattern.

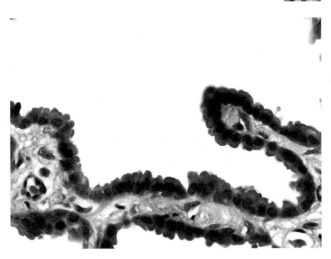

FIGURE 4-3 High power of Figure 4-2 demonstrates that the neoplastic columnar cells are cytologically bland and comparatively homogeneous. They are arranged adjacent to each other covering the surface of the septum with a row of single cells in a lepidic pattern without invasion of the septum or other structures.

Using the current definition of BAC as strictly noninvasive or in-situ carcinoma, only 2% to 6% of non–small cell carcinomas are pure BACs. About 40% to 50% of mixed pattern non–small cell carcinomas have a BAC component, however, and in 7% to 16% this is the dominant pattern in the tumor.[5,25,26] Surgical resection results in a 5-year survival rate of 100% for small, solitary peripheral BACs, consistent with their in-situ status.[6,16] Since invasion must not be present in order to meet the current diagnostic criteria for BAC, a final diagnosis of true BAC cannot be made on a small transbronchial biopsy, needle core biopsy, or cytology specimen. This is because the entire tumor is not sampled in these limited specimens and, therefore, invasion elsewhere in the tumor cannot be excluded.[2–15]

BAC has some unique demographic features compared to other lung cancers. Although approximately 75% of BACs are associated with tobacco smoking, about 25% of BACs occur in never smokers, a greater percentage than with any other lung cancer cell type. In addition, a majority (up to 63%) of patients with BAC are women.[4,10,14,17] Caution is required, however, in interpreting the literature in this area, since published data on BAC, even post-2000, do not necessarily concern tumors fulfilling the current strict definition of BAC.

NONMUCINOUS BRONCHIOLOALVEOLAR CARCINOMA, GROSS FEATURES

Nonmucinous BACs make up at least 60% to 75%, possibly almost 100% of true BAC.[2–15] Nonmucinous BACs are peripheral, ivory to tan lesions measuring a few millimeters to around 2 cm in size. It is extremely unusual to find a lesion over 2 cm in diameter that does not have invasion. Most are solitary, but they are occasionally multifocal. Nonmucinous BAC may have a spongy texture or be poorly defined from surrounding parenchyma due to the preservation of airspaces by tumor cells growing in a lepidic pattern along intact alveolar septa. In well-preserved specimens the alveolar spaces can be seen on the lesion cut surface with the naked eye. Collapse of fibrotic alveolar septa or a central scar may make the tumor firmer, but, by definition, invasion is not present in pure BAC. Therefore, there is no desmoplastic reaction, necrosis, or hemorrhage. Subpleural BAC may, however, have puckering of the overlying pleura.[2–15]

NONMUCINOUS BRONCHIOLOALVEOLAR CARCINOMA, HISTOLOGY

The tumor cells of nonmucinous BAC are cuboidal to columnar cells that, by definition, grow in lepidic pattern along intact alveolar septa (Fig. 4-4).[2–15] The tumor cells are usually relatively homogeneous with a uniform degree of mild to moderate cytologic atypia from one cell to another (Fig. 4-5). This uniformity helps distinguish BAC from benign hyperplastic pneumocytes with reactive atypia in which there are admixtures of normal cells and

FIGURE 4-4 Uniform columnar cells with bland basal nuclei are arranged in a lepidic pattern along the surface of intact, mildly thickened alveolar septa.

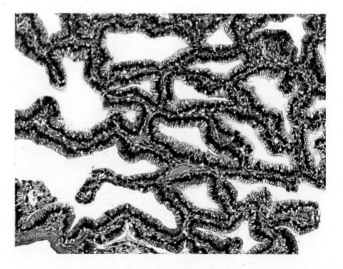

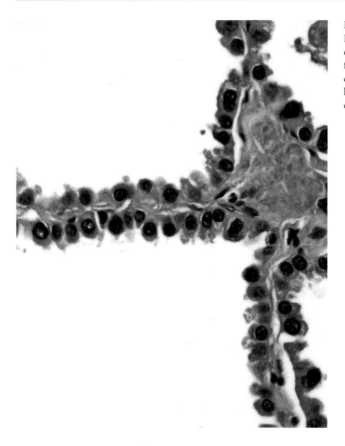

FIGURE 4-5 In this high power of a BAC/AIS, the malignant cells show mild cytologic atypia and minimal variation from one cell to another but lack the cytologic pleomorphism and cell-to-cell heterogeneity of most pulmonary adeno-carcinomas.

cells with varying degrees of atypia, lacking uniformity from one cell to another (Fig. 4-6). Likewise, AAH shows greater cytologic heterogeneity and lesser degrees of cytologic atypia than nonmucinous BAC. Criteria for the distinction between AAH and BAC are presented in Chapter 27.

The tumor cells may be cuboidal to columnar cells with basally or centrally located nuclei, often with nucleoli visible and eosinophilic to foamy cytoplasm (Fig. 4-7). The tumor cells may also be "hobnail" with apical nuclei (Fig. 4-8). Traditionally, based on histological, ultrastructural,

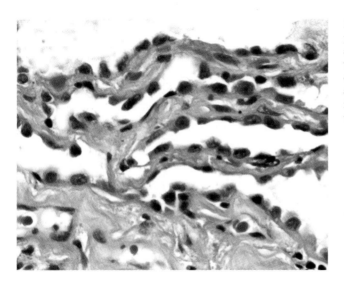

FIGURE 4-6 High power of hyperplastic pneumocytes with reactive atypia shows admixtures of flat type I pneumocytes with type II pneumocytes of varying degrees of reactive atypia from one cell to another. This proliferation lacks the uniformity of a BAC/AIS that has replaced the septal surface epithelium.

FIGURE 4-7 The cells of this BAC/AIS demonstrate central nuclei, prominent nucleoli, and foamy cytoplasm on high power.

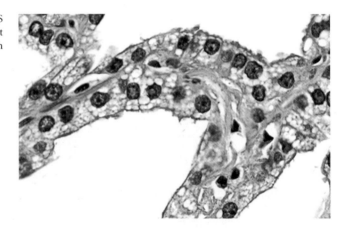

FIGURE 4-8 High power of BAC/AIS shows two "hobnail" cells with apical nuclei.

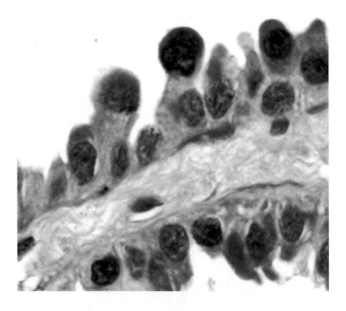

and immunohistochemical features, it was noted that 90% of nonmucinous BAC demonstrated Clara cell differentiation and that 10% displayed pneumocyte differentiation.[4,5]

Eosinophilic intranuclear inclusions may be present (Fig. 4-9) and are PAS (periodic acid Schiff)-positive. The tumor cells are often lined in a single row along the surface of the alveolar septa, but the cells may stratify and epithelial tufts may project into the alveolar space (Fig. 4-10). The alveolar septa may display fibrous thickening with or without lymphocytic infiltrates, but, by definition, invasion into the fibrous stroma must not be present. Detached tumor cells or clusters of tumor cells may be observed floating in the alveolar spaces (Fig. 4-10). BAC may have simple epithelial tufts that lack the complex secondary and tertiary branching architecture seen with papillary adenocarcinoma (Fig. 4-11). In addition, BAC tumor cells are less pleomorphic than tumor cells of papillary adenocarcinoma.[2–15]

Nonmucinous BACs often have collapse of the thickened fibrotic alveolar septa that compresses the alveolar spaces, creating elongated slitlike or tubulelike spaces lined by the BAC cells (Fig. 4-12). Such lesions may be referred to as Noguchi Type B lesions, as opposed to Noguchi Type A, which is without collapse.[16] This collapsed architecture may suggest acini of adenocarcinoma invasive within fibrous stroma, but the slitlike spaces have a regular distribution retaining

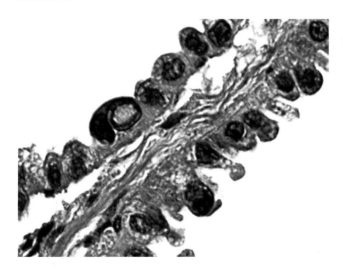

FIGURE 4-9 A neoplastic cell displays an eosinophilic intranuclear inclusion in this high power of a BAC/AIS.

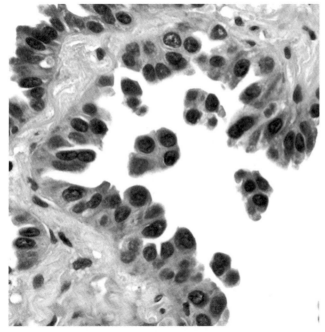

FIGURE 4-10 In this high power of BAC/AIS, there is focal stratification with tufting of the neoplastic cells and detached clusters of neoplastic cells floating in the adjacent alveolar space.

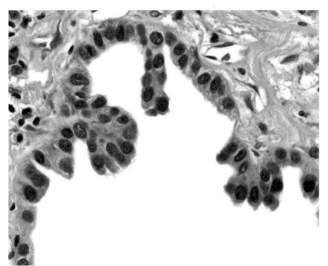

FIGURE 4-11 Simple epithelial tufts project from the surface of this BAC/AIS.

FIGURE 4-12 Collapse of thickened alveolar septa has compressed the alveolar spaces in this BAC/AIS, leaving elongated residual spaces lined by neoplastic cells.

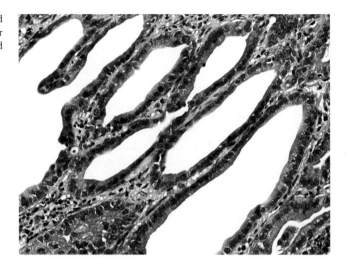

the basic alveolar architecture (Figs. 4-13–4-15). Collapse of fibrotic alveolar septa in BAC may be difficult to differentiate from invasion with desmoplastic reaction, and the presence of true new fibroblastic proliferation, as opposed to paucicellular fibroelastotic tissue, should raise suspicion of invasion. In collapsed BAC, alveolar spaces may retain alveolar macrophages in airspaces in continuity with the rest of the lung. Histologic features that favor invasion over collapse of fibrotic alveolar septa are listed in Table 4-1 (Figs. 4-16–4-19).[8,11,14]

Up to 50% of mixed type adenocarcinomas have a nonmucinous BAC component, at the periphery of the tumor (Fig. 4-20). A number of studies suggest that the greater the amount or percentage of BAC component in a mixed pattern adenocarcinoma, the better the prognosis.[22–29] It is a matter of some debate as to whether or not these BAC components truly represent "residual" AIS at the margins of the lesion (Figs. 4-21 and 4-22) or whether this pattern of disease is a particular form of invasion or progression of a more advanced malignant cell clone akin to that which is invading the tumor stroma (Fig. 4-23). Both scenarios are plausible and may even coexist.[19]

In addition, a number of studies suggest that BAC-predominant tumors with the so-called "minimal invasion" have as good of a prognosis as pure BAC, implying that they may likewise be

FIGURE 4-13 At low power, this neoplasm has a lepidic pattern with an area that probably represents collapsed thickened alveolar septa with residual alveolar spaces lined by BAC cells, although invasion must also be considered.

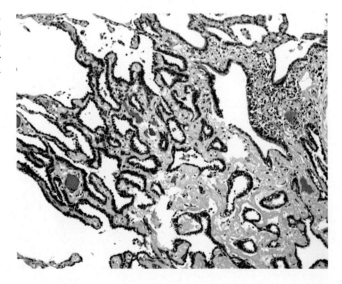

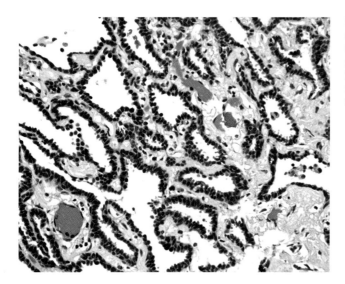

FIGURE 4-14 In this area, the elongated spaces display a morphology that suggests that they are distorted alveolar spaces rather than glands. It is possible to visualize that expansion of these spaces would result in a recognizable alveolar architecture.

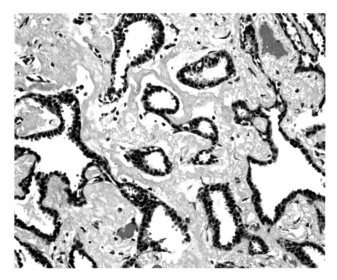

FIGURE 4-15 In this area, there are slitlike spaces that are elongated and regularly distributed, suggesting alveolar spaces that have been compressed by collapsed fibrotic alveolar septa. The neoplastic cells lining the spaces are identical to the uniform, relatively bland cells lining the areas of unequivocal lepidic growth. The stroma consists of poorly cellular fibroelastotic tissue and there is no fibroblastic proliferation to suggest desmoplasia. The smaller spaces, which are the most likely to suggest invasive glands, probably represent tangential cuts of compressed alveolar spaces.

cured by surgical excision.[16,18,19,30–32] Although invasion of ≤5 mm has been proposed as a definition for "minimal invasion" by some authors,[14,18,31,32] since studies have used different criteria for "minimal invasion," there is currently no consensus on the definition of "minimal invasion," which limits comparison between studies and inhibits reproducibility by other pathologists.[14,32] This issue is further discussed in Chapter 5.

Table 4-1	Histologic features favoring invasion over collapsed fibrotic alveolar septa in BAC
Small, irregular, angulated glands within fibroblastic stroma	
Haphazard distribution of glands within fibroblastic stroma	
Individual tumor cells, cords or nests of tumor cells within fibroblastic stroma	
Tumor cells are larger and more pleomorphic	
Tumor cells have more eosinophilic cytoplasm	

FIGURE 4-16 High power of an invasive focus within a predominantly lepidic adenocarcinoma consists of a small, irregularly shaped gland composed of malignant cells and an individual malignant cell within a desmoplastic stroma. The invasive cells show greater cytologic atypia than the in-situ cells of BAC/AIS. They have larger, more irregular nuclei, more prominent nucleoli, and more abundant eosinophilic cytoplasm. They are embedded in a loose, myxoid stroma containing numerous fibroblasts.

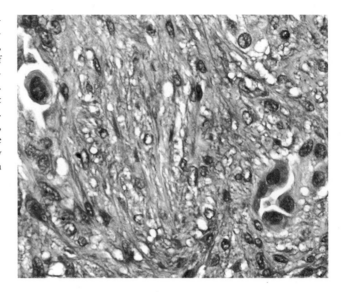

FIGURE 4-17 Invasive cells are seen in the stroma beneath a BAC/AIS. The cells of the BAC/AIS are relatively homogeneous columnar cells with very similar, relatively small nuclei with mild atypia. They are distributed in a single row of side-by-side cells in a lepidic pattern. The underlying invasive cells in the stroma have larger, more irregular nuclei and abundant eosinophilic cytoplasm. They are polygonal, rather than columnar. Although there are some resemblances between the in-situ and invasive cells, the invasive cells are clearly larger, more pleomorphic, and have more eosinophilic cytoplasm.

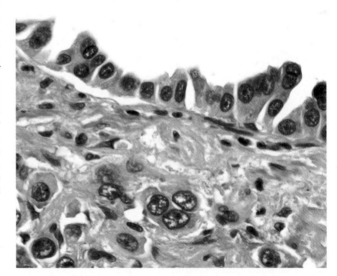

Solitary lesions with the architecture of true noninvasive BAC are described with mixtures of nonmucinous and mucinous cells but, in the authors' experience, definitive examples of such lesions are distinctly uncommon. Pure mucinous BAC, without invasion, is also very rare (see below).

NONMUCINOUS BRONCHIOLOALVEOLAR CARCINOMA, IMMUNOHISTOCHEMISTRY

Nonmucinous BACs have an immunostaining pattern that resembles the more frequently encountered invasive pulmonary adenocarcinomas. Similar to well-differentiated pulmonary adenocarcinomas, BACs are immunopositive for cytokeratin 7 (CK7) and thyroid transcription factor-1 (TTF-1) (Fig. 4-24), as well as surfactant proteins, and are immunonegative for CK20.[2–15]

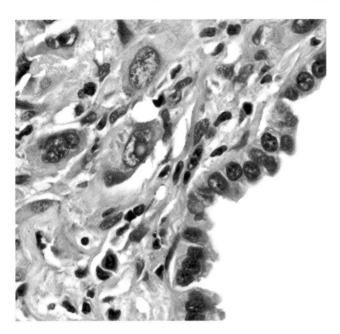

FIGURE 4-18 A striking contrast between BAC/AIS on the right and invasive cells on the left is observed in this figure. The columnar cells of the BAC/AIS display a consistent degree of mild atypia with very similar appearing nuclei. The polygonal invasive cells show much larger, much more pleomorphic vesicular nuclei and abundant eosinophilic cytoplasm.

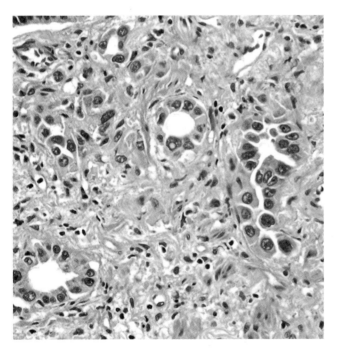

FIGURE 4-19 These glands are small and irregular and are haphazardly distributed within a fibroblastic stroma, indicating that they are invasive glands rather than compressed alveolar spaces lined by in-situ neoplasm. The degree of pleomorphism and abundant eosinophilic cytoplasm of the cells that line the lumens are also consistent with invasive glands. Individual invasive cells and clusters of invasive cells can also be observed in the surrounding stroma.

NONMUCINOUS BRONCHIOLOALVEOLAR CARCINOMA, DIFFERENTIAL DIAGNOSIS

The differential diagnosis of nonmucinous BAC includes its precursor lesion AAH, which is discussed in Chapter 27. Lambertosis (or peribronchiolar metaplasia) of the fibrotic alveolar septa with peribronchiolar fibrosis may be florid in some cases and BAC may enter into the differential diagnosis. Lambertosis is differentiated from nonmucinous BAC because it is confined to areas of peribronchiolar fibrosis and the metaplastic cells often have cilia (Figs. 4-25–4-27).

FIGURE 4-20 Low power shows an invasive adenocarcinoma with acinar pattern on the left and lepidic growth of malignant cells along intact fibrotic alveolar septa around its periphery.

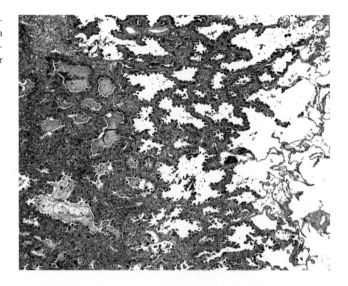

FIGURE 4-21 Medium power illustrates lepidic growth of malignant cells along intact fibrotic alveolar septa on the periphery of an invasive adenocarcinoma with solid and acinar patterns on the left of the figure.

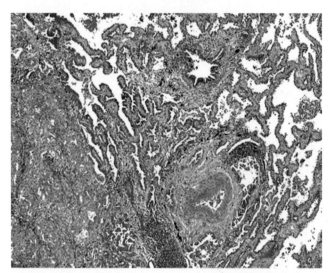

FIGURE 4-22 At higher power, the cells lining the thickened alveolar septa in Figure 4-21 are observed to be uniform and cytologically bland, in contrast to the invasive tumor cells, suggesting that they represent residual AIS at the margins of the lesion.

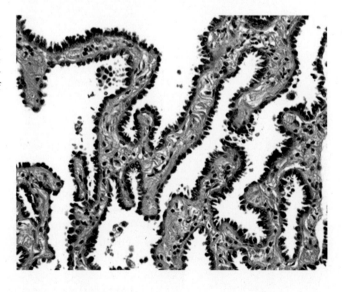

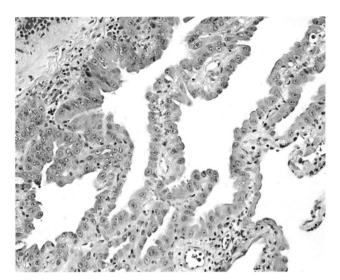

FIGURE 4-23 At the periphery of a different tumor, the malignant cells growing in a lepidic pattern are cytologically identical to the corresponding invasive cancer and show a greater degree of atypia than expected for BAC/AIS. This suggests that these cells may represent lepidic extension of the invasive cancer, as opposed to residual AIS.

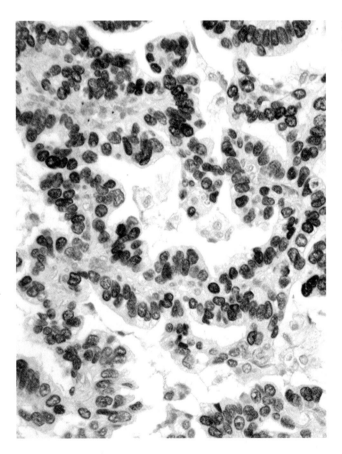

FIGURE 4-24 Immunostain for TTF-1 shows immunopositivity in the nuclei of this BAC/AIS.

Reactive type II pneumocyte hyperplasia may be seen in a wide range of diseases and conditions including acute lung injury (diffuse alveolar damage, acute fibrinous and organizing pneumonia, etc.), organizing lung injury, and pulmonary fibrosis. When reactive type II pneumocyte hyperplasia is florid and cytologically atypical, nonmucinous BAC may enter into the differential diagnosis (Fig. 4-6). Nonmucinous BACs display relative homogeny of the proliferating cells that

FIGURE 4-25 At low power, the alveolar septa around these bronchioles show mild fibrotic thickening and lining by metaplastic bronchiolar cells.

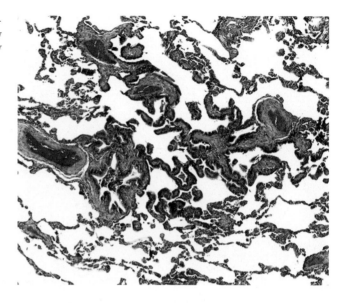

FIGURE 4-26 Medium power of Figure 4-25 shows the lining of metaplastic bronchiolar epithelium along fibrotic alveolar septa. This should not be mistaken for BAC/AIS. The findings should be interpreted within their context. Bronchiolar metaplasia (lambertosis) occurs in a peribronchiolar distribution in association with bronchiolar and/or peribronchiolar fibrosis.

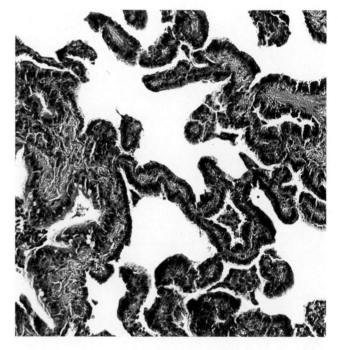

exhibit a comparatively uniform degree of cytologic atypia compared to reactive pneumocytes that show more variability with mixed degrees of cytologic atypia. Fibrotic thickening of the alveolar septa is limited to the areas lined by atypical cells in BAC, whereas areas of fibrosis and organizing or acute injury are typically more extensive than the areas with atypical epithelium in a reactive process. If present, intranuclear inclusions are typically large and numerous in nonmucinous BAC compared to the smaller, less frequent intranuclear inclusions in reactive type II pneumocytes.

Adenocarcinomas metastatic to the lung from other primary sites (colon, breast, pancreas, ovary, etc.) may grow in a lepidic pattern and mimic either nonmucinous or mucinous

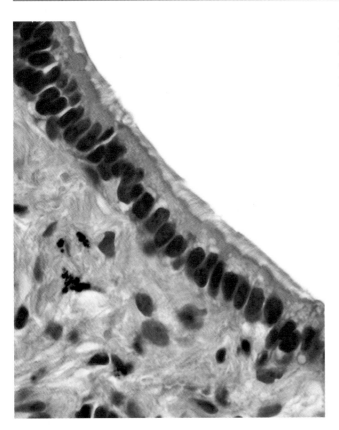

FIGURE 4-27 High power of bronchiolar metaplasia seen in Figures 4-25 and 4-26 shows well-formed terminal bars and surface cilia supporting a diagnosis of metaplastic epithelium rather than BAC/AIS.

BAC.[4,33] Histologic features, clinical history, imaging findings, and immunostaining pattern are helpful in differentiating a metastasis from BAC. Metastatic cancers are further discussed in Chapter 17.

NONMUCINOUS BRONCHIOLOALVEOLAR CARCINOMA, HISTOGENESIS

It is currently believed that most nonmucinous BACs arise from AAH and the nonmucinous BACs then progress to invasive peripheral adenocarcinomas.[3–15,24] The histogenesis of BAC from AAH is discussed in detail in Chapter 27.

MUCINOUS BRONCHIOLOALVEOLAR CARCINOMA, GROSS FEATURES

Mucinous BACs often have a soft, mucinous, gray cut surface. They may diffusely infiltrate a segment or lobe in a pneumonic pattern, filling the alveolar spaces with mucin (Fig. 4-28). This may actually make the margins of the tumor very difficult to discern since the fine granularity of the alveolar parenchyma may still be appreciated within these extensive areas of mucinous consolidation. Careful examination of what are usually quite large and irregular lesions often shows areas that are more solid, gray, and fibrotic with a collapsed, contracted scarlike appearance. This change may be associated with considerable pleural distortion. Such lesions are virtually always multifocal, although there may be one particular predominant mass with small satellite lesions. Solitary mucinous BAC is distinctly unusual (see below).

FIGURE 4-28 Gross of the so-called mucinous BAC shows cut surface of the lung with large, irregular, multifocal areas of mucinous consolidation.

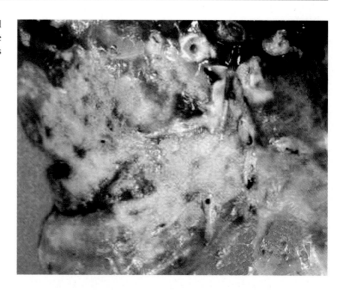

MUCINOUS BRONCHIOLOALVEOLAR CARCINOMA, HISTOLOGY

In mucinous BAC, uniform columnar cells typically with bland cytology and lacking increased mitoses grow in a lepidic pattern along thin alveolar septa with little or no fibrotic thickening (Fig. 4-29). The columnar cells may have relatively small, bland central nuclei, but they often have goblet cell morphology, and are cytologically very bland, with small, basal nuclei and abundant apical mucin (Fig. 4-30). The alveolar spaces are often filled with pools of mucin. The lepidic growth of the columnar cells is often discontinuous and intermittent along the septa, with the cells forming

FIGURE 4-29 Low power of mucinous BAC shows goblet cells growing in a lepidic pattern along intact alveolar septa.

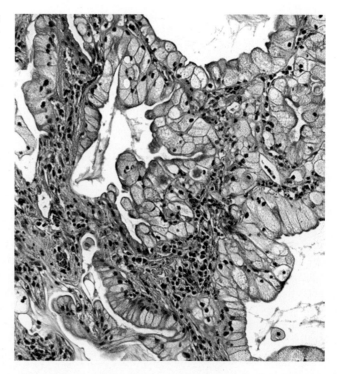

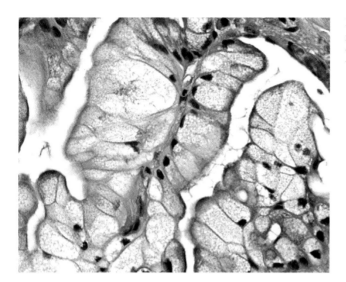

FIGURE 4-30 High power demonstrates goblet cells of mucinous BAC with abundant apical cytoplasmic mucin and small, very bland, basal nuclei.

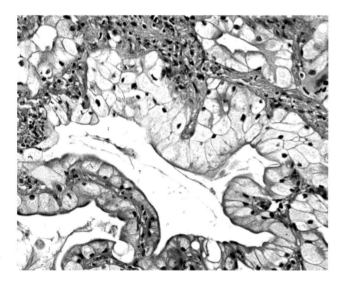

FIGURE 4-31 The so-called mucinous BAC with lepidic growth in lower portion of image shows invasion into stroma in the upper portion.

strips or tufts that may float free in the alveolar pools of mucin. Columnar cells in rows often form straight edges along the contiguous cell apices; hobnail cells are absent. There is a remarkable homogeneity in morphology between the numerous foci of disease present in the lung.

This is the typical *pattern* of the so-called mucinous BAC. It is arguable as to whether, given the rarity of a small, focal and localized true mucinous BAC, this represents mucinous AIS. In the authors' experience, extensive sampling (when possible) of tumor in cases with this histological pattern nearly always shows invasion of mucinous adenocarcinoma in those areas with fibrous scarring (Fig. 4-31). Once again, the multifocality of this disease may represent biologically relatively advanced mucinous adenocarcinoma spreading (metastasizing) in a particular (lepidic) fashion in the lung.

MUCINOUS BRONCHIOLOALVEOLAR CARCINOMA, IMMUNOHISTOCHEMISTRY

Mucinous BACs are typically immunopositive for CK7, immunonegative for TTF-1, and may sometimes be immunopositive for CK20. They are immunonegative for CDX2.[11,12,34]

MUCINOUS BRONCHIOLOALVEOLAR CARCINOMA, DIFFERENTIAL DIAGNOSIS

Mucinous adenocarcinomas from the colon and other sites may metastasize to the lung and grow in a lepidic pattern that mimics mucinous BAC. As noted above, TTF-1 and CK20 immunostaining may not be helpful in differentiating mucinous BAC from metastatic colon cancer, although CDX2 is likely to be helpful. Metastatic cancers are further discussed in Chapter 17.

MUCINOUS BRONCHIOLOALVEOLAR CARCINOMA, HISTOGENESIS

In children and young adults, mucinous BAC may arise from the mucinous cells of congenital cystic adenomatoid malformation, possibly from atypical goblet cell hyperplasia within these lesions.[35–38] In adults, in contrast to nonmucinous BAC, mucinous BAC may arise from metaplastic bronchiolar goblet cells rather than Clara cells or type II pneumocytes. Also, mucinous BACs typically show K-ras mutations rather than EGFR mutations. It has been suggested that they may possibly arise from AAH with K-ras mutations.[9,39,40]

References

1. Liebow AA. Bronchiolo-alveolar carcinoma. *Adv Intern Med*. 1960;10:329–358.
2. Travis WD, Colby TV, Corrin B, et al. In Collaboration with Sobin LH and Pathologists from 14 Countries. *World Health Organization International Histological Classification of Tumours. Histological Typing of Lung and Pleural Tumours*. 3rd ed. Berlin: Springer-Verlag; 1999.
3. Colby TV, Noguchi M, Henschke C, et al. Adenocarcinoma. In: Travis WD, Brambilla E, Muller-Hermelink HK, Harris CC, eds. *World Health Organisation Classification of Tumours. Pathology and Genetics of Tumours of the Lung, Pleura, Thymus and Heart*. Lyon: IARC Press; 2004:35–44.
4. Cagle PT. Carcinoma of the lung. In: Churg AM, Myers JL, Tazelaar HD, Wright JL, eds. *Pathology of the Lung*. 3rd ed. New York, NY: Thieme Medical Publishers; 2005:413–479.
5. Jackman DM, Chirieac LR, Jänne PR. Bronchioloalveolar carcinoma: a review of the epidemiology, pathology, and treatment. *Semin Respir Crit Care Med*. 2005;26:342–352.
6. Christiani DC, Pao W, DeMartini JC, et al. BAC consensus conference, November 4–6, 2004: epidemiology, pathogenesis, and preclinical models. *J Thorac Oncol*. 2006;1(9 suppl):S2–S7.
7. Travis WD, Garg K, Franklin WA, et al. Bronchioloalveolar carcinoma and lung adenocarcinoma: the clinical importance and research relevance of the 2004 World Health Organization pathologic criteria. *J Thorac Oncol*. 2006 Nov;1(9 suppl):S13–S19.
8. Yousem SA, Beasley MB. Bronchioloalveolar carcinoma: a review of current concepts and evolving issues. *Arch Pathol Lab Med*. 2007;131:1027–1032.
9. Garfield DH, Cadranel J, West HL. Bronchioloalveolar carcinoma: the case for two diseases. *Clin Lung Cancer*. 2008 Jan;9(1):24–29.
10. Laga AC, Allen T, Ostrowski M, et al. Adenocarcinoma. In: Cagle PT, editor-in-chief. *The Color Atlas and Text of Pulmonary Pathology*. 2nd ed. New York, NY: Lippincott Williams & Wilkins; 2008.
11. Flieder DB, Hammar SP. Common non-small cell carcinomas and their variants. In: Tomashefski J, editor-in-chief, Cagle PT, Farver C, Fraire A, eds. *Dail and Hammar's Pulmonary Pathology*. Vol 2, 3rd ed. New York, NY: Springer; 2008:216–307.
12. Jones KD. Malignant epithelial neoplasms. In: Cagle PT, Allen TC, Beasley MB, eds. *Diagnostic Pulmonary Pathology*. 2nd ed. New York, NY: Informa; 2008:611–626.
13. Kwon KY, Kerr KM, Ro JY. Non-small cell carcinomas. In: Cagle PT, Allen TC, Kerr KM, editors-in-chief. *Transbronchial and Endobronchial Biopsies*. New York, NY: Lippincott Williams & Wilkins; 2009:7–19.

14. Kerr KM. Pulmonary adenocarcinomas: classification and reporting. *Histopathology.* 2009;54(1): 12–27.

15. Gordon IO, Sitterding S, Mackinnon AC, et al. Update in neoplastic lung diseases and mesothelioma. *Arch Pathol Lab Med.* 2009;133(7):1106–1115.

16. Noguchi M, Morikawa A, Kawasaki M, et al. Small adenocarcinoma of the lung: histologic characteristics and prognosis. *Cancer.* 1995;75:2844–2852.

17. Zell JA, Ou SH, Ziogas A, et al. Epidemiology of bronchioloalveolar carcinoma: improvement in survival after release of the 1999 WHO classification of lung tumors. *J Clin Oncol.* 2005;23(33): 8396–8405.

18. Terasaki H, Niki T, Matsuno Y, et al. Lung adenocarcinoma with mixed bronchioloalveolar and invasive components: clinicopathological features, subclassification by extent of invasive foci, and immunohistochemical characterization. *Am J Surg Pathol.* 2003;27(7):937–951.

19. Sakurai H, Maeshima A, Watanabe S, et al. Grade of stromal invasion in small adenocarcinoma of the lung: histopathological minimal invasion and prognosis. *Am J Surg Pathol.* 2004;28(2):198–206.

20. Minami Y, Matsuno Y, Iijima T, et al. Prognostication of small-sized primary pulmonary adenocarcinomas by histopathological and karyometric analysis. *Lung Cancer.* 2005;48(3):339–348.

21. Okudera K, Kamata Y, Takanashi S, et al. Small adenocarcinoma of the lung: prognostic significance of central fibrosis chiefly because of its association with angiogenesis and lymphangiogenesis. *Pathol Int.* 2006;56(9):494–502.

22. Sakao Y, Miyamoto H, Sakuraba M, et al. Prognostic significance of a histologic subtype in small adenocarcinoma of the lung: the impact of nonbronchioloalveolar carcinoma components. *Ann Thorac Surg.* 2007;83(1):209–214.

23. Weydert JA, Cohen MB. Small peripheral pulmonary adenocarcinoma: morphologic and molecular update. *Adv Anat Pathol* 2007;14(2):120–128.

24. Soh J, Toyooka S, Ichihara S, et al. Sequential molecular changes during multistage pathogenesis of small peripheral adenocarcinomas of the lung. *J Thorac Oncol.* 2008;3(4):340–347.

25. Kerr KM, Fyfe MN, Nicolson MC, et al. Influence of tumour patterns in mixed-type adenocarcinoma on post-operative survival. *J Thorac Oncol.* 2007;2(suppl 4):S801–S802.

26. Motoi N, Szoke J, Riely GJ, et al. Lung Adenocarcinoma: Modification of the 2004 WHO mixed subtype to include the major histologic subtype suggests correlations between papillary and micropapillary adenocarcinoma subtypes, EGFR mutations and gene expression analysis. *Am J Surg Pathol.* 2008;32: 810–827.

27. Castro CY, Coffey DM, Medeiros LJ, et al. Prognostic significance of percentage of bronchioloalveolar pattern in adenocarcinomas of the lung. *Ann Diagn Pathol.* 2001;5(5):274–284.

28. Lin DM, Ma Y, Zheng S, et al. Prognostic value of bronchioloalveolar carcinoma component in lung adenocarcinoma. *Histol Histopathol.* 2006;21(6):627–632.

29. Anami Y, Iijima T, Suzuki K, et al. Bronchioloalveolar carcinoma (lepidic growth) component is a more useful prognostic factor than lymph node metastasis. *J Thorac Oncol.* 2009;4(8):951–958.

30. Noguchi M, Minami Y, Iijima T, et al. Reproducibility of the diagnosis of small adenocarcinoma of the lung and usefulness of an educational program for the diagnostic criteria. *Pathol Int.* 2005;55:8–13.

31. Yim J, Zhu L-C, Chiriboga L, et al. Histologic features are important prognostic indicators in early stages lung adenocarcinomas. *Mod Pathol.* 2007;20:233–241.

32. Dacic S. Minimally invasive adenocarcinomas of the lung. *Adv Anat Pathol.* 2009;16(3):166–171.

33. Rosenblatt MB, Lisa JR, Collier F. Primary and metastatic bronchiolo-alveolar carcinoma. *Dis Chest.* 1967;52:147–152.

34. Saad RS, Cho P, Silverman JF, et al. Usefulness of Cdx2 in separating mucinous bronchioloalveolar adenocarcinoma of the lung from metastatic mucinous colorectal adenocarcinoma. *Am J Clin Pathol.* 2004;122(3):421–427.

35. Sheffield EA, Addis BJ, Corrin B, et al. Epithelial hyperplasia and malignant change in congenital lung cysts. *J Clin Pathol.* 1987;40(6):612–614.

36. Stacher E, Ullmann R, Halbwedl I, et al. Atypical goblet cell hyperplasia in congenital cystic adenomatoid malformation as a possible preneoplasia for pulmonary adenocarcinoma in childhood: a genetic analysis. *Hum Pathol.* 2004;35(5):565–570.

37. Lantuejoul S, Ferretti GR, Goldstraw P, et al. Metastases from bronchioloalveolar carcinomas associated with long-standing type 1 congenital cystic adenomatoid malformations. A report of two cases. *Histopathology.* 2006;48(2):204–206.

38. Lantuejoul S, Nicholson AG, Sartori G, et al. Mucinous cells in type 1 pulmonary congenital cystic adenomatoid malformation as mucinous bronchioloalveolar carcinoma precursors. *Am J Surg Pathol.* 2007;31(6):961–969.

39. Marchetti A, Buttitta F, Pellegrini S, et al. Bronchioloalveolar lung carcinomas: K-ras mutations are constant events in the mucinous subtype. *J Pathol.* 1996;179(3):254–259.

40. Garfield D. Can K-ras-mutated atypical adenomatous hyperplasia be another precursor lesion for mucinous bronchioloalveolar carcinoma? *Am J Clin Pathol.* 2008;130(2):315–316.

Proposed Revisions to the Classification of Adenocarcinoma

5

▶ Philip T. Cagle
▶ Keith M. Kerr

The International Association for the Study of Lung Cancer (IASLC) in collaboration with the American Thoracic Society and the European Respiratory Society is proposing an International Multidisciplinary Classification of Lung Adenocarcinoma.[1] This effort is led by William Travis, chair of the 1999 and 2004 World Health Organization thoracic tumor classifications,[2,3] with integrated clinical, radiologic, molecular, and surgical inputs in addition to histologic criteria. The proposed revisions to the classification of pulmonary adenocarcinomas, including bronchioloalveolar carcinomas (BACs), are partly derived from pathologic correlation with recent observations in radiology and clinical behavior and are partly in response to the needs of oncologists who are using and investigating new therapeutic protocols, including targeted molecular therapy. The observations of Noguchi and other investigators in Japan have led to the concepts of pure lepidic tumors (BAC or adenocarcinoma in situ [AIS]) and minimal invasion, which is a foundation for the new classification.[4–17] A more precise, clinically relevant terminology is also an objective. In addition to this specific proposal, a number of authors have addressed similar issues of classification of lung cancers, particularly adenocarcinoma, in the past few years.[18,19] In particular, some authors have noted that it is likely that the atypical adenomatous hyperplasia-BAC/AIS/invasive carcinoma pathway is not the only sequence of changes leading to the development of invasive adenocarcinomas.[20,21]

Another motivation to reconsider the classification of adenocarcinomas is the current inconsistency and multiplicity of uses of the term "bronchioloalveolar," either as a descriptive term for a particular pattern of tumor or as an actual diagnosis, viz, bronchioloalveolar carcinoma. The term BAC is used correctly to describe localized, noninvasive, and usually nonmucinous lesions (see below and Chapters 4 and 27) but is still also frequently used in the context of both mixed pattern invasive adenocarcinomas of usual type when a BAC pattern is present and less common, multifocal advanced forms of adenocarcinoma of nonmucinous, but more often mucinous, type, where there is widespread "pneumonic consolidation" in one or both lungs by a predominantly lepidic-pattern spreading adenocarcinoma, for example, so-called "mucinous BAC."

The increasing interest in these patterns of disease among pulmonologists and oncologists, driven by the emergence of targeted therapies that appear especially effective in some such tumors, brought the existence of widespread confusion around terminology and pathology into sharp focus. A solution was required.

Finally, the molecular, as well as morphological, heterogeneity of lung adenocarcinomas was emphasized by a number of important publications looking at global gene expression in these tumors. A number of studies suggested subgroups of adenocarcinoma defined by common gene expression.[22–26] These data were commensurate with the prospect of selecting subgroups of adenocarcinomas for specific molecular targeted therapy.

PREINVASIVE LESIONS

Atypical adenomatous hyperplasia is recognized as a preinvasive lesion that may, in some cases, be the precursor to AIS (BAC) and, eventually, to invasive adenocarcinomas. Atypical adenomatous hyperplasia is discussed in detail in Chapter 27.

As noted in Chapter 4, it has been recommended that the term adenocarcinoma-in-situ replace bronchioloalveolar carcinoma. Therefore, AIS is a localized and small, usually 2 cm or less in diameter, lesion in which the cells grow only along preexisting alveolar septa (lepidic pattern) without invasion into stroma, vessels, or pleura. The alveolar septa may be widened by fibrosis but, by definition, are not invaded by tumor cells. Virtually all cases of AIS are nonmucinous. Mucinous variants are extremely rare. Nuclear atypia is absent or inconspicuous, and complex papillary and micropapillary patterns should be absent. In the current WHO classification, small simple epithelial tufts may be seen in pure localized nonmucinous BAC. Obviously, to exclude invasion, the entire tumor must be examined. Patients with AIS have a nearly 100% 5-year survival rate if their tumors are completely resected.

MINIMALLY INVASIVE ADENOCARCINOMA

As mentioned in Chapter 4, the definition of minimal invasion requires further study. However, the proposed definition for minimally invasive adenocarcinoma (MIA) is a solitary, discrete adenocarcinoma, usually 2 cm or less, with a predominantly lepidic pattern and 5 mm or less of invasion in any one focus (Figs. 5-1 and 5-2). An invasive focus can be recognized as histologic subtypes other than lepidic pattern (acinar, papillary, micropapillary, and/or solid) or myofibroblastic (desmoplastic) stroma associated with invasive cancer cells (see also Chapter 4). If there is lymphovascular invasion, pleural invasion, tumor necrosis, or metastases from the cancer, minimal invasion is excluded. As with AIS, most MIAs are nonmucinous and are only very rarely mucinous. If a cancer has more than one focus of invasion, the size of the largest focus of invasion determines whether the cancer is minimally invasive, rather than the sum of the sizes of the invasive foci. Once again, to confirm the amount of invasion, the entire tumor must be examined. Patients with MIA also have a nearly 100% 5-year survival rate if their tumors are completely resected.

FIGURE 5-1 On scanning power, this adenocarcinoma consists predominantly of in-situ lepidic pattern. There are a couple of small foci that, on higher power, disclose invasion of less than 5 mm in diameter, making this an MIA by proposed criteria.

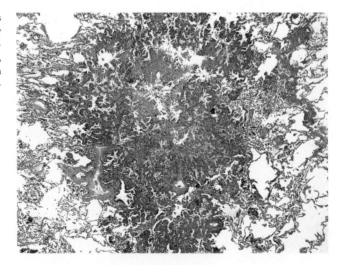

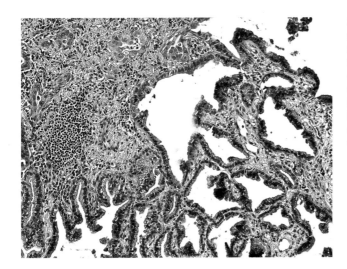

FIGURE 5-2 High power of a focus of minimal invasion from the MIA in Figure 5-1. The lepidic growth of the majority of the tumor along intact fibrotic alveolar septa is seen on the right and lower portions of the image. In the upper left, there is invasion of the fibrous stroma by small, irregular glands lined by cells with greater cytologic atypia and more abundant eosinophilic cytoplasm than the AIS cells.

INVASIVE ADENOCARCINOMA

The vast majority of pulmonary adenocarcinomas are of mixed histologic subtypes, and rather than "mixed subtype" as a separate histologic category, as it is in the 2004 WHO classification, it is proposed that adenocarcinomas should be classified according to their predominant histologic subtype. In addition, a semiquantitative percentage of the various subtypes within a single tumor should be estimated in 5% increments for clinical and molecular correlations. The micropapillary subtype has been added to the major histologic subtypes and is associated with a poor prognosis in early-stage disease. The proposed histologic subtypes are lepidic predominant, acinar predominant, papillary predominant, micropapillary predominant, and solid predominant. These changes are appropriate given the fact that the vast majority of cases fall into the current "mixed subtype" category and that tumors with predominantly lepidic histology have a relatively good prognosis while those that are predominantly micropapillary or solid pattern appear to be more aggressive.

VARIANTS

The striking differences between nonmucinous BAC and mucinous BAC are discussed in Chapter 4. Tumors that would have previously been classified as mucinous BAC have an invasive component in most cases, and, therefore, it is now recommended that these tumors be called mucinous adenocarcinomas with a predominant lepidic pattern. As already noted, mucinous AIS and mucinous MIA are extremely rare.

In addition to mucinous adenocarcinoma, other variants currently being proposed include colloid adenocarcinoma, fetal adenocarcinoma, and enteric adenocarcinoma. Colloid adenocarcinoma, and fetal adenocarcinoma are described in Chapter 3. Enteric adenocarcinoma consists of columnar cells (with or without apical mucin) in a cribriform pattern and "dirty" necrosis that histologically mimics adenocarcinoma of the colon (Fig. 5-3). In addition, enteric adenocarcinomas have an immunostaining pattern similar to colon cancer.

It is proposed that clear cell adenocarcinoma and signet ring cell adenocarcinoma no longer be recognized as separate subtypes or variants because there are currently no significant clinical associations identified. Instead, these are recognized as cytologic changes that may occur in multiple histologic subtypes, although they are especially associated with the solid predominant subtype.

LEPIDIC-PATTERN LESIONS

Discontinuance of the term "Bronchioloalveolar carcinoma" is a positive move that should help to provide a more meaningful and accurate classification. Although in some contexts, it is still a valid descriptive terminology, to retain its use in some instances would be likely to perpetuate confusion. Nevertheless, discontinuance of this long-standing term is expected to be controversial.

The term adenocarcinoma-in-situ fits well with the morphology and biology of those small, localized, cytologically low-grade lesions of pure lepidic growth that lack any evidence of pleural, stromal, or lymphatic invasion. The cell populations in such lesions are growing in their native epithelial compartment and have not (yet) acquired the genetic and, therefore, the morphological or biological characteristics of a malignant (invasive) cell population. The recognition of MIA underpins the place of AIS as a recognizable stage in this particular pathway of adenocarcinoma development.

Does this mean that every instance of glandular neoplastic cells growing in a lepidic fashion represents AIS? In a small adenocarcinoma of predominantly lepidic growth pattern, as the invasive focus grows and exceeds the 5-mm dimension defining MIA, the peripheral lepidic component of the lesion remains, biologically speaking, noninvasive AIS. The cells here are of lower grade and are genetically different from those in the invasive area. Ultimately, as the invasive clone progresses and expands, it will overgrow and replace the preexisting AIS in most cases.

In larger, mixed-pattern adenocarcinomas, a lepidic component is often also present. Morphologically, this may, at least in part, resemble the low-grade cell population typical of AIS and be quite different from the cytologically higher grade invasive patterns also present, in other words residual AIS. In many instances, however, the lepidic pattern may be cytologically high grade, similar to the cells in the invasive component of the tumor, and exist at the periphery of a

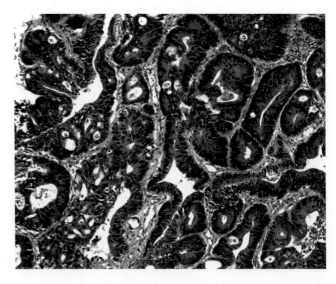

FIGURE 5-3 Pulmonary enteric adenocarcinoma consists of malignant columnar cells arranged in cribriform pattern resembling colorectal carcinoma.

large lesion, much larger than true AIS lesions ever are. While this pattern of tumor is technically "in situ" in the sense that it is within the alveolar epithelial compartment, it is hard to accept that this is biologically the same as true AIS. The same questions arise in the context of multifocal lepidic-pattern adenocarcinomas, most often of mucinous type. These latter scenarios may well represent a particular form of invasive adenocarcinoma, biologically more advanced than AIS but, for whatever reason, having a propensity to grow and spread within the lung in this very particular way.

More research, especially on the genetic characteristics of these lesions, is required to clarify our understanding of this still complex area.

ADENOCARCINOMA VERSUS SQUAMOUS CELL CARCINOMA

About 70% of lung cancers are diagnosed on small biopsies or cytology specimens alone. The majority of lung cancers are inoperable, mostly due to advanced stage at diagnosis or significant patient comorbidity.

For various treatment protocols, including clinical trials, oncologists require pathologists to distinguish specific cell types (adenocarcinoma or squamous cell carcinoma) on lung cancer biopsies and cytology specimens. This is a change from the past when treatment options and responses were much more limited and a simple diagnosis of "non–small cell lung carcinoma" (NSCLC) often sufficed. There is substantial evidence that patients with nonsquamous NSCLC have better outcomes when treated with pemetrexed in combination with platinum-based cytotoxics, as opposed to other so-called platinum doublets. Patients with squamous cell carcinoma have been reported to experience life-threatening hemorrhage when treated with bevacizumab. These findings are now reflected in the licensed prescribing conditions for these drugs in many countries. Smarter strategies for the selection of NSCLC cases for *EGFR* mutation testing could be based upon NSCLC subtyping. Specific molecular targeted agents are emerging, which may be more efficacious in squamous cell carcinomas.

All this means that distinguishing squamous cell carcinoma from adenocarcinoma is much more important than in the past. The IASLC recommendation is that the specific cell type of an NSCLC should be diagnosed whenever possible, and the use of NSCLC, not otherwise specified (NOS), as a diagnosis should be minimized.

If the histologic features do not permit a definitive diagnosis of adenocarcinoma or squamous cell carcinoma, then the morphological diagnosis is NSCLC, NOS. Special stains and immunostains may, however, help in *suggesting* a likely tumor subtype. Thyroid transcription factor-1 (TTF-1) is the best widely available marker for adenocarcinoma. Napsin A is another more recently described marker for pulmonary adenocarcinoma that is gaining in popularity. Periodic acid Schiff with diastase stain, possibly combined with Alcian blue, may also be used to stain mucin for diagnosing adenocarcinoma. The best markers for squamous cell carcinoma are p63 and CK 5/6. The adenocarcinoma markers and squamous cell carcinoma markers are usually mutually exclusive. Therefore, in a biopsy or cytology specimen where H&E morphology is not definitive, a tumor that is positive for TTF-1 and/or mucin and negative for p63 and CK 5/6 should be diagnosed as "NSCLC, favor adenocarcinoma." Likewise, a tumor that is positive for p63 and/or CK 5/6 and negative for adenocarcinoma markers should be diagnosed as "NSCLC, favor squamous cell carcinoma."[27]

It should be emphasized that interpretation of immunostains should be carried out with care. Clearly defined thresholds for what constitutes a "positive" or "negative" stain need to be strictly observed, and it should be realized that antibodies supplied from different sources may have different specificities and may not demonstrate identical predictive ability.

References

1. Travis WD, Brambilla E, Noguchi M, et al. The new IASLC/ATS/ERS international multidisciplinary lung adenocarcinoma classification. *J Thorac Oncol.* 2009;4(Suppl. 1):s86–s89.
2. Travis WD, Colby TV, Corrin B, et al. In collaboration with Sobin LH and pathologists from 14 countries. *World Health Organization International Histological Classification of Tumours. Histological Typing of Lung and Pleural Tumours.* 3rd ed. Berlin: Springer-Verlag; 1999.
3. Travis WD, Brambilla E, Muller-Hermelink HK, et al., eds. *World Health Organisation Classification of Tumours. Pathology and Genetics of Tumours of the Lung, Pleura, Thymus and Heart.* Lyon: IARC Press; 2004:35–44.
4. Noguchi M, Morikawa A, Kawasaki M, et al. Small adenocarcinoma of the lung: histologic characteristics and prognosis. *Cancer.* 1995;75:2844–2852.
5. Zell JA, Ou SH, Ziogas A, et al. Epidemiology of bronchioloalveolar carcinoma: improvement in survival after release of the 1999 WHO classification of lung tumors. *J Clin Oncol.* 2005;23(33): 8396–8405.
6. Terasaki H, Niki T, Matsuno Y, et al. Lung adenocarcinoma with mixed bronchioloalveolar and invasive components: clinicopathological features, subclassification by extent of invasive foci, and immunohistochemical characterization. *Am J Surg Pathol.* 2003;27(7):937–951.
7. Sakurai H, Maeshima A, Watanabe S, et al. Grade of stromal invasion in small adenocarcinoma of the lung: histopathological minimal invasion and prognosis. *Am J Surg Pathol.* 2004;28(2):198–206.
8. Minami Y, Matsuno Y, Iijima T, et al. Prognostication of small-sized primary pulmonary adenocarcinomas by histopathological and karyometric analysis. *Lung Cancer.* 2005;48(3):339–348.
9. Noguchi M, Minami Y, Iijima T, et al. Reproducibility of the diagnosis of small adenocarcinoma of the lung and usefulness of an educational program for the diagnostic criteria. *Pathol Int.* 2005;55:8–13.
10. Okudera K, Kamata Y, Takanashi S, et al. Small adenocarcinoma of the lung: prognostic significance of central fibrosis chiefly because of its association with angiogenesis and lymphangiogenesis. *Pathol Int.* 2006;56(9):494–502.
11. Sakao Y, Miyamoto H, Sakuraba M, et al. Prognostic significance of a histologic subtype in small adenocarcinoma of the lung: the impact of nonbronchioloalveolar carcinoma components. *Ann Thorac Surg.* 2007;83(1):209–214.
12. Weydert JA, Cohen MB. Small peripheral pulmonary adenocarcinoma: morphologic and molecular update. *Adv Anat Pathol.* 2007;14(2):120–128.
13. Soh J, Toyooka S, Ichihara S, et al. Sequential molecular changes during multistage pathogenesis of small peripheral adenocarcinomas of the lung. *J Thorac Oncol.* 2008;3(4):340–347.
14. Castro CY, Coffey DM, Medeiros LJ, et al. Prognostic significance of percentage of bronchioloalveolar pattern in adenocarcinomas of the lung. *Ann Diagn Pathol.* 2001;5(5):274–284.
15. Lin DM, Ma Y, Zheng S, et al. Prognostic value of bronchioloalveolar carcinoma component in lung adenocarcinoma. *Histol Histopathol.* 2006;21(6):627–632.
16. Yim J, Zhu L-C, Chiriboga L, et al. Histologic features are important prognostic indicators in early stages lung adenocarcinomas. *Mod Pathol.* 2007;20:233–241.
17. Anami Y, Iijima T, Suzuki K, et al. Bronchioloalveolar carcinoma (lepidic growth) component is a more useful prognostic factor than lymph node metastasis. *J Thorac Oncol.* 2009;4(8):951–958.
18. Kerr KM. Pulmonary adenocarcinomas: classification and reporting. *Histopathology.* 2009;54(1): 12–27.
19. Dacic S. Minimally invasive adenocarcinomas of the lung. *Adv Anat Pathol.* 2009;16(3):166–171.
20. Bach PB. Is our natural-history model of lung cancer wrong? *Lancet Oncol.* 2008;9(7):693–697.
21. Chirieac LR, Flieder DB. High-resolution computed tomography screening for lung cancer: unexpected findings and new controversies regarding adenocarcinogenesis. *Arch Pathol Lab Med.* 2010;134(1):41–48.
22. Garber ME, Troyanskaya OG, Schluens K et al. Diversity in gene expression in adenocarcinoma of the lung. *Proc Natl Acad Sci USA.* 2001;98:13784–13789.
23. Bhattacharjee A, Richards WG, Staunton J, et al. Classification of human lung carcinomas bt mRNA expression profiling reveals distinct adenocarcinoma subgroups. *Proc Natl Acad Sci USA.* 2001;98: 13790–13795.

24. Beer DG, Kardia SLR, Huang C-C, et al. Gene-expression profiles predict survival of patients with lung adenocarcinoma. *Nat Med.* 2002;8:816–824.

25. Takeuchi T, Tomida S, Yatabe Y, et al. Expression profile-defined classification of lung adenocarcinoma shows close relationship with underlying major genetic changes and clinicopathologic behaviour. *J Clin Oncol* 2006;24:1679–1688.

26. Hayes DN, Monti S, Parmigiani G, et al. Gene expression profiling reveals reproducible human lung adenocarcinoma subtypes in multiple independent patient cohorts. *J Clin Oncol.* 2006;24:5079–5090.

27. Loo PS, Thomas SC, Nicolson MC, et al. Subtyping of undifferentiated non-small cell carcinomas in bronchial biopsy specimens. *J Thorac Oncol.* 2010;5(4):442–447.

6

Squamous Cell Carcinoma

▶ Timothy Craig Allen

Squamous cell lung cancer remains the most common histologic type of lung cancer worldwide; however, in the United States, Canada, Japan, and China, due to differences in smoking behavior and cigarette designs, adenocarcinoma has replaced squamous cell carcinoma as the histologic type of lung cancer with the highest incidence.[1,2] In the United States, squamous cell lung cancer peaked in incidence in 1981 in men; however, it continues to rise in incidence in women.[1] Currently, squamous cell carcinoma makes up approximately 30% of lung cancer diagnoses in the United States.[3]

Cigarette smoking is the primary etiology of squamous cell lung cancer; however, other associations have been identified, including radiation, arsenic, and chloromethyl ether exposures. A diet high in fruits and vegetables may have a protective effect on the development of squamous cell lung cancer.[1] Because squamous cell lung cancer is frequently central, that is, arising within the mainstem bronchi, lobar bronchi, or segmental bronchi, sputum cytology for preneoplasia and early invasive tumors has been attempted; however, currently bronchoscopy detects fewer than 40% of in-situ lesions. While autofluorescence bronchoscopy is more sensitive, it has a high false-positive rate caused by goblet cell hyperplasia and inflammatory lesions.[1,4]

Clinically, patients with centrally located squamous cell carcinoma often present with obstructive symptoms including cough, wheezing, increased amounts of sputum production, or hemoptysis. Many centrally placed tumors present symptomatically while still relatively small due to their propensity to obstruct, with associated postobstructive pneumonia and mucostasis. Central necrosis is frequently a feature of squamous cell lung cancers, especially larger tumors.[1–3,5] Peripheral squamous cell carcinomas are more likely to be associated with dyspnea and chest pain.[1–3,5,6] Radiologically, central squamous cell carcinomas may exhibit lung collapse, mediastinal shifting toward the side involved with tumor, and, in cases with perihilar and mediastinal extension of tumor, perihilar and mediastinal masses. Peripheral tumors often radiologically exhibit solitary tumor nodules and masses, many of which may show central cavitation and lucency. Pleural effusions may occur. So-called Pancoast tumors, arising in the superior sulcus, often radiologically exhibit posterior rib destruction and clinically Horner syndrome.[2–4,7,8]

The specific histological diagnosis of the non–small cell carcinomas of the lung, including accurate diagnosis of squamous cell lung carcinoma, has become increasingly important as new, novel therapies have evolved that depend upon accurate differentiation of non–small cell lung carcinomas as squamous cell carcinoma, adenocarcinoma, or large cell carcinoma.[9–15] Limited, including frequently cytologic, sampling of lung tumors and lung cancer heterogeneity are confounding factors in accurate diagnostic typing of non–small cell carcinomas.[16] Second-line treatments with bevacizumab, pemetrexed, erlotinib, or docetaxel may be of benefit in some patients who have lung cancers with "predominantly nonsquamous histology."[17] Indeed, differentiating adenocarcinoma from squamous cell carcinoma is extremely important prior to beginning pemetrexed or bevacizumab therapy (see Chapter 22).

SQUAMOUS CELL CARCINOMA, CYTOLOGY

Sputum cytology may contain single tumor cells or small clusters of tumor cells, and bronchial brushings and fine-needle aspiration specimens may contain sheets of tumor cells (Fig. 6-1).[3] Tumor cell nuclei may be hyperchromatic, with an "ink dot" appearance, and poorly differentiated tumors may contain prominent nucleoli. Some tumor cells may have irregular shapes such as "tadpole" cells (Fig. 6-2). Cytoplasm may be densely orangophilic, or, on Pap stain, cyanophilic (Fig. 6-3).[3]

SQUAMOUS CELL CARCINOMA, GROSS FEATURES

About two thirds of squamous cell carcinomas are centrally located tumors.[3] Excised tumors are variably fibrotic, ranging from white to gray-tan, and may be centrally cavitated. Central tumors may show polypoid luminal tumor growth with associated infiltration of tumor into bronchial wall and surrounding lung parenchyma and hilum (Figs. 6-4 and 6-5). Partial or complete luminal

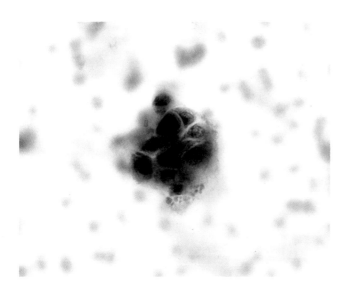

FIGURE 6-1 High power of Pap stain of sputum specimen containing squamous cell carcinoma showing a three-dimensional cluster of tumor cells with enlarged, hyperchromatic nuclei and dense cytoplasm.

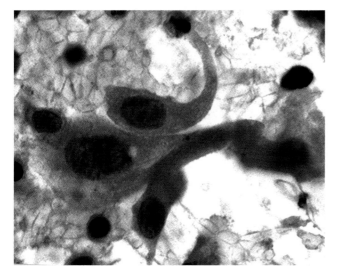

FIGURE 6-2 High power of Pap-stained cytology of pulmonary squamous cell carcinoma showing a tadpole cell and some "inkblot" nuclei.

FIGURE 6-3 High power of Pap-stained squamous cell carcinoma cytology showing a tumor cell with an enlarged atypical nucleus and dense keratinized cytoplasm.

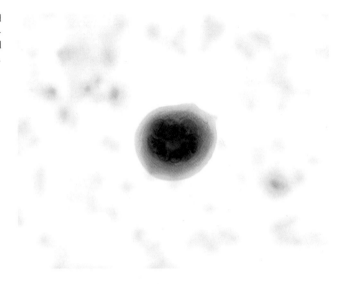

FIGURE 6-4 Gross image of lung containing squamous cell carcinoma with widespread necrosis and a large area of central cavitation.

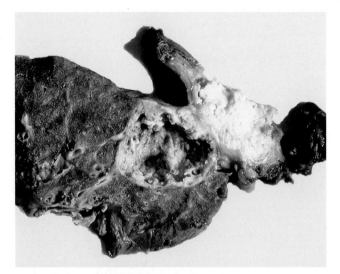

FIGURE 6-5 Gross image of bronchial squamous cell carcinoma showing tumor protruding into the bronchiolar lumen.

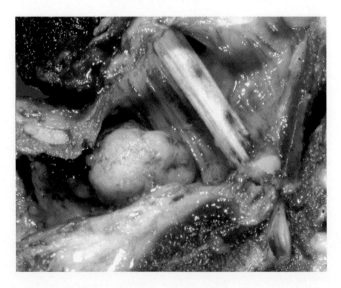

obstruction is frequent, with associated postobstructive pneumonia and mucostasis. Peripheral tumors are variably sized nodules or masses that may show an expansile or stellate growth pattern, with or without central necrosis.[1–3,18–20] Pulmonary squamous cell carcinoma is defined by the WHO as "a malignant epithelial tumor showing keratinization and/or intercellular bridges that arises from bronchial epithelium."[4]

SQUAMOUS CELL CARCINOMA, HISTOLOGY

Squamous cell carcinomas histologically contain intercellular bridges or keratinization in the form of keratin pearls or single-cell keratinization (Figs. 6-6–6-8).[2,3] Although the amount varies with the degree of tumor differentiation, single-cell keratinization, squamous pearl formation, or intercellular bridges are required for the diagnosis of squamous cell carcinoma. In poorly differentiated squamous cell carcinomas, careful inspection may be required to make the diagnosis.

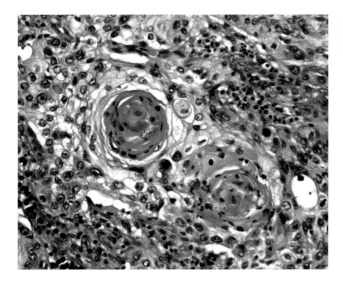

FIGURE 6-6 High power showing squamous cell carcinoma with keratin pearl formation.

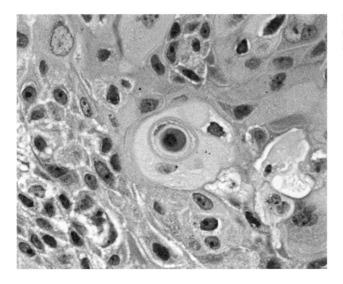

FIGURE 6-7 High power of squamous cell carcinoma showing single-cell keratinization.

FIGURE 6-8 High power of an area of squamous cell carcinoma containing intercellular bridges.

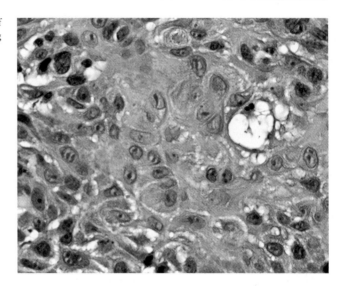

Tumors that show squamoid features but without single-cell keratinization, squamous pearl formation, or intercellular bridges, should be diagnosed as large cell carcinoma and not as poorly differentiated squamous cell carcinoma.[1-4,20] With transbronchial biopsy, extension of squamous cell carcinoma in situ from the bronchial surface into underlying bronchial glands, with replacement of those glands, may mimic invasive squamous cell carcinoma, and care must be taken to distinguish these two situations (Fig. 6-9) (see Chapter 26). Focal residual glands and identifiable lobular architecture may help in distinguishing glandular involvement with squamous cell carcinoma in situ. Care must be taken not to misinterpret residual or entrapped bronchial glands as adenosquamous carcinoma (Fig. 6-10) (see Chapter 7). Repeat biopsy may be of benefit in making the correct diagnosis. Another potential risk with transbronchial biopsy is that squamous metaplasia within alveolar spaces, in reaction to inflammatory or other disease, may be sampled and may mimic squamous cell carcinoma. Strict adherence to diagnostic criteria will help reduce this risk.[2]

FIGURE 6-9 High power of squamous cell carcinoma in situ showing superficial gland involvement beneath surface mucosa entirely made up of squamous cell carcinoma in situ.

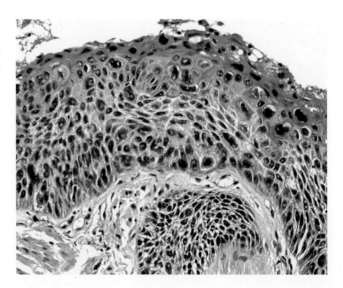

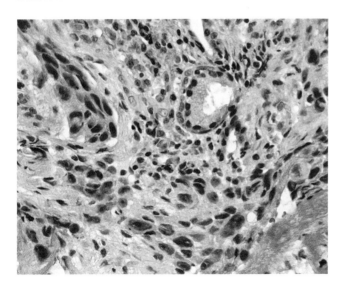

FIGURE 6-10 High power of squamous cell carcinoma showing an entrapped bronchial gland, not to be confused with adenosquamous carcinoma. Note the benign features of the glandular cells as compared with the malignant squamous cells.

SQUAMOUS CELL CARCINOMA, IMMUNOHISTOCHEMISTRY

Tumor cells are generally immunopositive with cytokeratins, including AE1/AE3, CK5, CK6, 34BE12, EMA, HMFG-2; often immunopositive with CEA; occasionally immunopositive with vimentin; and generally immunonegative with CK7 and TTF-1 (Figs. 6-11 and 6-12).[3,20] As noted above and discussed in Chapter 5, differentiating squamous cell carcinoma from adenocarcinoma has become increasingly important for therapeutic purposes, and immunostains play a role in differential diagnosis. Where the histologic features of a non–small cell lung cancer are not definitively diagnostic of squamous cell carcinoma or adenocarcinoma, such as in limited biopsies, immunostains with TTF-1, p63, and CK5/6, and periodic acid-Schiff with Diastase (PAS-D), possibly combined with Alcian blue stain, may assist is suggesting the tumor subtype. Squamous cell carcinomas typically show immunopositivity with p63 and CK5/6, immunonegativity with TTF-1, and no mucin staining with PAS-D stain, whereas adenocarcinomas generally show the opposite. According to the International Association for the Study of Lung Cancer recommendation, therefore, a biopsy or cytology specimen for which H&E morphology is not

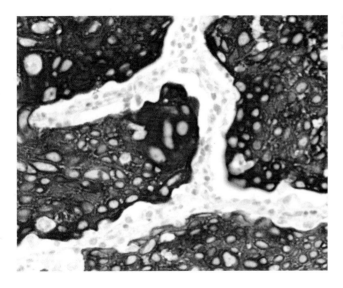

FIGURE 6-11 This poorly-differentiated squamous cell carcinoma shows strong cytoplasmic immunopositivity with CK5.

FIGURE 6-12 This poorly-differentiated squamous cell carcinoma shows strong nuclear immunopositivity with p63.

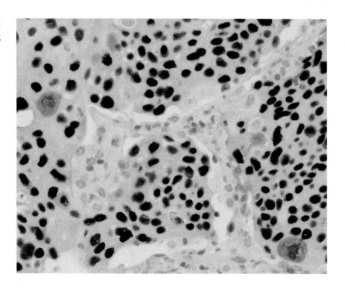

definitive, but where there is tumor cell immunopositivity with p63 and/or CK5/6, along with tumor cell immunonegativity with TTF-1 and negative mucin staining with PAS-D, the tumor should be diagnosed as "non–small cell lung carcinoma, favor squamous cell carcinoma"; and in cases that are p63 and CK5/6 immunonegative, but show TTF-1 immunopositivity and/or mucin positivity with PAS-D, the tumor should be diagnosed as "non–small cell lung carcinoma, favor adenocarcinoma."

SQUAMOUS CELL CARCINOMA, VARIANTS

Squamous cell carcinomas are often heterogeneous, and clear cell, basaloid, papillary, and small cell variants have been recognized by the WHO.[2,3,20,21] Basaloid squamous cell carcinoma is an uncommon variant of squamous cell carcinoma that exhibits prominent peripheral palisading of tumor cell nuclei (Figs. 6-13 and 6-14). If such peripheral palisading is identified in a poorly differentiated tumor that does not exhibit diagnostic features of squamous cell carcinoma such as single-cell keratinization, keratin pearl formation, or intercellular bridges, then the diagnosis of basaloid large cell carcinoma is appropriate.[1–4,20,22,23] Papillary variant of squamous cell carcinoma is a rare variant that exhibits a unique exophytic papillary endobronchial growth pattern, often with invasion of underlying bronchial wall and lung parenchyma. Histologically, fibrovascular cores lined by squamous epithelium protrude into the bronchial lumen (Fig. 6-15). While these cases often occur in adult smokers, they may arise in patients with squamous papillomatosis. Care must be taken to differentiate papillary squamous cell carcinoma without invasion from squamous papilloma. Some cases of squamous papilloma show bronchial gland extension of the lesion that may mimic invasion. The clear cell variant of squamous cell carcinoma exhibits tumor cells with clear cytoplasm that make up almost all or the vast majority of the tumor (Fig. 6-16). Care must be taken to not overdiagnose squamous cell carcinoma that contains only focal areas of cytoplasmic clearing, and to not misdiagnose adenocarcinoma or large cell carcinoma with clear cell change. Metastatic renal cell carcinoma must also be considered in the differential diagnosis.[1–4,20] The small cell variant of squamous cell carcinoma is a rare variant that shows small cells with focal areas of squamous cell differentiation. The small cells have nuclear features of non–small cell carcinoma rather than small cell carcinoma (Fig. 6-17). The small cells have generally vesicular rather than "salt and pepper" chromatin, typically conspicuous nucleoli, and relatively abundant cytoplasm. Immunostains with p63, p16, high-molecular-weight keratin, and TTF-1, may assist in making the correct diagnosis.[1–4,20,24–26]

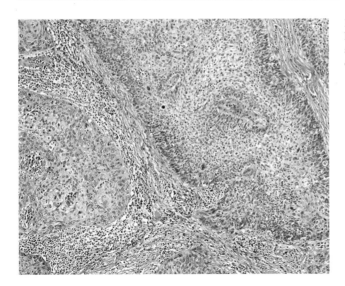

FIGURE 6-13 Medium power of basaloid variant of squamous cell carcinoma showing peripheral palisading of tumor cells and focal areas of keratinization.

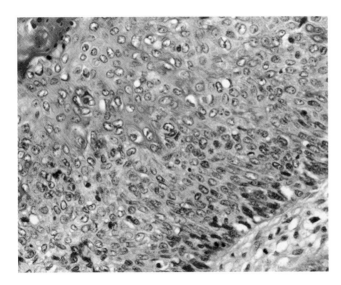

FIGURE 6-14 High power image of basaloid variant of squamous cell carcinoma showing peripheral palisading at the edge of the tumor cell nest. Focal keratinization is present at the upper left.

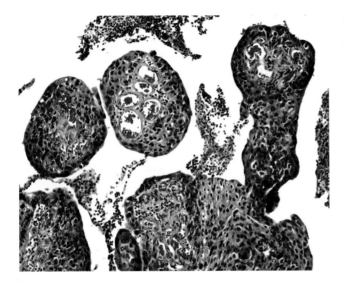

FIGURE 6-15 High power of papillary variant of squamous cell carcinoma showing tumor cells lining fibrovascular cores.

FIGURE 6-16 High power of clear cell variant of squamous cell carcinoma showing nests of tumor cells with abundant clear cytoplasm.

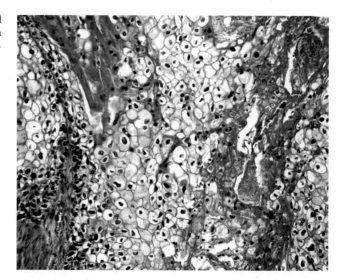

FIGURE 6-17 High power of small cell variant of squamous cell carcinoma showing small tumor cells in the upper part of the image, with nuclear features similar to those of the larger tumor cells in the lower part of the image.

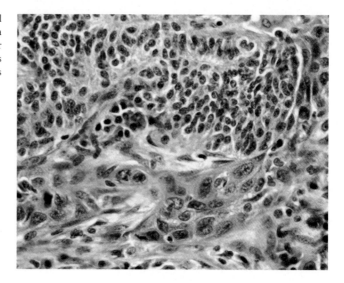

While most squamous cell carcinomas arise centrally, peripheral squamous cell carcinomas do occur, with studies showing peripheral tumors in between 15% and 30% of pulmonary squamous cell carcinomas.[27] Peripheral squamous cell carcinomas may be increasing in incidence.[4,19] Peripheral squamous cell carcinomas have been generally considered to be smaller, earlier stage, slower growing tumors with a tendency to remain localized when compared with squamous cell carcinomas arising within the central airways.[27] Yousem[18] examined 62 peripheral squamous cell carcinomas and found them to range from 1.2 to 8.5 cm (range: 4.23 cm) in size.[18] Some studies have shown a lower rate of lymph node involvement with pulmonary squamous cell carcinomas that are peripheral and <2 cm in size; however, Sakurai et al.[27] did not find a statistically significant lower risk, with 14% of tumors <2 cm showing nodal metastases and 33% of tumors >2 cm showing nodal metastases.[27] This rate of nodal metastasis is higher than rates reported by other authors, ranging from 0% to 7.4%.[27] Mediastinal metastases without hilar or intraparenchymal lymph node metastases, which occur in approximately 255 of N2 peripheral non–small cell carcinomas, a not uncommon finding with peripheral adenocarcinomas, occur rarely with peripheral squamous cell carcinomas.[27] Yousem[18] has described four marginal growth

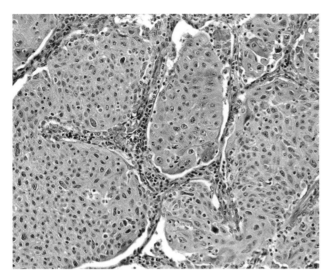

FIGURE 6-18 High power of alveolar filling pattern in a peripheral squamous cell carcinoma showing intact alveolar septa and tumor cells filling alveolar spaces.

patterns of peripheral squamous cell carcinomas, including pushing, infiltrative, alveolar filling, and pseudoalveolar filling patterns. The pushing pattern has a well-defined expansile border compressing surrounding lung parenchyma. The infiltrative pattern consists of nests of tumor cells that infiltrate septal connective tissue collagen and elastic lamina, lifting alveolar pneumocytes from the basement membrane that form elongated or tubular structures that are CK7 and TTF-1 positive, surrounded by tumor cells. The alveolar filling pattern is characterized by cohesive aggregates of tumor cells filling airspaces and leaving intact alveolar septa (Fig. 6-18). The pseudoalveolar filling pattern displays a similar appearance to the alveolar filling pattern except that TTF-1 and CK7 stains show fragmented alveolar lining epithelium and fragmented alveolar septal elastic, with insinuation of tumor cells into septal structures.[18] Tumors can show a mixture of marginal growth patterns. In some cases with alveolar filling pattern, the tumor size may be downgraded to take into account this noninvasive component.[18]

SQUAMOUS CELL CARCINOMA, DIFFERENTIAL DIAGNOSIS

Poorly differentiated, solid-type squamous cell carcinoma of the lung may be difficult to distinguish from large cell carcinoma or poorly differentiated, solid-type adenocarcinoma. As noted above, differentiation of solid-type squamous cell carcinoma from solid-type adenocarcinoma is very important in selecting the appropriate therapeutic agents, as, for example, bevacizumab may potentially cause fatal hemorrhage in patients with squamous cell carcinoma (see Chapters 3 and 22). Strict adherence to diagnostic criteria will assist in making the correct diagnosis. In the variants of squamous cell carcinoma, other differential diagnoses must be considered, as discussed above. Determining whether squamous cell carcinoma in the lung is a primary tumor or whether it is metastatic may be problematic. This situation frequently arises in patients with prior squamous cell carcinoma of the head and neck, but may also occur with other primary squamous cell carcinomas, such as uterine cervix.[20] When clinical indicators suggest metastatic disease, molecular analysis might be of benefit in selected cases[20] (see chapter 22).

SQUAMOUS CELL CARCINOMA, HISTIOGENESIS

Squamous cell carcinomas arise from progressive squamous epithelial dysplasia, which itself is a continuum generally divided into mild, moderate, and severe dysplasia, and carcinoma in situ based on both cytologic atypia and the distribution of the atypical cells within the bronchial epithelium.[28] Squamous preneoplasia is discussed in detail in Chapter 26.

References

1. Flieder DB, Hammar SP. Common non-small-cell carcinomas and their variants. In: Tomashefski JF, Cagle PT, Farver CF, Fraire AE, ed. *Dail and Hammar's Pulmonary Pathology*. 3rd ed. New York, NY: Springer; 2008.

2. Kwon KY, Kerr KM, Ro JY. Non-small cell carcinomas. In: Cagle PT, Allen TC, Kerr K.M., ed. *Transbronchial and Endobronchial Biopsies*. Philadelphia, PA: Lippincott Williams & Wilkins; 2009:7–20.

3. Zeren EH, Laga AC, Allen TC, et al. Squamous-Cell Carcinoma. In: Cagle PT, ed. *Color Atlas and Text of Pulmonary Pathology*. 2nd ed. Philadelphia, PA: Lippincott Williams & Wilkins; 2008:42–45.

4. Hammar SP, Brambilla C, Pugatch B, et al. Squamous cell carcinoma. In: Travis WD, Brambilla E, Muller-Hermelink HK, Harris CC, ed. *Tumours of the Lung, Pleura, Thumus and Heart*. Lyon: IARC Press; 2004:26–30.

5. Blackmon S. Clinical diagnosis of pulmonary neoplasms. In: Cagle PT. Allen TC, Beasley MB, ed. *Diagnostic Pulmonary Pathology*. 2nd ed. New York, NY: Informa; 2008:539–556.

6. Tomashefski JF, Connors AF, Rosenthal ES, et al. Peripheral vs central squamous cell carcinoma of the lung. A comparison of clinical features, histopathology, and survival. *Arch Pathol Lab Med*. 1990;114:468–474.

7. Byrd RB, Miller WE, Carr DT, et al. The roentgenographic appearance of squamous cell carcinoma of the bronchus. *Mayo Clin Proc*. 1968;43:327–332.

8. Roggli VL, Vollmer RT, Greenberg SD, et al. Lung cancer heterogeneity: a blinded and randomized study of 100 consecutive cases. *Hum pathol*. 1985;16:569–579.

9. Felip E, Rosell R. Pemetrexed as second-line therapy for advanced non-small-cell lung cancer (NSCLC). *Ther Clin Risk Manag*. 2008;4:579–585.

10. Rossi A, Ricciardi S, Maione P, et al. Pemetrexed in the treatment of advanced non-squamous lung cancer. *Lung Cancer*. 2009.

11. Longo-Sorbello GS, Chen B, Budak-Alpdogan T, et al. Role of pemetrexed in non-small cell lung cancer. *Cancer Invest*. 2007;25:59–66.

12. Vokes EE, Senan S, Treat JA, et al. PROCLAIM: a phase III study of pemetrexed, cisplatin, and radiation therapy followed by consolidation pemetrexed versus etoposide, cisplatin, and radiation therapy followed by consolidation cytotoxic chemotherapy of choice in locally advanced stage III non-small-cell lung cancer of other than predominantly squamous cell histology. *Clin Lung Cancer*. 2009;10:193–198.

13. Scagliotti GV, Parikh P, von Pawel J, et al. Phase III study comparing cisplatin plus gemcitabine with cisplatin plus pemetrexed in chemotherapy-naive patients with advanced-stage non-small-cell lung cancer. *J Clin Oncol*. 2008;26:3543–3551.

14. Downey P, Cummins R, Moran M, et al. If it's not CK5/6 positive, TTF-1 negative it's not a squamous cell carcinoma of lung. *APMIS*. 2008;116:526–529.

15. Pirker R, Filipits, M. Targeted therapies in lung cancer. *Curr Pharm Design*. 2009;15:188–206.

16. Roggli VL, Vollmer RT, Greenberg SD, et al. Lung cancer heterogeneity: a blinded and randomized study of 100 consecutive cases. *Hum Pathol*. 1985;16:569–579.

17. D'Addario G, Felip E. Non-small-cell lung cancer: ESMO clinical recommendations for diagnosis, treatment and follow-up. *Ann Oncol*. 2009;20 Suppl 4:68–70.

18. Yousem SA. Peripheral squamous cell carcinoma of lung: patterns of growth with particular focus on airspace filling. *Hum Pathol*. 2009;40:861–867.

19. Funai K, Yokose T, Ishii G, et al. Clinicopathologic characteristics of peripheral squamous cell carcinoma of the lung. *Am J Surg Pathol*. 2003;27:978–984.

20. Jones KD. Malignant epithelial neoplasms. In: Cagle PT, Allen, TC, Beasley MB, ed. *Diagnostic Pulmonary Pathology*. 2nd ed. New York, NY: Informa; 2008:611–626.

21. Laga AC, Allen TC, Cagle PT. Adenosquamous carcinoma. In: Cagle PT, ed. *Color Atlas and Text of Pulmonary Pathology*. 2nd ed. Philadelphia, PA: Lippincott Williams & Wilkins; 2008:62.

22. Moro-Sibilot D, Lantuejoul S, Diab S, et al. Lung carcinomas with a basaloid pattern: a study of 90 cases focusing on their poor prognosis. *Eur Respir J*. 2008;31:854–859.

23. Cakir E, Demirag F, Ucoluk GO, et al. Basaloid squamous cell carcinoma of the lung: a rare tumour with a rare clinical presentation. *Lung Cancer*. 2007;57:109–111.

24. Brambilla E, Lantuejoul S, Strum N. Divergent differentiation in nertoendocrine lung tumors. *Semin Diagn Pathol*. 2000;17:138–148.

25. Churg A, Johnston WH, Stulbarg M. Small cell squamous and mixed small cell squamous-small cell anaplastic carcinomas of the lung. *Am J Surg Pathol.* 1980;4:255–263.

26. Zhang H, Liu J, Cagle PT, et al. Distinction of pulmonary small cell carcinoma from poorly differentiated squamous cell carcinoma: an immunohistochemical approach. *Mod Pathol.* 2005;18:111–118.

27. Sakurai H, Asamura H, Watanabe S, et al. Clinicopathologic features of peripheral squamous cell carcinoma of the lung. *Ann Thorac Surg.* 2004;78:222–227.

28. Kerr KM. Preinvasive lesions. In: Cagle PT, Allen TC, Kerr KM, ed. *Transbronchial and Endobronchial Biopsies.* Philadelphia, PA: Lippincott Williams & Wikins; 2009:35–38.

7

Adenosquamous Carcinoma

▶ Timothy Craig Allen

Adenosquamous carcinoma is an uncommon, mixed subtype of non–small cell lung cancer that makes up approximately 2% to 5% of lung cancers.[1-4] The incidence of adenosquamous carcinoma may be increasing, however, along with adenocarcinoma.[5] Clinically, patients with adenosquamous carcinoma are usually smokers and typically exhibit symptoms similar to patients with tumors of other histologies, including cough and dyspnea, chest pain, and hemoptysis.[6] Radiographically, adenosquamous carcinoma is characterized on CT scan as a solid, lobulated mass, usually peripheral, and typically exhibits heterogeneous soft tissue attenuation after intravenous injection of positive contrast medium.[7,8] There may be central scarring and peripheral ground glass opacification, as well as puckering of the overlying pleura.[9-11] Adenosquamous carcinomas generally exhibit earlier metastases and have a poorer prognosis than squamous cell carcinomas or adenocarcinomas.[4,9-16] Metastatic tumors often show both adenocarcinomatous and squamous cell carcinomatous differentiation, as with the primary tumor.[17]

ADENOSQUAMOUS CARCINOMA, GROSS FEATURES

Adenosquamous carcinoma is grossly similar to other major lung cancers. The tumors are typically peripheral and associated with a central scar (Fig. 7-1).[3,18]

ADENOSQUAMOUS CARCINOMA, HISTOLOGY

Histologically, adenosquamous carcinoma is characterized by exhibiting areas both of adenocarcinoma and squamous cell carcinoma, each involving 10% or more of the tumor (Fig. 7-2).[9-11,17] Diagnostic criteria for squamous cell carcinoma and adenocarcinoma, specifically single-cell keratinization, keratin pearls, or intercellular bridges; and acinar, tubular, or papillary structures, respectively, must be clearly and unequivocally identified in order to make the diagnosis (Figs. 7-3 and 7-4).[9-11,17] Papillary and acinar patterns of adenocarcinoma may be easily recognizable; however, solid pattern adenocarcinoma with mucin formation may be more difficult to recognize, and some squamous cell carcinomas may show focal mucin positivity. In order to diagnose solid pattern adenocarcinoma, more than 5 mucin droplets per high-power field are required on mucin stain for the diagnosis of adenocarcinoma.[17] The different tumor types are independently, and may be variably, differentiated. The different tumor types may be arranged separately or may be mixed with each other. Areas of large cell carcinoma may also be present in adenosquamous carcinoma. Because of the diagnostic requirement that 10% or more of each component be present in order to make the diagnosis, adenosquamous carcinoma cannot definitively be diagnosed by transbronchial biopsy or core needle biopsy.[11]

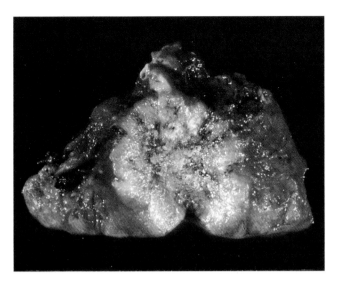

FIGURE 7-1 Gross image of a wedge resection of adenosquamous carcinoma showing a peripheral, well-circumscribed tumor mass with a central scar.

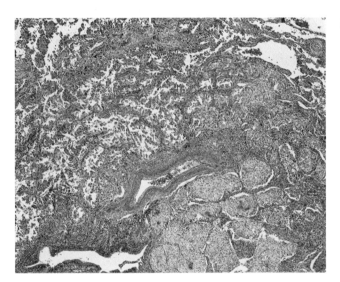

FIGURE 7-2 Low-power image of adenosquamous carcinoma showing predominantly bronchioloalveolar pattern adenocarcinoma at the upper left and predominantly clear cell pattern squamous cell carcinoma in the lower right. Lung parenchyma is identified in the upper right and a bronchiole in the lower left.

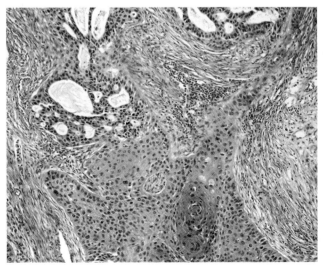

FIGURE 7-3 Medium-power image of adenosquamous carcinoma showing both adenocarcinoma, predominantly in the upper portion of the image, and squamous cell carcinoma, predominantly in the lower portion of the image, within the tumor. Each of the histologies made up more than 10% of the overall tumor, as required to render the diagnosis of adenosquamous carcinoma.

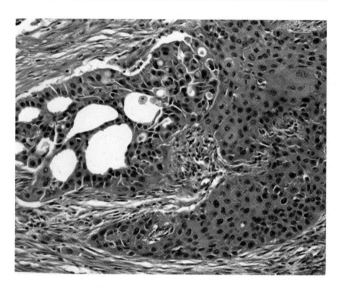

FIGURE 7-4 High-power image of adenosquamous carcinoma showing adenocarcinoma on the left abutting squamous cell carcinoma on the right.

ADENOSQUAMOUS CARCINOMA, IMMUNOHISTOCHEMISTRY

Immunostaining of adenosquamous carcinomas typically shows immunopositivity with AE1/AE3, CK7, and CAM 5.2, and immunonegativity with C20. TTF-1 immunopositivity is usually limited to the adenocarcinomatous component.[9–11,17]

ADENOSQUAMOUS CARCINOMA, DIFFERENTIAL DIAGNOSIS

The major differential diagnoses of adenosquamous carcinoma are squamous cell carcinoma with associated entrapped lung parenchymal acinar structures, and adenocarcinoma with associated squamous metaplasia (Figs. 7-5 and 7-6).[3,4,9–11,14,17,18] Mucoepidermoid carcinoma may also show histologic similarities to adenosquamous carcinoma. Low-grade mucoepidermoid carcinoma

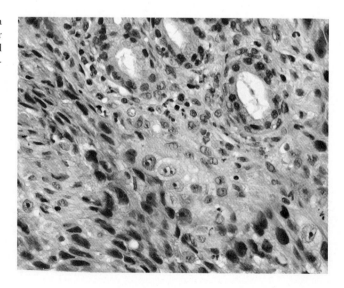

FIGURE 7-5 High-power image of a large cell carcinoma showing tumor cells encompassing entrapped bronchial mucosa which exhibits smaller, more uniform, less atypical nuclei.

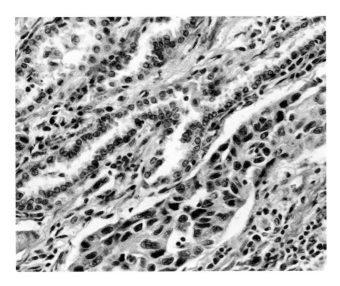

FIGURE 7-6 High-power image of another large cell carcinoma showing entrapped airway mucosa with smaller, more uniform nuclei adjacent to nests of enlarged tumor cells with contrasting larger, atypical neoplastic cells.

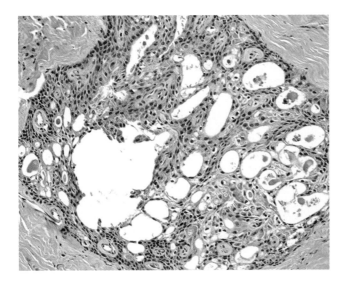

FIGURE 7-7 High-power image of low-grade pulmonary mucoepidermoid carcinoma showing glandular spaces and surrounding relatively bland squamous cells. The histologic criteria of adenosquamous carcinoma are not present.

typically shows little nuclear atypia; however, high-grade mucoepidermoid carcinoma may be more difficult to differentiate from adenosquamous carcinoma. Identification of areas of low-grade mucoepidermoid carcinoma may help differentiate the tumors (Fig. 7-7).[9–11,17,19,20]

ADENOSQUAMOUS CARCINOMA, HISTIOGENESIS

Niho and colleagues examined pulmonary adenosquamous carcinoma clonally based on an X-chromosome-linked polymorphic marker, the human androgen receptor gene (HUMARA), and found that both the squamous cell component and adenocarcinoma component in the cases showed identical monoclonal patterns, suggesting that both components originate from the same cell.[21] Kang et al.,[22] noting that epidermal growth factor receptor (EGFR) mutations generally occur in pulmonary adenocarcinomas and not in squamous cell carcinomas, found that the frequency of EGFR mutations and clinicopathologic characteristics of the EGFR mutants in adenosquamous carcinoma are similar to those of Asian patients with adenocarcinomas, suggesting monoclonality in the histiogenesis of adenosquamous carcinoma.

References

1. Nakagawa K, Yasumitu T, Fukuhara K, et al. Poor prognosis after lung resection for patients with adenosquamous carcinoma of the lung. *Ann Thorac Surg.* 2003;75:1740–1744.
2. Hsia JY, Chen CY, Hsu CP, et al. Adenosquamous carcinoma of the lung. Surgical results compared with squamous cell and adenocarcinoma. *Scand Cardiovasc J.* 1999;33:29–32.
3. Takamori S, Noguchi M, Morinaga S, et al. Clinicopathologic characteristics of adenosquamous carcinoma of the lung. *Cancer.* 1991;67:649–654.
4. Kamiyoshihara M, Hirai T, Kawashima O, et al. A clinicopathologic study of the resected cases of adenosquamous carcinoma of the lung. *Oncol Rep.* 1998;5:861–865.
5. Sridhar KS, Raub WA Jr, Duncan RC, et al. The increasing recognition of adenosquamous lung carcinoma (1977–1986). *Am J Clin Oncol.* 1992;15:356–362.
6. Sridhar KS, Bounassi MJ, Raub W Jr, et al. Clinical features of adenosquamous lung carcinoma in 127 patients. *Am Rev Respir Dis.* 1990;142:19–23.
7. Yu JQ, Yang ZG, Austin JH, et al. Adenosquamous carcinoma of the lung: CT-pathological correlation. *Clin Radiol.* 2005;60:364–369.
8. Kazerooni EA, Bhalla M, Shepard JA, et al. Adenosquamous carcinoma of the lung: radiologic appearance. *Am J Roentgenol.* 1994;163:301–306.
9. Jones KD. Malignant epithelial neoplasms. In: Cagle PT, Allen TC, Beasley MB, ed. *Diagnostic Pulmonary Pathology.* 2nd ed. New York, NY: Informa; 2008:611–626.
10. Laga AC, Allen TC, Cagle PT. Adenosquamous carcinoma. In: Cagle PT, ed. *Color Atlas and Text of Pulmonary Pathology.* 2nd ed. Philadelphia, PA: Lippincott, Williams & Wilkins; 2008:62.
11. Kwon KY, Kerr KM, Ro JY. Non-small cell carcinomas. In: Cagle PT, Allen TC, Kerr KM, ed. *Transbronchial and Endobronchial Biopsies.* Philadelphia, PA: Lippincott Williams & Wilkins; 2009:7–20.
12. Gawrychowski J, Brulinski K, Malinowski E, et al. Prognosis and survival after radical resection of primary adenosquamous lung carcinoma. *Eur J Cardiothorac Surg.* 2005;27:686–692.
13. Ben Y, Yu H, Wang Z, et al. Adenosquamous lung carcinoma: clinical characteristics, surgical treatment and prognosis. *Chin Med Sci J.* 2000;15:238–240.
14. Shimizu J, Oda M, Hayashi Y, et al. A clinicopathologic study of resected cases of adenosquamous carcinoma of the lung. *Chest.* 1996;109:989–994.
15. Hofmann HS, Knolle J, Neef H. The adenosquamous lung carcinoma: clinical and pathological characteristics. *J Cardiovasc Surg (Torino).* 1994;35:543–547.
16. Naunheim KS, Taylor JR, Skosey C, et al. Adenosquamous lung carcinoma: clinical characteristics, treatment, and prognosis. *Ann Thorac Surg.* 1987;44:462–466.
17. Brambilla E, Travis WD. Adenosquamous carcinoma. In: Travis WD, Brambilla E, Muller-Hermelink HK, Harris CC, ed. *Tumours of the Lung, Pleura, Thymus and Heart.* Lyon: IARC Press; 2004:51–52.
18. Ishida T, Kaneko S, Yokoyama H, et al. Adenosquamous carcinoma of the lung. Clinicopathologic and immunohistochemical features. *Am J Clin Pathol.* 1992;97:678–685.
19. Yousem SA, Hochholzer L. Mucoepidermoid tumors of the lung. *Cancer.* 1987;60:1346–1352.
20. Mooi WJ. Common lung cancers. In: Hasleton PS, ed. *Spencer's Pathology of the Lung.* 5th ed. New York, NY: McGraw-Hill; 1996:1009–1064.
21. Niho S, Yokose T, Kodama T, et al. Clonal analysis of adenosquamous carcinoma of the lung. *Jpn J Cancer Res.* 1999;90:1244–1247.
22. Kang SM, Kang HJ, Shin JH, et al. Identical epidermal growth factor receptor mutations in adenocarcinomatous and squamous cell carcinomatous components of adenosquamous carcinoma of the lung. *Cancer.* 2007;109:581–587.

Large Cell Carcinoma

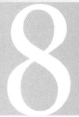

▶ Timothy Craig Allen

arge cell carcinoma of the lung is defined as "an undifferentiated non–small cell carcinoma that lacks the cytological and architectural features of small cell carcinoma and glandular or squamous differentiation."[1–5] Making up fewer than 10% of lung carcinomas, these poorly differentiated, generally large peripheral carcinomas often invade the pleura and chest wall.[1–5] More frequently identified in men, large cell carcinomas are smoking related and present clinically and radiologically as do other non–small cell carcinomas.[1–5] Besides basaloid carcinoma and large cell neuroendocrine carcinoma, there are three other extremely uncommon variants of large cell carcinoma, including clear cell carcinoma, lymphoepithelioma-like carcinoma, and large cell carcinoma with rhabdoid phenotype.[1–6] Prior terms used to designate large cell carcinoma, such as large cell undifferentiated carcinoma and large cell anaplastic carcinoma, should be avoided.[1–3] Clinically and radiologically, large cell carcinomas present in a similar manner as other non–small cell lung cancers.[1–3,7] Although large cell carcinomas are generally peripheral tumors and may undergo core needle biopsy, the criteria for diagnosis require extensive tissue sampling to be fulfilled. As such, the diagnosis of large cell carcinoma is one that is reliably rendered only upon excision of, and close pathologic examination of, the tumor mass.[1,5] Cytology and small biopsy specimens are generally not suitable for the diagnosis. The more general diagnosis of non–small cell carcinoma should be rendered for small biopsies or cytology specimens containing tumor cells containing features of large cell carcinoma.[5] Prognostically, large cell carcinomas behave similarly to other non–small cell carcinomas.

LARGE CELL CARCINOMA, CYTOLOGY

Cytologically, large cell carcinomas usually show features that are not specific for the diagnosis of large cell carcinoma, including tumor cells arranged singly and in syncytial groups, with indistinct but generally abundant cytoplasm and large round to oval nuclei with irregular course nuclear chromatin (Fig. 8-1).[1,3,4] Tumor cells often contain large, often multiple, nucleoli.

LARGE CELL CARCINOMA, GROSS FEATURES

Grossly, large cell carcinomas are similar to other non–small cell carcinomas, with off-white to tan-gray and occasionally hemorrhagic cut surface (Fig. 8-2). Large cell carcinomas generally do not cavitate as do some squamous cell carcinomas (Fig. 8-3).

LARGE CELL CARCINOMA, HISTOLOGY

Histologically, tumor cells are generally arranged in nests and sheets of large polygonal cells with a moderate amount of cytoplasm and nuclear features similar to the cytologic description above.[1–5] Large cell carcinoma tumor cells are generally large, polygonal cells with large, hyperchromatic nuclei and conspicuous nucleoli (Fig. 8-4). H&E stain shows no adenocarcinomatous or squamous differentiation, specifically, no single-cell keratinization, keratin pearls, intercellular bridges, or acinar, papillary, or tubular structures.[1–5] Mucin stain is typically negative (Fig. 8-5). While

71

FIGURE 8-1 High-power image of Pap-stained fine-needle aspiration cytology of a patient who on surgical resection was found to have large cell carcinoma showing a group of tumor cells with a moderate amount of indistinct cytoplasm and large round to oval nuclei containing irregular course nuclear chromatin and occasional large nucleoli. Some benign ciliated mucosal cells are present and provide size comparison. These cytologic features are not specific for large cell carcinoma and would be appropriately diagnosed as non–small cell carcinoma.

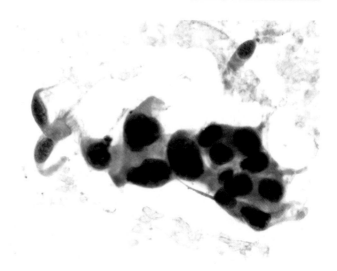

FIGURE 8-2 Gross image of a wedge resection of large cell carcinoma, showing an off-white to gray subpleural mass without areas of necrosis.

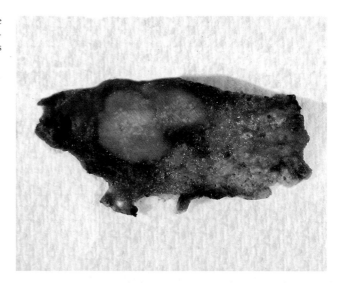

FIGURE 8-3 Gross image of a lobectomy specimen containing large cell carcinoma, with focal hemorrhage, but no cavitation seen in this large tumor mass.

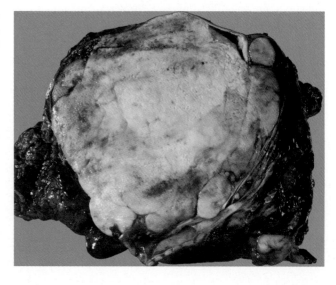

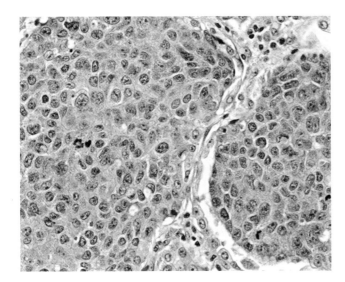

FIGURE 8-4 High-power image of large cell carcinoma showing nests of large polygonal cells with a moderate amount of cytoplasm and large, hyperchromatic nuclei with conspicuous nucleoli.

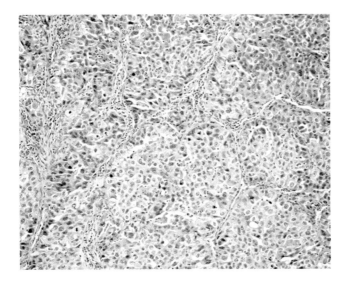

FIGURE 8-5 Medium-power image of mucicarmine stain of large cell carcinoma showing no cellular staining for mucin.

occasional mucin droplets may be identified by mucin stain, if by PAS with diastase digestion or mucicarmine stain there are >5 mucin droplets per 2 high-power fields, then the diagnosis of solid adenocarcinoma with mucin formation is appropriate.[4]

LARGE CELL CARCINOMA, IMMUNOHISTOCHEMISTRY

The current WHO classification of non–small cell lung cancers is histology based and does not require immunostains for the diagnosis of adenocarcinoma, squamous cell carcinoma, and large cell carcinoma, and the use of immunostains to further characterize non–small cell carcinomas is controversial. Nonetheless, the institution of newer, molecular-based lung cancer therapies necessitates the differentiation of squamous cell carcinomas from other non–small cell carcinomas in order to avoid serious drug-related injuries. As such, the diagnosis of large cell carcinoma may decline in the future with the development of the use of immunostains to better characterize non–small cell lung cancers.[7] Pardo et al.[7] noted that the use of seven immunostains—TTF-1, CK7, CK19, p63, 34βE12, thrombomodulin, and CD44v6—dramatically reduced the number of non–small cell lung cancers characterized as large cell carcinoma in a study of 101 lung cancer cases previously diagnosed as large cell carcinoma. Pardo et al.[7] found that large cell carcinomas characteristically exhibit CK5/6 and CK14 immunonegativity, immunostains that are typically positive in squamous cell carcinomas; and MOC31 immunonegativity, an immunostain typically positive in adenocarcinomas. Large cell carcinomas also exhibited immunopositivity with EGFR, PDGFR-alpha, and c-kit.[7] Pardo et al.[7] reclassified over two thirds of the cases as adenocarcinomas or poorly differentiated squamous cell carcinomas (32.9% and 37.8%, respectively) based on immunopositivity with TTF-1, CK7, and CK19; and immunonegativity with p63 (adenocarcinomas) or immunopositivity with 34βE12, p63, thrombomodulin, and CD44v6 (poorly differentiated squamous cell carcinomas). Almost one fifth (19.5%) of large cell carcinomas were reclassified by the authors as adenosquamous carcinomas based on their exhibiting positivity with immunostains typically found to be positive in both adenocarcinoma and squamous cell carcinoma.[7] Further studies will be of benefit in determining whether immunostain patterns in non–small cell lung cancers can successfully assist in categorizing poorly differentiated non–small cell carcinomas as adenocarcinomas or squamous cell carcinomas, thereby reducing the numbers of non–small cell lung cancers diagnosed as large cell carcinomas. The International Association for the Study of Lung Cancer suggests that in small biopsies containing non–small cell carcinoma without diagnostic features of adenocarcinoma or squamous cell carcinoma, and for which immunostains are noncontributory, the term "large cell carcinoma" not be used, and instead the term "non–small cell carcinoma, not otherwise specified" be used.

LARGE CELL CARCINOMA, DIFFERENTIAL DIAGNOSIS

Large cell carcinoma of the lung must be differentiated from poorly differentiated solid-type squamous cell carcinoma and solid-type adenocarcinoma primary in the lung, and from metastatic poorly differentiated carcinomas. Poorly differentiated squamous cell carcinomas contain foci of keratinization or intercellular bridges; and poorly differentiated adenocarcinomas contain foci of acinar formation or focal mucin (see Chapters 3, 6, and 17). Other differential diagnostic considerations include primary and metastatic lymphoma, sarcoma, and melanoma. Differential diagnoses of the variants of large cell carcinoma are discussed below.

LARGE CELL CARCINOMA, HISTIOGENESIS

Large cell carcinomas are believed to arise from a pleuripotent progenitor cell that is able to differentiate multidirectionally. As such, an in situ component is not characteristic of large cell carcinoma. The variants of large cell carcinoma, discussed below, most likely are a reflection of the tumor cells' pleuripotentiality.[1]

LARGE CELL CARCINOMA, VARIANTS

Clear cell carcinoma is a rare variant of large cell carcinoma that consists histologically of large polygonal cells with clear or foamy cytoplasm (Fig. 8-6). Areas of clear cell change may be identified in up to two thirds of non–small cell lung cancers, and clear cell variants of adenocarcinoma and squamous cell carcinoma exist and must be distinguished from clear cell carcinoma. Other differential diagnoses include clear cell (sugar) tumor of the lung, clear cell carcinoid tumor, and metastatic carcinomas that may have a prominent clear cell component such as renal cell carcinoma, salivary gland carcinomas, and thyroid carcinoma.[1,2,4,8–12] Clear cell (sugar) tumor is generally immunopositive with HMB45 and immunonegative with cytokeratin, whereas clear cell carcinoma is typically HMB-45 immunonegative and cytokeratin positive.[2]

Large cell carcinoma with rhabdoid phenotype is another rare variant of large cell carcinoma that is an aggressive neoplasm. The diagnosis of large cell carcinoma with rhabdoid phenotype requires that at least 10% of the tumor be composed of rhabdoid tumor cells, which

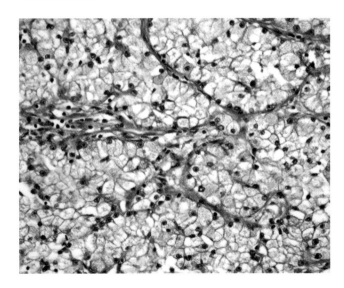

FIGURE 8-6 High-power image of clear cell carcinoma showing large polygonal cells with clear or foamy cytoplasm. In a case with these histologic features, care must be taken to exclude histologically similar metastatic tumors such as metastatic renal cell carcinoma.

are characterized by having large globular eosinophilic cytoplasmic inclusions, ultrastructurally shown to be composed of large intracytoplasmic paranuclear intermediate filaments (Fig. 8-7). The rhabdoid cells may be interspersed within the tumor, or arranged near the periphery of the tumor. Tumor cells generally grow in nests and sheets, and may exhibit an alveolar filling pattern. Nuclei show features of large cell carcinoma, including large, hyperchromatic nuclei and prominent nucleoli. The rhabdoid tumor cells are generally immunopositive with CK7, EMA, and vimentin; and immunonegative with CK20, TTF-1, muscle specific actin, and desmin. Some cases show immunopositivity with neuroendocrine marker, especially chromogranin. Differential diagnosis includes metastatic tumors with rhabdoid features.[1–4,6,13]

Lymphoepithelioma-like carcinoma is another rare variant of large cell carcinoma and is the only one that is not strongly related to smoking. Identified predominantly in Asians, often in middle-aged women, where it comprises up to 1% of lung tumors, lymphoepithelioma-like carcinoma is a variant of large cell carcinoma that is characterized histologically by syncytial sheets of large tumor cells with large vesicular nuclei, prominent nucleoli, numerous mitoses, and an associated marked inflammatory cell infiltrate made up of lymphocytes with admixed plasma cells and histiocytes, as well as interspersed eosinophils and neutrophils (Fig. 8-8). Amyloid may be identified occasionally. The inflammatory cell infiltrate is identified in metastatic

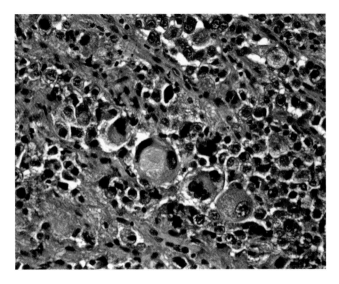

FIGURE 8-7 High-power image of large cell carcinoma with rhabdoid phenotype showing rhabdoid tumor cells, with large globular eosinophilic cytoplasmic inclusions and large hyperchromatic nuclei, some of which have prominent nucleoli.

FIGURE 8-8 Medium-power image of lymphoepithelioma-like carcinoma showing syncytial sheets of large cell carcinoma tumor cells and an associated marked mixed chronic inflammatory cell infiltrate.

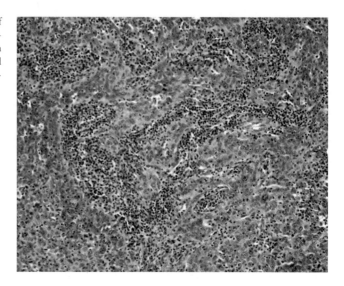

sites as well. Tumor often shows a pushing border. There is a strong association with Epstein-Barr virus in Asians, but the association is not strong in Western populations. Adenocarcinomatous or squamous cell differentiation is not found in lymphoepithelioma-like carcinomas. Information regarding prognosis is limited, but some patients may have a better prognosis than other non–small cell carcinoma patients. Differential diagnosis includes inflammatory pseudotumor, thymoma, melanoma, lymphoma, and metastatic nasopharyngeal carcinoma.[1–4,14–19]

LARGE CELL NEUROENDOCRINE CARCINOMA

Large cell neuroendocrine carcinoma of the lung is a variant of large cell carcinoma, the diagnosis of which requires that the large cell carcinoma show morphologic and ultrastructural or immunohistochemical features of neuroendocrine differentiation.[1–3,20–29] Large cell neuroendocrine carcinoma is a relatively uncommon, smoking-related, aggressive lung cancer that makes up approximately 2% to 5% of all lung tumors.[20,22,28,29] They frequently arise peripherally, but may arise centrally.[20,30] Radiographically, large cell neuroendocrine carcinomas are usually solid masses with irregular on CT scan, and cannot generally be distinguished from other non–small cell carcinomas or atypical carcinoid tumor. Central cavitation, as seen in squamous cell carcinomas, is infrequent. They may show associated emphysema, calcification, and pleural indentation.[30–32]

Grossly, large cell neuroendocrine carcinomas have features similar to other non–small cell carcinomas. Histologically, features of neuroendocrine morphology, including organoid, trabecular, or nesting patterns of tumor architecture, peripheral palisading of tumor cells, and rosette formation are identified. Central necrosis of tumor cell nests may be present, and large areas of necrosis may occur (Fig. 8-9).[1,21] Large cell neuroendocrine carcinomas characteristically have >10 mitoses per 10 high-power fields, and average approximately 70 to 75 mitoses per 10 high-power fields.[1–3,20,21,28] Some tumors may have up to 200 mitoses per 10 high-power fields.[28] Tumor cells are characterized by cells larger than small cell carcinoma cells, with generally polygonal shape, abundant cytoplasm, course or vesicular nuclear chromatin, and prominent nucleoli (Figs. 8-10 and 8-11).[20,21] Large cell neuroendocrine carcinomas are not characterized by having foci of adenocarcinoma, squamous cell carcinoma, or small cell carcinoma; however, combined large cell neuroendocrine carcinoma is recognized by the WHO as a large cell carcinoma variant that contains both large cell neuroendocrine carcinoma along with areas of adenocarcinoma, squamous cell carcinoma, or pleomorphic carcinoma tumor morphology.[1,2,28] Because of the specific morphological and immunohistochemical criteria that must be met, large cell neuroendocrine carcinoma is an extremely difficult diagnosis to render cytologically (Fig. 8-12).[33]

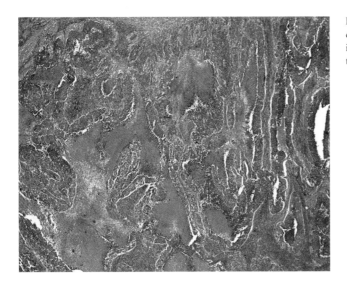

FIGURE 8-9 Low-power image of large cell neuroendocrine carcinoma showing diffuse areas of necrosis within the tumor.

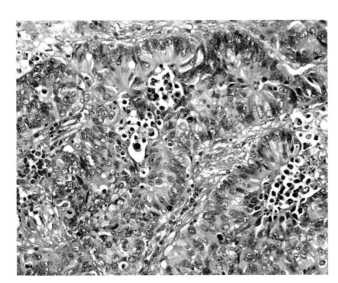

FIGURE 8-10 High-power image of large cell neuroendocrine carcinoma showing peripheral palisading and rosette formation within nests of tumor cells.

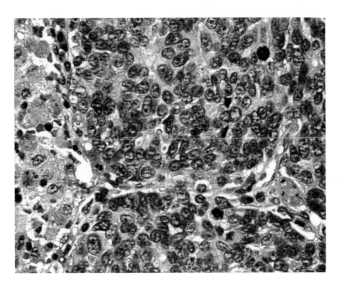

FIGURE 8-11 High-power image of nests of large cell neuroendocrine carcinoma showing enlarged vesicular nuclei with conspicuous nucleoli, abundant pink cytoplasm, and scattered mitoses. Pigment-laden macrophages lie within airspaces adjacent to the tumor.

FIGURE 8-12 High-power image of cytology smear of large cell neuroendocrine carcinoma showing abundant cytoplasm, large nuclei, obvious nucleoli, and a mitosis. Immunostains on cell block material showed neuroendocrine marker positivity, and the differential diagnosis on cytology included atypical carcinoid tumor and large cell neuroendocrine carcinoma. On surgical excision, the diagnosis of large cell neuroendocrine carcinoma was rendered.

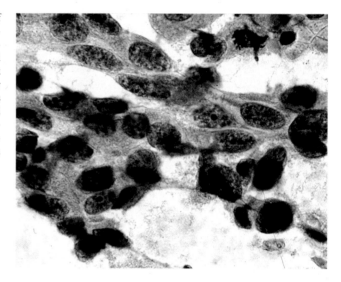

Currently, almost all diagnoses of large cell neuroendocrine carcinoma are confirmed by showing, along with neuroendocrine morphology on H&E staining, strong immunopositivity with at least two neuroendocrine markers, CD56 (NCAM), chromogranin, and synaptophysin.[20,28] The WHO criteria require that, along with neuroendocrine morphology, at least one neuroendocrine marker show clear-cut immunopositivity within viable tumor to appropriately render diagnosis of large cell neuroendocrine carcinoma (Fig. 8-13).[1,21] Large cell neuroendocrine carcinomas are typically immunopositive with CK7, and pankeratin, and approximately half are immunopositive with TTF-1; however, unlike other non–small cell lung cancers, large cell neuroendocrine carcinomas are generally immunonegative with high molecular weight cytokeratins 34βE12 (CK1, CK5, CK10, and CK14).[1,20,21] Prognostically, large cell neuroendocrine carcinomas are considered aggressive tumors with lower 5-year survival than other non–small cell carcinomas.[1,20,22,26,28,34–36] Currently, surgery is the therapy of choice, and radiotherapy is often used in advanced cases. While some cases have shown chemotherapeutic responses, there is no consensus on the best chemotherapeutic regime for treatment of large cell neuroendocrine carcinomas.[29,37–39]

Differential diagnosis includes large cell carcinoma with neuroendocrine morphology, large cell carcinoma with neuroendocrine differentiation, basaloid carcinoma and basaloid variant of

FIGURE 8-13 Medium-power image of synaptophysin immunostain showing strong diffuse positivity within viable large cell neuroendocrine carcinoma tumor cells.

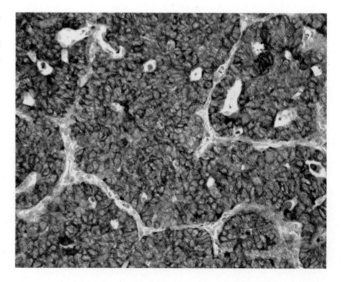

squamous cell carcinoma, as well as small cell carcinoma and atypical carcinoid tumor. Large cell carcinomas showing neuroendocrine morphology but immunonegativity with neuroendocrine markers are designated large cell carcinoma with neuroendocrine features. Also, large cell carcinomas that do not exhibit morphologic features of neuroendocrine differentiation on H&E stain, but which show immunopositivity with neuroendocrine markers, are termed large cell carcinoma with neuroendocrine differentiation. Little is currently known regarding these tumors' relationship with large cell neuroendocrine carcinoma. Large cell neuroendocrine carcinomas generally exhibit larger tumor cell size, increased mitoses, and increased nuclear pleomorphism compared to basaloid carcinoma and basaloid variant of squamous cell carcinoma; and are generally immunonegative with high molecular weight cytokeratins 34βE12 (CK1, CK5, CK10, and CK14), a valuable feature in distinguishing them from histologically similar-appearing basaloid carcinomas.[1,20,21] Basaloid carcinomas are not characterized by having immunopositivity with neuroendocrine markers; however, up to 10% of cases may show immunopositivity with one neuroendocrine marker in 5% to 20% of tumor cells.[28] Atypical carcinoid tumors share similar histologic features to large cell neuroendocrine carcinomas, including trabecular, nesting, or organoid architecture, peripheral palisading, and rosette formation. One important feature in differentiating atypical carcinoid tumor from large cell neuroendocrine carcinoma is mitotic rate. Whereas the diagnosis of large cell neuroendocrine carcinoma requires >10, averages 70 to 75, may show up to 200 mitoses per 10 high-power fields, atypical carcinoid tumors are defined as having between 2 and 10 mitotic figures per 10 high-power fields.[1,21,28] Large cell carcinomas also generally exhibit more tumor necrosis than atypical carcinoid tumors.[28] Care must be taken when examining small pieces of transbronchial or core biopsy tissue, as an accurate number of mitoses may be difficult to determine on those pieces.[28] Small cell carcinoma typically exhibits small tumor cell size, less conspicuous nucleoli, more finely granular chromatin, and less cytoplasm than large cell neuroendocrine carcinomas; however, there is broad overlap between the two diagnoses in terms of cell size. Nuclear features such as course and vesicular versus finely granular chromatin, conspicuous versus inconspicuous nucleoli, and polygonal versus more fusiform tumor cell shape help in differentiating large cell neuroendocrine carcinoma from small cell carcinoma, respectively.[1,2,20,28,40–42] Both small cell carcinoma and large cell neuroendocrine carcinoma show similar immunostaining patterns, so immunostaining is of no benefit in differentiating the two tumors.[2,28] Metastatic medullary carcinoma may be histologically and immunohistochemically similar to large cell neuroendocrine carcinoma; however, metastatic medullary carcinoma is typically associated with high serum calcitonin levels.[28]

BASALOID CARCINOMA

Basaloid carcinoma, described in various body sites including tongue, hypopharynx, larynx, gastrointestinal tract, thymus, skin, anal canal, and cervix, was first identified in the lung as a rare variant of large cell carcinoma by Brambilla et al. in 1992 and first included in the WHO classification of lung tumors in 1999.[2,3,5,43–49] Many nonpulmonary basaloid carcinomas contain histologic features of squamous cell carcinoma, and some pulmonary basaloid carcinomas contain features of squamous differentiation and are termed basaloid variant of squamous cell carcinoma.[5,44,45,50,51] These tumors are discussed in Chapter 6.

Basaloid large cell lung cancers are typically central in location, and have been characterized as having a significantly poorer prognosis than other non–small cell lung cancers, with frequent brain metastases and an approximately 15% 5-year survival in patients with stage I or stage II disease.[1,2,44,45,50–54] The tumors are typically large, measuring up to 7 cm. Approximately 85% exhibit an endobronchial growth pattern in addition to invasive tumor, and approximately 70% of resected tumors are diagnosed as stage I or stage II tumors.[1,2,44,45,50,51,53–57]

Histologically, basaloid variant of large cell carcinoma exhibits lobular or trabecular growth of small cuboidal or fusiform cells with characteristic peripheral palisading of tumor cells. Small cuboidal, fusiform, or spindle tumor cells generally exhibit a high nuclear-cytoplasm ratio and have a small amount of cytoplasm and small, hyperchromatic nuclei with granular cytoplasm and inconspicuous nucleoli. Central comedonecrosis within lobules of tumor is usually identified. There are usually numerous mitotic figures present within the tumor (Figs. 8-14 and 8-15). Nuclear molding, a feature of small cell carcinoma, is not characteristic of basaloid carcinoma. Occasionally, papillary architecture, small cystic spaces, rosettes, and myxoid change may be present; and rarely, chondroid or osseous metaplasia may be identified.[1,2,5,43-45,49-58]

In about half of basaloid carcinomas, the above-described histologic features comprise 90% or more of the tumor. The diagnosis of basaloid carcinoma is appropriate if the features comprise more than 50% of a large cell carcinoma. As noted above and described in Chapter 6, for tumors with features of squamous cell carcinoma present along with >50% basaloid carcinoma, the diagnosis of basaloid variant of squamous cell carcinoma is appropriate. In cases of non–small cell cancers that contain some, but <50%, basaloid component, the diagnosis of the predominant nonbasaloid component followed by "with basaloid features" or a similar descriptive phrase is appropriate.[1,2,44,45,49]

Basaloid carcinomas typically are immunopositive with high molecular weight cytokeratins 34βE12 (CK1, CK5, CK10, and CK14), CK7, CK8, CK18, and CK19, and are often immunopositive with CK5/6, CK13, CK14, and CK16. Basaloid carcinoma is characteristically immunonegative

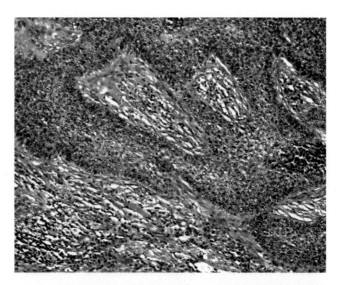

FIGURE 8-14 Medium-power image of basaloid carcinoma showing cords and nests of tumor cells with small nuclei and peripheral palisading, with surrounding desmoplastic stroma and inflammatory cells.

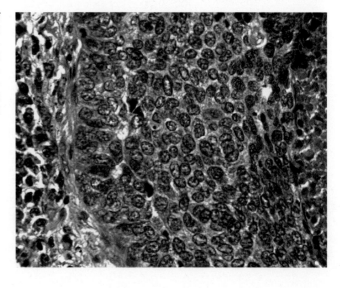

FIGURE 8-15 High-power image of basaloid carcinoma showing peripheral palisading of tumor cells, with comedonecrosis at the edge of the image. Small cuboidal to fusiform cells with hyperchromatic nuclei containing finely granular chromatin and inconspicuous nuclei have a high nuclear-cytoplasm ratio and mitotic figures at the top of the image.

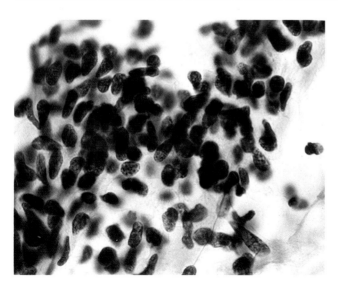

FIGURE 8-16 High-power image of Pap stained cytology smear of basaloid carcinoma showing cytologic features similar to small cell carcinoma, including small cuboidal to spindle cells with finely granular chromatin, inconspicuous nucleoli, and scant cytoplasm. However, unlike small cell carcinoma, the nuclei are generally uniform and there is not prominent nuclear molding.

with TTF-1. Neuroendocrine markers chromogranin and synaptophysin are generally negative; however, approximately one third of basaloid carcinomas may show focal neuroendocrine immunopositivity, and approximately 10% of tumors express CD56 (NCAM).[1,2,44,45,49–51,57] While histologic features suggestive of basaloid carcinoma may be identified on transbronchial or core lung biopsy, these features may not be representative of the entire tumor; therefore, the definitive diagnosis of basaloid carcinoma (and basaloid variant of squamous cell carcinoma) is reserved for the resected tumor.[5]

Differential diagnosis of basaloid carcinoma includes large cell neuroendocrine carcinoma, which may also exhibit peripheral palisading. Basaloid carcinoma may contain occasional rosettes, which are a frequently identified histologic feature of large cell neuroendocrine carcinoma; however, large cell neuroendocrine carcinoma generally has tumor cells with more prominent nuclei and increased amounts of cytoplasm as compared to basaloid carcinoma, express immunopositivity with neuroendocrine markers, and are immunonegative with high molecular weight cytokeratins.[5] Small cell carcinoma may also occasionally be confused with basaloid carcinoma; however, basaloid carcinoma is not characterized by nuclear molding, and small cell carcinoma is typically immunopositive with neuroendocrine markers and does not typically exhibit the lobulated growth pattern of basaloid carcinoma.[5] Diagnosis based solely on cytology may be misdiagnosed as small cell carcinoma or poorly differentiated squamous cell carcinoma (Fig. 8-16).[51,55]

References

1. Brambilla E, Pugach B, Geisinger K, et al. Large cell carcinoma. In: Travis WD, Brambilla, E, Muller-Hermelink HK, Harris CC, ed. *Pathology & Genetics: Tumours of the Lung, Pleura, Thymus and Heart*. Lyon: AIRC Press; 2004:45–50.
2. Flieder DB, Hammar SP. Common non-small cell carcinomas and their variants. In: Tomashefski JF, Cagle PT, Farver CF, Fraire AE, ed. *Dail and Hammar's Pulmonary Pathology*. 3rd ed. New York, NY: Springer; 2008:216–307.
3. Jones KD. Malignant epithelial neoplasms. In: Cagle PT, Allen TC, Beasley MB, ed. *Diagnostic Pulmonary Pathology*. 2nd ed. New York, NY: Informa; 2008:611–626.
4. Laga AC, Allen TC, Bedrossian C, et al. Large-Cell Carcinoma. In: Cagle PT, ed. *Color Atlas and Text of Pulmonary Pathology*. 2nd ed. Philadelphia, PA: Lippincott Williams & Wilkins; 2008:47–49.
5. Kwon KY, Kerr KM, Ro JY. Non-small cell carcinomas. In: Cagle PT, Allen TC, Kerr KM, ed. *Transbronchial and Endobronchial Biopsies*. Philadelphia, PA: Lippincott Williams & Wilkins; 2009:7–20.

6. Kaneko T, Honda T, Fukushima M, et al. Large cell carcinoma of the lung with a rhabdoid phenotype. *Pathol Int.* 2002;52:643–647.

7. Pardo J, Martinez-Penuela AM, Sola JJ, et al. Large cell carcinoma of the lung: an endangered species? *Appl Immunohistochem Mol Morphol.* 2009;17:383–392.

8. Katzenstein AL, Prioleau PG, Askin FB. The histologic spectrum and significance of clear-cell change in lung carcinoma. *Cancer.* 1980;45:943–947.

9. Hsu AA, Yeo CT, Ang HK, et al. Clear cell carcinoma of the lung—a case report. *Ann Acad Med Singapore.* 1992;21:827–829.

10. McNamee CJ, Simpson RH, Pagliero KM, et al. Primary clear-cell carcinoma of the lung. *Respir Med.* 1993;87:471–473.

11. Yamamato T, Yazawa T, Ogata T, et al. Clear cell carcinoma of the lung: a case report and review of the literature. *Lung Cancer.* 1993;10:101–106.

12. Garzon JC, Lai FM, Mok TS, et al. Clear cell carcinoma of the lung revisited. *J Thorac Cardiovasc Surg.* 2005;130:1198–1199.

13. Cavazza A, Colby TV, Tsokos M, et al. Lung tumors with a rhabdoid phenotype. *Am J Clin Pathol.* 1996;105:182–188.

14. Hernandez Vazquez J, de Miguel Diez J, Llorente Inigo D, et al. Large cell lymphoepithelioma-like carcinoma of the lung. *Arch Bronconeumol.* 2004;40:381–383.

15. Castro CY, Ostrowski ML, Barrios R, et al. Relationship between Epstein-Barr virus and lymphoepithelioma-like carcinoma of the lung: a clinicopathologic study of 6 cases and review of the literature. *Hum Pathol.* 2001;32:863–872.

16. Han AJ, Xiong M, Gu YY, et al. Lymphoepithelioma-like carcinoma of the lung with a better prognosis. A clinicopathologic study of 32 cases. *Am J Clin Pathol.* 2001;115:841–850.

17. Chen FF, Yan JJ, Lai WW, et al. Epstein-Barr virus-associated nonsmall cell lung carcinoma: undifferentiated "lymphoepithelioma-like" carcinoma as a distinct entity with better prognosis. *Cancer.* 1998;82:2334–2342.

18. Chang YL, Wu CT, Shih JY, et al. New aspects in clinicopathologic and oncogene studies of 23 pulmonary lymphoepithelioma-like carcinomas. *Am J Surg Pathol.* 2002;26:715–723.

19. Butler AE, Colby TV, Weiss L, et al. Lymphoepithelioma-like carcinoma of the lung. *Am J Surg Pathol.* 1989;13:632–639.

20. Kerr KM, Kwon KY, Ro JY. Neuroendocrine tumors. In: Cagle PT, Allen, TC, Kerr KM, ed. *Transbronchial and Endobronchial Biopsies.* Philadelphia, PA: Lippincott Williams & Wilkins; 2009:21–28.

21. Beasley MB. Large-cell neuroendocrine carcinoma. In: Cagle PT, ed. *Color Atlas and Text of Pulmonary Pathology.* 2nd ed. Philadelphia, PA: Lippincott Williams & Wilkins; 2008:60–61.

22. Veronesi G, Morandi U, Alloisio M, et al. Large cell neuroendocrine carcinoma of the lung: a retrospective analysis of 144 surgical cases. *Lung Cancer.* 2006;53:111–115.

23. Peng WX, Sano T, Oyama T, et al. Large cell neuroendocrine carcinoma of the lung: a comparison with large cell carcinoma with neuroendocrine morphology and small cell carcinoma. *Lung Cancer.* 2005;47:225–233.

24. Battafarano RJ, Fernandez FG, Ritter J, et al. Large cell neuroendocrine carcinoma: an aggressive form of non-small cell lung cancer. *J Thorac Cardiovasc Surg.* 2005;130:166–172.

25. Paci M, Cavazza A, Annessi V, et al. Large cell neuroendocrine carcinoma of the lung: a 10-year clinicopathologic retrospective study. *Ann Thorac Surg.* 2004;77:1163–1167.

26. Takei H, Asamura H, Maeshima A, et al. Large cell neuroendocrine carcinoma of the lung: a clinicopathologic study of eighty-seven cases. *J Thorac Cardiovasc Surg.* 2002;124:285–292.

27. Hammond ME, Sause WT. Large cell neuroendocrine tumors of the lung. Clinical significance and histopathologic definition. *Cancer.* 1985;56:1624–1629.

28. Brambilla E. Differential diagnosis of neuroendocrine lung neoplasms. In: Cagle PT, Allen TC, Beasley MB, ed. *Diagnostic Pulmonary Pathology.* 2nd ed. New York, NY: Informa; 2008:627–646.

29. Filosso PL, Ruffini E, Oliaro A, et al. Large-cell neuroendocrine carcinoma of the lung: a clinicopathologic study of eighteen cases and the efficacy of adjuvant treatment with octreotide. *J Thorac Cardiovasc Surg.* 2005;129:819–824.

30. Akata S, Okada S, Maeda J, et al. Computed tomographic findings of large cell neuroendocrine carcinoma of the lung. *Clin Imaging.* 2007;31:379–384.

31. Tanaka K, Tsuboi M, Kato H. Large cell neuroendocrine carcinoma of the lung with a cystic appearance on computed tomography. *Jpn J Thorac Cardiovasc Surg.* 2006;54:174–177.

32. Shin AR, Shin BK, Choi JA, et al. Large cell neuroendocrine carcinoma of the lung: radiologic and pathologic findings. *J Comput Assist Tomogr.* 2000;24:567–573.

33. Jimenez-Heffernan JA, Lopez-Ferrer P, Vicandi B, et al. Fine-needle aspiration cytology of large cell neuroendocrine carcinoma of the lung: a cytohistologic correlation study of 11 cases. *Cancer.* 2008;114: 180–186.

34. Fernandez FG, Battafarano RJ. Large-cell neuroendocrine carcinoma of the lung. *Cancer Control.* 2006;13:270–275.

35. Fernandez FG, Battafarano RJ. Large-cell neuroendocrine carcinoma of the lung: an aggressive neuro-endocrine lung cancer. *Semin Thorac Cardiovasc Surg.* 2006;18:206–210.

36. Mazieres J, Daste G, Molinier L, et al. Large cell neuroendocrine carcinoma of the lung: pathological study and clinical outcome of 18 resected cases. *Lung Cancer.* 2002;37:287–292.

37. Yamazaki S, Sekine I, Matsuno Y, et al. Clinical responses of large cell neuroendocrine carcinoma of the lung to cisplatin-based chemotherapy. *Lung Cancer.* 2005;49:217–223.

38. Fujiwara Y, Sekine I, Tsuta K, et al. Effect of platinum combined with irinotecan or paclitaxel against large cell neuroendocrine carcinoma of the lung. *Jpn J Clin Oncol.* 2007;37:482–486.

39. Gounaris I, Rahamim J, Shivasankar S, et al. Marked response to a cisplatin/docetaxel/temozolomide combination in a heavily pretreated patient with metastatic large cell neuroendocrine lung carcinoma. *Anticancer Drugs.* 2007;18:1227–1230.

40. Marmor S, Koren R, Halpern M, et al. Transthoracic needle biopsy in the diagnosis of large-cell neuro-endocrine carcinoma of the lung. *Diagn Cytopathol.* 2005;33:238–243.

41. Hiroshima K, Iyoda A, Shida T, et al. Distinction of pulmonary large cell neuroendocrine carcinoma from small cell lung carcinoma: a morphological, immunohistochemical, and molecular analysis. *Mod Pathol.* 2006;19:1358–1368.

42. Masuya D, Liu D, Ishikawa S, et al. Large cell carcinoma with neuroendocrine morphology of the lung. *Jpn J Thorac Cardiovasc Surg.* 2006;54:31–34.

43. Brambilla E, Moro D, Veale D, et al. Basal cell (basaloid) carcinoma of the lung: a new morphologic and phenotypic entity with separate prognostic significance. *Hum Pathol.* 1992;23:993–1003.

44. Laga AC, Allen TC, Ostrowski ML, et al. Basaloid Carcinoma. In: Cagle PT, ed. *Color Atlas and Text of Pulmonary Pathology.* 2nd ed. Philadelphia, PA: Lippincott Williams & Wilkins; 2008:63–64.

45. Ohori NP. Uncommon endobronchial neoplasms. In: Cagle PT, Allen TC, Beasley MB, ed. *Diagnostic Pulmonary Pathology.* 2nd ed. New York, NY: Informa; 2008:705–730.

46. Benisch B, Toker C. Esophageal carcinomas with adenoid cystic differentiation. *Arch Otolaryngol.* 1972;96:260–263.

47. McKay MJ, Bilous AM. Basaloid-squamous carcinoma of the hypopharynx. *Cancer.* 1989;63: 2528–2531.

48. Wain SL, Kier R, Vollmer RT, et al. Basaloid-squamous carcinoma of the tongue, hypopharynx, and larynx: report of 10 cases. *Hum Pathol.* 1986;17:1158–1166.

49. Travis W, Colby T, Corrin B, et al., eds. *Histological typing of lung and pleural tumors. International histo-logical classification of tumors. World Health Organization* 3rd ed. Berlin, Heidelberg, New York, Tokyo: Springer; 1999.

50. Kim DJ, Kim KD, Shin DH, et al. Basaloid carcinoma of the lung: a really dismal histologic variant? *Ann Thorac Surg.* 2003;76:1833–1837.

51. Nagakawa H, Hiroshima K, Takiguchi Y, et al. Basaloid squamous-cell carcinoma of the lung in a young woman. *Int J Clin Oncol.* 2006;11:66–68.

52. Moro D, Brichon PY, Brambilla E, et al. Basaloid bronchial carcinoma. A histologic group with a poor prognosis. *Cancer.* 1994;73:2734–2739.

53. Ro YS, Park JH, Park CK, et al. Basaloid carcinoma of the lung presenting concurrently with cutaneous metastasis. *J Am Acad Dermatol.* 2003;49:523–526.

54. Hirai K, Koizumi K, Hirata T, et al. Basaloid carcinoma of the lung. *Jpn J Thorac Cardiovasc Surg.* 2005;53:263–265.

55. Foroulis CN, Iliadis KH, Mauroudis PM, et al. Basaloid carcinoma, a rare primary lung neoplasm: report of a case and review of the literature. *Lung Cancer.* 2002;35:335–338.

56. Cakir E, Demirag F, Ucoluk GO, et al. Basaloid squamous cell carcinoma of the lung: a rare tumour with a rare clinical presentation. *Lung Cancer.* 2007;57:109–111.

57. Bhagavathi S, Chang CH. Multicentric basaloid carcinoma of lung clinically mimicking metastatic car-cinoma: a case report. *Int J Surg Pathol.* 2009;17:68–71.

58. Geddy PM, Gouldesbrough DR. Basal cell (basaloid) carcinoma of the lung. *Hum Pathol.* 1993;24:452–453.

9 Small Cell Carcinoma

▶ Mary Beth Beasley

Small cell lung carcinoma (SCLC) comprises approximately 20% of all lung carcinomas, classically presenting as a hilar mass with extensive adenopathy, although approximately 20% of SCLC are peripherally located.[1–3] The incidence of SCLC appears to have decreased slightly in the past decade.[3] SCLC frequently presents at an advanced stage and has a poor prognosis with a 5-year survival rate of 10% and a 10-year survival rate of <5%.[1,2,4] Less than 10% of patients with SCLC have stage 1 disease.[3] SCLC is seen almost exclusively in cigarette smokers and is more common in males. Depending on the location, size, and extent of spread, symptoms may include cough, dyspnea, hemoptysis, weight loss, or other constitutional symptoms. Superior vena cava syndrome is a presenting finding in 10% of patients. Associated paraneoplastic syndromes such as syndrome of inappropriate antidiuretic hormone, Cushing syndrome, autoimmune neuropathies, and encephalomyelitis, among others, may be encountered.[4,5] SCLC has typically been regarded as distinct from other lung carcinomas due to its responsiveness to chemotherapy; however, some studies have shown that surgery is of potential benefit in low-stage disease.[6–9] SCLC has been historically divided into limited (confined to the thorax) and extensive stage disease; however, in the 7th edition of the AJCC staging guidelines it is recommended that SCLC be staged using the same criteria as non–small cell lung carcinoma (NSCLC).[10,11]

SMALL CELL CARCINOMA, CYTOLOGY

Cytologically, SCLCs exhibit cells that are approximately three to four times the size of a resting lymphocyte, generally arranged singly and in small clusters. Tumor cells show a finely granular ("salt and pepper") chromatin pattern, with scant cytoplasm. Small nucleoli may be present occasionally, but do not predominate. Typically, there are frequent mitotic figures and nuclear molding is common. Necrotic cells or necrotic debris may be found in the background (Figs. 9-1 and 9-2).

SMALL CELL CARCINOMA, GROSS FEATURES

SCLCs are typically centrally located tumors, often not involving the bronchus but frequently involving hilar lymph nodes. The surface is typically off-white to tan-gray, and frequently areas of tumor necrosis or hemorrhage are present (Fig. 9-3).

SMALL CELL CARCINOMA, HISTOLOGY

The World Health Organization (WHO) classification of lung tumors defines SCLC as a tumor with >10 mitoses per10 high-power fields (HPF) and small cell cytologic features.[2] Histologically, SCLC is characterized by oval to spindle shaped cells approximately three to four times the size of a resting lymphocyte, as noted above. The cells have very high nuclear/cytoplasmic ratios and scant, almost indiscernible cytoplasm. Nuclear molding may be observed, and cytoplasmic borders are usually indistinct. Nuclear chromatin is finely granular and nucleoli are typically absent

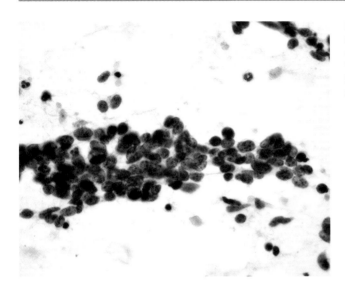

FIGURE 9-1 High-power image of Pap-stained cytology preparation showing a cluster of SCLC tumor cells, exhibiting "salt and pepper" nuclear chromatin, inconspicuous nuclei, scant cytoplasm, and nuclear molding.

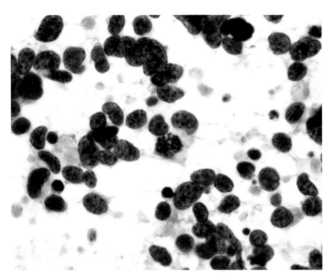

FIGURE 9-2 High-power image of Pap-stained cytology preparation of SCLC showing predominantly single cells exhibiting "salt and pepper" chromatin and a central mitotic figure. Note the occasional resting lymphocyte for size comparison.

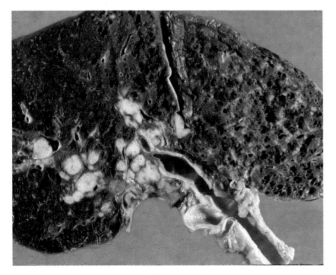

FIGURE 9-3 Gross image of lung with SCLC, showing off-white central tumor nodules that abut but do not involve the bronchi, and associated more peripheral intrapulmonary metastatic tumor nodules.

or inconspicuous (Fig. 9-4). While the mitotic rate is by definition >10 per 10 HPF, the mitotic rate is generally in excess of 50 to 60 per 10 HPF, with a median of 80 mitotic figures per 10 HPF.[2,12] Necrosis, both infarct like and single cell, is usually present (Fig. 9-5). Encrustation of blood vessels with basophilic material, the so-called Azzopardi phenomenon, may also be encountered. SCLC may occur in combination with large cell neuroendocrine carcinoma (LCNEC) or with other NSCLCs such as adenocarcinoma or squamous cell carcinoma (Figs. 9-6 and 9-7).[2,13] Such tumors are termed "combined SCLC" in the WHO classification, and the histology of the additional component should be specified. Pure SCLC may exhibit a range of cell sizes and it is recommended that any second component comprise at least 10% of the tumor before assigning the designation of combined SCLC.[2]

On small transbronchial biopsies (TBBX), SCLC may exhibit significant crush artifact. Such cases should be interpreted with caution as other tumors such as lymphoma, squamous cell carcinoma, and carcinoid tumors may also show considerable crush artifact (Figs. 9-8 and 9-9). In needle core biopsies and larger or resected specimens, the cells of SCLC may appear larger in comparison to their appearance on a TBBX and have slightly more discernable cytoplasm; however, in comparison to lymphocytes the cells remain proportionally small and nuclear cytoplasmic ratios

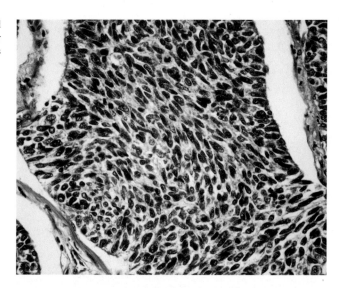

FIGURE 9-4 SCLC is comprised of oval to spindle cells with granular nuclear chromatin, absent or inconspicuous nucleoli, and scant cytoplasm.

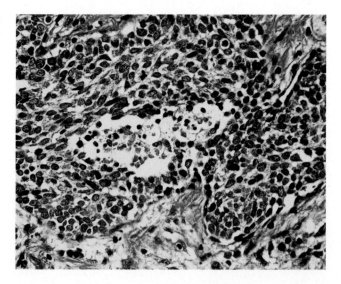

FIGURE 9-5 SCLC is characterized by a very high mitotic rate and areas of necrosis are frequently present.

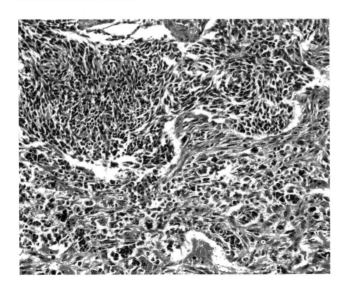

FIGURE 9-6 Combined SCLC. In this unusual case, SCLC (top) is combined with a pleomorphic/spindle cell carcinoma (bottom).

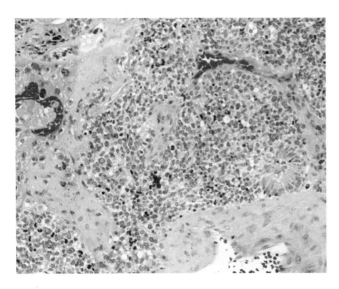

FIGURE 9-7 High-power image of a lung tumor composed of combined SCLC and large cell carcinoma. Large cells with abundant cytoplasm and enlarged nuclei are present on the left, and SCLC with abundant mitoses and focal rosette formation is identified in the center and on the right.

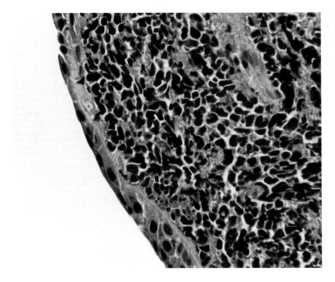

FIGURE 9-8 High-power image of SCLC showing typical crush artifact. Crush artifact is frequently seem in biopsies of SCLC but should be interpreted with caution.

FIGURE 9-9 High-power image of a typical carcinoid tumor with extensive crush artifact mimicking SCLC. The case was initially misdiagnosed as SCLC.

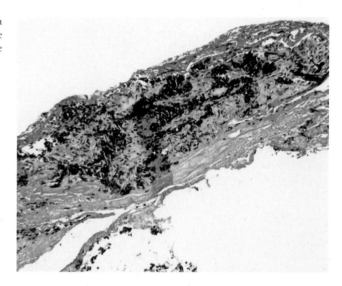

FIGURE 9-10 SCLC may show more obvious neuroendocrine growth patterns in larger specimens that should not be mistaken as evidence of large cell neuroendocrine carcinoma or carcinoid tumor.

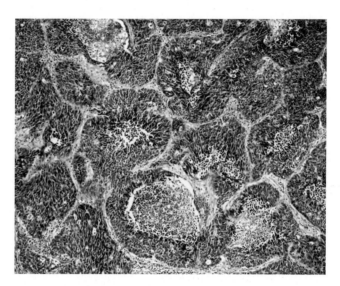

remain very high. Additionally, a more obvious neuroendocrine growth pattern with organoid morphology and rosette formation may be seen in larger specimens (Fig. 9-10).[13]

SMALL CELL CARCINOMA, IMMUNOHISTOCHEMISTRY

SCLC is positive for cytokeratins such as AE1/AE3 or CAM 5.2 and characteristically exhibits a "dot-like" pattern (Fig. 9-11). Cytokeratin 7 is frequently negative, but may be positive in a significant minority of cases, whereas cytokeratin 20 is consistently negative.[14] Other cytokeratins such as CK 34βE12 and CK5/6 are also typically negative.[15] Neuroendocrine markers such as chromogranin, synaptophysin, and CD56 (NCAM) are positive in the majority of cases; however, it should be noted that individual markers may be negative in up to 30% of cases and multiple markers may be negative in 10% to 15% of cases (Fig. 9-12).[13,16] As such, negative neuroendocrine markers do not necessarily militate against a diagnosis of SCLC in the presence of otherwise appropriate morphologic features. Thyroid transcription factor-1 (TTF-1) is also positive in the majority of SCLC but, unlike TTF-1 expression in adenocarcinoma, TTF-1 expression in SCLC does not definitively support a pulmonary origin and may be found in SCLC arising in other locations (Fig. 9-13).[17–19] Napsin A has thus far been negative in SCLC but needs to be evaluated in a larger number of cases at this time.[20]

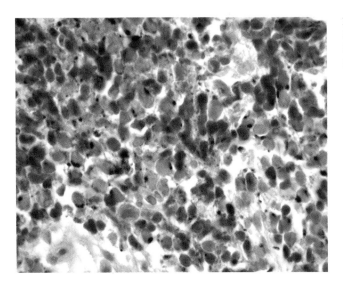

FIGURE 9-11 High-power image of SCLC with AE1/AE3 immunostain showing punctuate or "dot-like" cytoplasmic positivity.

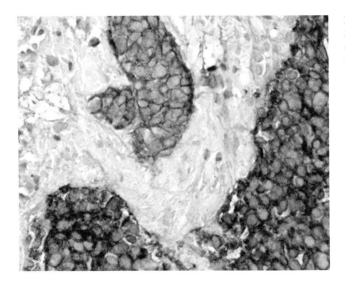

FIGURE 9-12 High-power image of SCLC stained with one of the neuroendocrine markers, CD56 (NCAM), showing strong cytoplasmic immunopositivity.

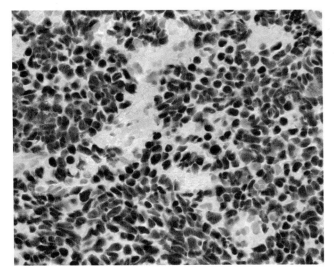

FIGURE 9-13 High-power image of SCLC immunostained with TTF-1 showing characteristic strong nuclear immunopositivity. Unlike pulmonary non-SCLCs such as adenocarcinoma, TTF-1 immunopositivity in SCLC is not in and of itself suggestive of a lung primary.

SCLC is also typically positive for bcl-2 and c-kit.[21] More recently, PAX-5, a marker typically seen in some lymphomas, has been reported to be positive in the majority of high-grade neuroendocrine carcinomas and negative in carcinoids.[22] Estrogen receptor and progesterone receptor expression has also been reported in SCLC.[23] Molecular studies have shown that SCLC, in contrast to typical (TC) and atypical carcinoid tumors (AC), typically exhibits a very high frequency of p53 mutations and Rb inactivation. Rb inactivation demonstrates an inverse correlation with p16 and cyclin D1.[24–27] SCLC also typically has a high frequency of deletions on chromosomes 3p and 17p and has an inverted bcl-2/Bax ratio.[24–26] SCLC also has a high level of telomerase activity.[28] Loss of heterozygosity for 3p, 5q21, and 9p has also been found.[25,26] Mutations of the MEN1 gene, as seen in TC and AC, are not seen in SCLC.[29] SCLC has not been shown to harbor EGFR mutations.[30]

SMALL CELL CARCINOMA, DIFFERENTIAL DIAGNOSIS

The differential diagnosis of SCLC primarily includes other neuroendocrine carcinomas, as well as NSCLCs (particularly squamous cell carcinoma), basaloid carcinoma, lymphoma, and Merkel cell carcinoma (Figs. 9-14–9-16). Primitive neuroectodermal tumor (PNET) and desmoplastic

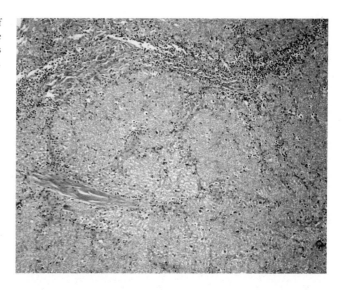

FIGURE 9-14 Medium-power image of Merkel cell carcinoma metastatic to the lung. There are sheets of small blue cells present, without obvious areas of necrosis.

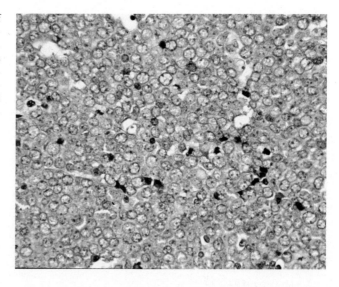

FIGURE 9-15 High-power image of Merkel cell carcinoma showing somewhat cleared nuclei and scant cytoplasm. Immunostains may be of benefit in cases of suspected metastatic Merkel cell carcinoma, as metastatic Merkel cell is generally immunopositive with CK20, and primary pulmonary SCLC typically is not.

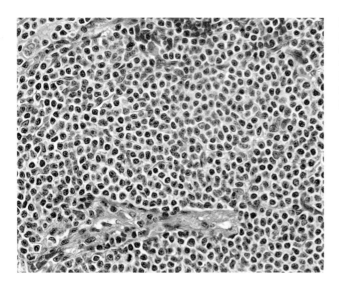

FIGURE 9-16 High-power image of well-differentiated B-cell lymphoma metastatic to the lung. Although the cells are small blue cells, there is less nuclear overlapping and nuclear molding than is typical for SCLC. Also, mitotic figures are not prominent and no necrosis is evident.

small round cell tumor (DSRCT) might also be considerations on morphologic grounds, but typically occur in a much younger patient population (Fig. 9-17).[31,32]

SCLC can be distinguished from typical TC and AC tumors largely by the nuclear morphology and mitotic rate (Figs. 9-18 and 9-19). Standard immunohistochemical stains such as keratins and neuroendocrine markers are not especially useful in discriminating these two tumors. Proliferation markers such as Ki-67 show nuclear staining in the majority of cells of SCLC (range 60%–96%) while TC is either negative or has a low proliferative index (<5%), which may be of aid in preventing misdiagnosis of TC as SCLC or vice versa in small biopsies.[33] Similarly, while AC, on average, has a higher proliferation rate than TC, it has not been reported as exceeding 20%, and thus an extremely high Ki-67 index would militate against a diagnosis of AC.[33–36] More recently, PAX-5 has been shown to stain high-grade neuroendocrine carcinomas but not carcinoid tumors.[22] High-grade neuroendocrine carcinomas have also been shown to express K homology domain containing protein whereas TC and AC have not.[37]

Discriminating SCLC and LCNEC may be particularly problematic, particularly on larger specimens or needle core biopsies where the cells of SCLC may appear larger than expected in comparison to the usual appearance on a transbronchial biopsy. The discriminating features of

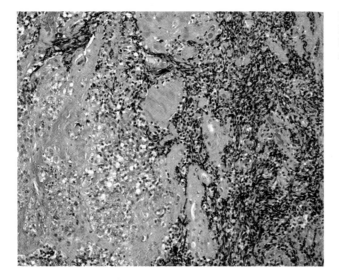

FIGURE 9-17 Medium-power image of DSRCT showing nests and cords of small blue cells within a background of fibrous stroma.

FIGURE 9-18 High-power image of typical carcinoid tumor showing generally uniform bland nuclei without areas of necrosis or mitotic figures.

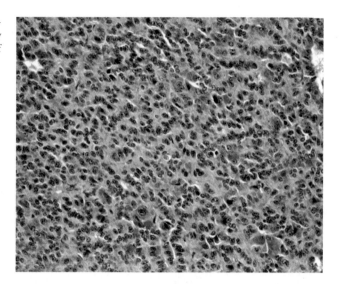

FIGURE 9-19 High-power image of an atypical carcinoid tumor showing generally uniform nuclei with a mitotic figure identified centrally. No necrosis is identified.

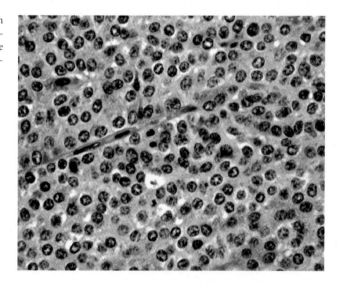

these two tumors are summarized in Table 9-1. As noted above, in larger specimens, SCLC may have a more obvious neuroendocrine growth pattern including prominent organoid patterns and rosette formation, findings that should not be taken as evidence of LCNEC. Peripheral SCLCs are often surprisingly well circumscribed. Further, LCNEC and SCLC have an essentially identical immunohistochemical profile, so this modality is not helpful in discriminating these two tumors, and therefore distinction must be based on cellular morphology. As such, a good-quality H&E stain is essential for proper classification. SCLC is composed of cells with oval to spindle nuclei with finely granular nuclear chromatin. Occasional small chromocenters or inconspicuous nucleoli may be encountered, but frequent large nucleoli should not be seen. While in larger specimens, SCLC may have more discernable cytoplasm than is appreciable on a small biopsy, the nuclear/cytoplasmic ratio is still extremely high and nuclear molding may be encountered, even in large specimens. Cell borders are often indistinct. In contrast, LCNEC tends to be composed of polygonal cells with moderately abundant cytoplasm. Nuclear chromatin tends to be vesicular and prominent nucleoli are often present (Fig. 9-20).[2,4,12,13]

Table 9-1	Comparison of SCLC and LCNEC	
	SCLC	Large Cell Neuroendocrine Carcinoma
Cell size	Smaller	Larger
Cell shape	Oval/spindle	**Polygonal**
Nuclear chromatin	Hyperchromatic, granular	Vesicular
Nucleoli	Inconspicuous or absent	Usually present, often large
Cytoplasm	Scant, may be visible in large specimens	Moderately abundant
Nuclear molding	Common	Absent/uncommon

Poorly differentiated squamous cell carcinoma may resemble SCLC, particularly in poorly preserved specimens. Individual neuroendocrine markers may be positive in a small percentage (up to 20%) of squamous cell carcinomas, which is an important pitfall. Studies have demonstrated that SCC is typically positive for CK5/6 and p63 and negative for TTF-1, while SCLC showed the opposite staining pattern in the majority of cases.[38–40] A study by Au et al.[41] however showed positive staining for p63 in 50% of SCLC, which suggests caution should be used with this marker alone.

Basaloid carcinoma (Figs. 9-21 and 9-22) may occur in either a pure form or may show areas of squamous differentiation, so-called basaloid squamous cell carcinoma (Fig. 9-23) (see Chapter 6). Basaloid carcinomas are typically composed of cells with more abundant cytoplasm and are characteristically positive for cytokeratin 34βE12, which should be negative in SCLC.[15] Basaloid carcinomas may occasionally be positive for neuroendocrine markers but the majority are negative, and they are typically negative for TTF-1.[42]

On small biopsies, it may be difficult to separate SCLC from poorly differentiated NSCLC regardless of subtype. As stated, crushed biopsies should be evaluated with extreme caution, and a definitive diagnosis should be made only when at least some preserved areas are present where cytologic features can be clearly evaluated. Comparison with any concurrent cytology specimens may be useful if available. SCLC is first and foremost an H&E diagnosis, but immunostains may be of some utility, with the staining patterns and pitfalls discussed in the preceding paragraphs and immunohistochemistry section.

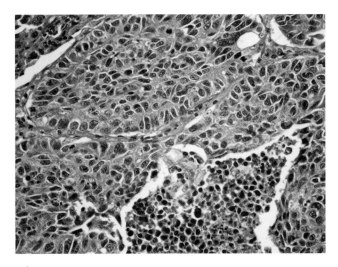

FIGURE 9-20 Large cell neuroendocrine carcinoma is comprised of large cells with vesicular nuclear chromatin. The cells have moderately abundant cytoplasm are often polygonal in shape, in contrast to the features of SCLC depicted in Figure 9-1.

FIGURE 9-21 Medium-power image of basaloid carcinoma showing a sheet of small blue cells, with focal necrosis at the left. Peripheral palisading is identified.

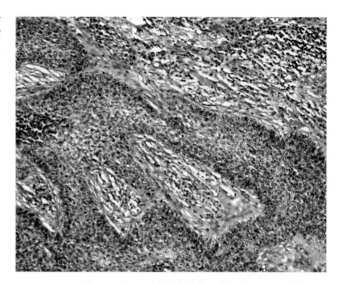

FIGURE 9-22 High-power image of basaloid carcinoma showing necrosis at the right and peripheral palisading at the left. Mitotic figures are present centrally. In difficult cases, immunostains help to make the correct diagnosis.

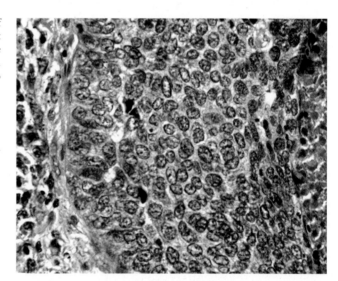

FIGURE 9-23 Basaloid squamous cell carcinoma has a nested growth pattern and cytologic features overlapping with those of neuroendocrine tumors. In this case, squamous differentiation is evident (upper left).

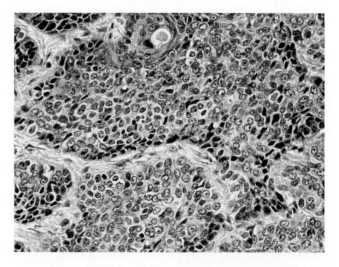

Lymphomas may be difficult to distinguish from SCLC on morphologic grounds, particularly on small distorted biopsies on poorly preserved specimens where cellular discohesion may be present. Immunohistochemical staining for lymphoid markers and cytokeratin generally resolves this dilemma.

Merkel cell carcinoma may occasionally be a consideration in the differential diagnosis. Merkel cell carcinoma, unlike SCLC, is positive for CK20 and negative for TTF-1, which is helpful in discriminating these two tumors.[43] Interestingly, Merkel cell polyoma virus was identified in 4 of 15 primary SCLC and 3 of 4 metastatic SCLC in one study, suggesting a possible causative link between the tumors.[44] However, these findings were not duplicated in subsequent studies by Duncavage et al.[45] and Busam et al.,[46] who failed to demonstrate the virus in SCLC.

PNET and DSRCT are rare in the thorax, typically occur in a much younger patient population than SCLC, and usually involve the pleura or chest wall. The "round blue cell" nature of these tumors has overlapping morphologic features with SCLC, so these tumors may occasionally be a diagnostic consideration in the differential of SCLC. Immunohistochemistry is useful in this differential and molecular analysis may resolve difficult cases. PNET is negative for cytokeratins and positive for neuroendocrine markers and CD99.[31] A small percentage of SCLC are also CD99 positive, but SCLC is positive for keratin. PNET is characterized by a t(11;22)(q24;q12) translocation involving EWS/FLI-1 gene fusion. DSRCT is positive for keratin, desmin, and WT-1 with only a small percentage staining for neuroendocrine markers. DSRCT is characterized by t(11;22) (p13;q12) involving WT-1/EWS fusion.[2,32,47]

Rarely, a malignant melanoma may mimic SCLC or other neuroendocrine tumors, an issue that is generally resolved with immunohistochemical staining.

SMALL CELL CARCINOMA, HISTIOGENESIS

SCLCs are tumors of the Amine Precursor Uptake and Decarboxylation system, and presumably arise from remnants of the neural crest.

References

1. Travis WD. Lung tumours with neuroendocrine differentiation. *Eur J Cancer*. 2009;45(suppl 1):251–266.
2. Travis WD, Brambilla E, Muller-Hermelink K, et al. *Pathology and Genetics. Tumours of the Lung, Pleura, Thymus and Heart*. Lyon: IARC Press; 2004.
3. Govindan R, Page N, Morgensztern D, et al. Changing epidemiology of small-cell lung cancer in the United States over the last 30 years: analysis of the surveillance, epidemiologic, and end results database. *J Clin Oncol*. 2006;1;24(28):4539–4544.
4. Lim E, Goldstraw P, Nicholson AG, et al. Proceedings of the IASLC international workshop on advances in pulmonary neuroendocrine tumors 2007. *J Thorac Oncol*. 2008;3(10):1194–201.
5. Gustafsson BI, Kidd M, Chan A. Bronchopulmonary neuroendocrine tumors. *Cancer* 2008;113(1):5–21.
6. Quoix E, Fraser R, Wolkove N, et al. Small cell lung cancer presenting as a solitary pulmonary nodule. *Cancer*. 1990;66(3):577–582.
7. Koletsis EN, Prokakis C, Karanikolas M, et al. Current role of surgery in small cell lung carcinoma. *J Cardiothorac Surg*. 2009;4:30.
8. Badzio A, Kurowski K, Karnicka-Mlodkowska H, et al. A retrospective comparative study of surgery followed by chemotherapy vs. non-surgical management in limited-disease small cell lung cancer. *Eur J Cardiothorac Surg*. 2004;26(1):183–188.
9. Lim E, Belcher E, Yap YK, et al. The role of surgery in the treatment of limited disease small cell lung cancer: time to reevaluate. *J Thorac Oncol*. 2008;3(11):1267–1271.
10. Vallieres E, Shepherd FA, Crowley J, et al. The IASLC Lung Cancer Staging Project: proposals regarding the relevance of TNM in the pathologic staging of small cell lung cancer in the forthcoming (seventh) edition of the TNM classification for lung cancer. *J Thorac Oncol*. 2009;4(9):1049–1059.

11. Shepherd FA, Crowley J, Van HP, et al. The International Association for the Study of Lung Cancer lung cancer staging project: proposals regarding the clinical staging of small cell lung cancer in the forthcoming (seventh) edition of the tumor, node, metastasis classification for lung cancer. *J Thorac Oncol.* 2007;2(12):1067–1077.

12. Travis WD, Linnoila RI, Tsokos MG, et al. Neuroendocrine tumors of the lung with proposed criteria for large-cell neuroendocrine carcinoma. An ultrastructural, immunohistochemical, and flow cytometric study of 35 cases. *Am J Surg Pathol.* 1991;15(6):529–553.

13. Nicholson SA, Beasley MB, Brambilla E, et al. Small cell lung carcinoma (SCLC): a clinicopathologic study of 100 cases with surgical specimens. *Am J Surg Pathol.* 2002;26(9):1184–1197.

14. Chu P, Wu E, Weiss LM. Cytokeratin 7 and cytokeratin 20 expression in epithelial neoplasms: a survey of 435 cases. *Mod Pathol.* 2000;13(9):962–972.

15. Sturm N, Rossi G, Lantuejoul S, et al. 34BetaE12 expression along the whole spectrum of neuroendocrine proliferations of the lung, from neuroendocrine cell hyperplasia to small cell carcinoma. *Histopathology.* 2003;42(2):156–166.

16. Guinee DG Jr, Fishback NF, Koss MN, et al. The spectrum of immunohistochemical staining of small-cell lung carcinoma in specimens from transbronchial and open-lung biopsies. *Am J Clin Pathol.* 1994;102(4):406–414.

17. Jerome MV, Mazieres J, Groussard O, et al. Expression of TTF-1 and cytokeratins in primary and secondary epithelial lung tumours: correlation with histological type and grade. *Histopathology.* 2004;45(2):125–134.

18. Agoff SN, Lamps LW, Philip AT, et al. Thyroid transcription factor-1 is expressed in extrapulmonary small cell carcinomas but not in other extrapulmonary neuroendocrine tumors. *Mod Pathol.* 2000;13(3):238–242.

19. Jones TD, Kernek KM, Yang XJ, et al. Thyroid transcription factor 1 expression in small cell carcinoma of the urinary bladder: an immunohistochemical profile of 44 cases. *Hum Pathol.* 2005;36(7):718–723.

20. Bishop JA, Sharma R, Illei PB. Napsin A and thyroid transcription factor-1 expression in carcinomas of the lung, breast, pancreas, colon, kidney, thyroid, and malignant mesothelioma. *Hum Pathol.* 2009;41:20–25

21. LaPoint RJ, Bourne PA, Wang HL, et al. Coexpression of c-kit and bcl-2 in small cell carcinoma and large cell neuroendocrine carcinoma of the lung. *Appl Immunohistochem Mol Morphol.* 2007;15(4):401–406.

22. Sica G, Vazquez MF, Altorki N, et al. PAX-5 expression in pulmonary neuroendocrine neoplasms: its usefulness in surgical and fine-needle aspiration biopsy specimens. *Am J Clin Pathol.* 2008;129(4):556–562.

23. Sica G, Wagner PL, Altorki N, et al. Immunohistochemical expression of estrogen and progesterone receptors in primary pulmonary neuroendocrine tumors. *Arch Pathol Lab Med.* 2008;132(12):1889–1895.

24. Brambilla E, Negoescu A, Gazzeri S, et al. Apoptosis-related factors p53, Bcl2, and Bax in neuroendocrine lung tumors. *Am J Pathol.* 1996;149(6):1941–1952.

25. Kobayashi Y, Tokuchi Y, Hashimoto T, et al. Molecular markers for reinforcement of histological subclassification of neuroendocrine lung tumors. *Cancer Sci.* 2004;95(4):334–341.

26. Onuki N, Wistuba II, Travis WD, et al. Genetic changes in the spectrum of neuroendocrine lung tumors. *Cancer.* 1999;85(3):600–607.

27. Beasley MB, Lantuejoul S, Abbondanzo S, et al. The P16/cyclin D1/Rb pathway in neuroendocrine tumors of the lung. *Hum Pathol.* 2003;34(2):136–142.

28. Zaffaroni N, De PD, Villa R, et al. Differential expression of telomerase activity in neuroendocrine lung tumours: correlation with gene product immunophenotyping. *J Pathol.* 2003;201(1):127–133.

29. Debelenko LV, Swalwell JI, Kelley MJ, et al. MEN1 gene mutation analysis of high-grade neuroendocrine lung carcinoma. *Genes Chromosomes Cancer.* 2000;28(1):58–65.

30. Sartori G, Cavazza A, Sgambato A, et al. EGFR and K-ras mutations along the spectrum of pulmonary epithelial tumors of the lung and elaboration of a combined clinicopathologic and molecular scoring system to predict clinical responsiveness to EGFR inhibitors. *Am J Clin Pathol.* 2009;131(4):478–489.

31. Askin FB, Perlman EJ. Neuroblastoma and peripheral neuroectodermal tumors. *Am J Clin Pathol.* 1998;109(4 suppl 1):S23–S30.

32. Zhang PJ, Goldblum JR, Pawel BR, et al. Immunophenotype of desmoplastic small round cell tumors as detected in cases with EWS-WT1 gene fusion product. *Mod Pathol.* 2003;16(3):229–235.

33. Pelosi G, Rodriguez J, Viale G, et al. Typical and atypical pulmonary carcinoid tumor overdiagnosed as small-cell carcinoma on biopsy specimens: a major pitfall in the management of lung cancer patients. *Am J Surg Pathol.* 2005;29(2):179–187.

34. Aslan DL, Gulbahce HE, Pambuccian SE, et al. Ki-67 immunoreactivity in the differential diagnosis of pulmonary neuroendocrine neoplasms in specimens with extensive crush artifact. *Am J Clin Pathol*. 2005;123(6):874–878.

35. Lin O, Olgac S, Green I, et al. Immunohistochemical staining of cytologic smears with MIB-1 helps distinguish low-grade from high-grade neuroendocrine neoplasms. *Am J Clin Pathol*. 2003;120(2):209–216.

36. Costes V, Marty-Ane C, Picot MC, et al. Typical and atypical bronchopulmonary carcinoid tumors: a clinicopathologic and KI-67-labeling study. *Hum Pathol*. 1995;26(7):740–745.

37. Xu H, Bourne PA, Spaulding BO, et al. High-grade neuroendocrine carcinomas of the lung express K homology domain containing protein overexpressed in cancer but carcinoid tumors do not. *Hum Pathol*. 2007;38(4):555–563.

38. Wu M, Wang B, Gil J, et al. p63 and TTF-1 immunostaining. A useful marker panel for distinguishing small cell carcinoma of lung from poorly differentiated squamous cell carcinoma of lung. *Am J Clin Pathol*. 2003;119(5):696–702.

39. Kalhor N, Zander DS, Liu J. TTF-1 and p63 for distinguishing pulmonary small-cell carcinoma from poorly differentiated squamous cell carcinoma in previously pap-stained cytologic material. *Mod Pathol*. 2006;19(8):1117–1123.

40. Zhang H, Liu J, Cagle PT, et al. Distinction of pulmonary small cell carcinoma from poorly differentiated squamous cell carcinoma: an immunohistochemical approach. *Mod Pathol*. 2005;18(1):111–118.

41. Au NH, Gown AM, Cheang M, et al. P63 expression in lung carcinoma: a tissue microarray study of 408 cases. *Appl Immunohistochem Mol Morphol*. 2004;12(3):240–247.

42. Sturm N, Lantuejoul S, Laverriere MH, et al. Thyroid transcription factor 1 and cytokeratins 1, 5, 10, 14 (34betaE12) expression in basaloid and large-cell neuroendocrine carcinomas of the lung. *Hum Pathol*. 2001;32(9):918–925.

43. Kaufmann O, Dietel M. Expression of thyroid transcription factor-1 in pulmonary and extrapulmonary small cell carcinomas and other neuroendocrine carcinomas of various primary sites. *Histopathology*. 2000;36(5):415–420.

44. Helmbold P, Lahtz C, Herpel E, et al. Frequent hypermethylation of RASSF1A tumour suppressor gene promoter and presence of Merkel cell polyomavirus in small cell lung cancer. *Eur J Cancer*. 2009;45(12):2207–2211.

45. Duncavage EJ, Le BM, Wang D, et al. Merkel cell polyomavirus: a specific marker for Merkel cell carcinoma in histologically similar tumors. *Am J Surg Pathol*. 2009;33(12):1771–1777.

46. Busam KJ, Jungbluth AA, Rekthman N, et al. Merkel cell polyomavirus expression in merkel cell carcinomas and its absence in combined tumors and pulmonary neuroendocrine carcinomas. *Am J Surg Pathol*. 2009;33(9):1378–1385.

47. Parkash V, Gerald WL, Parma A, et al. Desmoplastic small round cell tumor of the pleura. *Am J Surg Pathol*. 1995;19(6):659–665.

10

Typical Carcinoid Tumor

▶ Mary Beth Beasley

Carcinoid tumors as a whole make up approximately 1% to 2% of all pulmonary malignancies and consist of typical and atypical subtypes. Atypical carcinoid tumor (AC) is discussed in detail in Chapter 11. Typical carcinoid tumor (TC) is defined in the 2004 World Health Organization (WHO) classification of lung tumors as a carcinoid tumor with fewer than 2 mitoses per 10 HPF and lacking necrosis.[1] By definition, TC is >5 mm in size, which is currently the only feature discriminating TC from carcinoid tumorlet (Fig. 10-1). While a definitive precursor lesion has not been consistently identified, at least some cases, particularly peripheral TCs, appear to arise in a background of diffuse idiopathic pulmonary neuroendocrine cell hyperplasia, which is discussed in chapter 28.[2–4]

TC classically presents as a central endobronchial mass, although approximately a third of TC are peripheral and may not have an obvious associated airway.[1,5] TCs tend to occur with a slightly higher frequency in the right lung. Central tumors in particular may be associated with stridor or obstructive symptoms, while peripheral tumors may be asymptomatic. TC occurs in a younger population than conventional lung cancers and has an average age of presentation of 45 years. Fewer than half of patients with TC are current or former cigarette smokers, and while many studies indicate approximately equal gender incidence, some studies indicate that the disease occurs slightly more frequently in women. Carcinoid syndrome is uncommon and generally occurs in the presence of liver metastases. Cushing syndrome may also be encountered and rare cases may be associated with acromegaly.[1,6–10]

Radiographically, features characteristic of TCs are the presence of a well-defined tumor associated with an airway, occasionally associated with punctuate or diffuse calcification. Evaluation of TCs with positron emission tomography (PET) has yielded variable results, with most studies indicating that PET has low sensitivity for detecting carcinoid tumors. TCs generally have low metabolic activity and most studies indicate that PET results often demonstrate only low or equivocal uptake.[11] Octreotide scanning (somatostatin receptor scintigraphy) plays a role in imaging of carcinoid tumors due to the presence of somatostatin receptors on the tumor cells, and at least one study has reported a sensitivity of 90% and specificity of 83%.[8,10]

TC is generally associated with a favorable prognosis, with a 5-year survival rate of 85% to 90%, although patients with widely metastatic disease generally have a poor prognosis (14%–25% reported 5-year survival rate).[8,10] The presence of lymph node metastases also impacts prognosis, although some studies have found that the prognosis is generally still highly favorable or in keeping with that of tumors without nodal metastases.[12] The true incidence of nodal disease has been difficult to assess from the literature due to variable classification practices, although a number of 15% is frequently cited. A 2009 study by Wurtz et al.,[13] evaluating the presence of lymph node metastases in resected TC and AC using current WHO criteria, found nodal disease in 14.3% of TC cases ($N = 42$). A study by Ferolla et al.[14] also reported a 14% incidence of lymph node metastases in 100 TCs. In the Wurtz series, 4.8% of these cases were classified as N1 and 9.5% as N2. Interestingly, four of the N2 cases had so-called skip metastases without identification of metastatic disease in N1 nodes. All of the TCs with nodal metastases in that study were centrally located. Nodal metastases were seen more frequently in patients under age 35 and in tumors

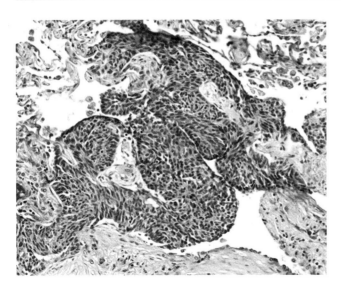

FIGURE 10-1 Medium power image of an approximately 3-mm carcinoid tumorlet. The histologic and immunohistochemical features of a carcinoid tumorlet are similar to those of a TC; however, the carcinoid tumorlet measures 5 mm in size.

larger than 3 cm, although N2 disease was observed in one case with a 0.7-cm tumor.[13] These findings, in combination with other studies, stress the importance of lymph node dissection in TC. Treatment of carcinoid is generally surgical, most frequently lobectomy or pneumonectomy, although lung sparing procedures have been used with success.[7,15,16] Chemotherapy and radiation therapy have generally been of limited value.[7,10,17] Several potential therapeutic targets have been identified that are discussed in the molecular section below.

Another issue in regard to outcome that has recently been investigated in several studies is the issue of multiple carcinoid tumors and/or tumorlets and whether there is an impact on prognosis. Peripheral carcinoid tumors in particular may be associated with multiple tumorlets or multiple carcinoid tumors.[18] Several studies have evaluated this issue and all have concluded that behavior is governed by the dominant carcinoid tumor and that the presence of additional carcinoid tumors does not impact prognosis.[3,19] A study by Ferolla et al.,[14] which identified multicentric carcinoid tumorlets in 12/100 TCs and 3/23 ACs, reported a negative impact on survival in univariate analysis; however, the significance in multivariate analysis is not stated in the paper.

Carcinoid tumors were not technically included in the 6th edition AJCC TNM Staging System of lung carcinomas, although in practice this staging system was generally applied to these tumors. Carcinoid tumors are included in the AJCC 7th Additional TNM Staging System and should therefore be staged according to the same guidelines as other lung carcinomas.[20]

TYPICAL CARCINOID TUMOR, CYTOLOGY

Cytologically, TCs show a monotonous population of small cells with round, uniform nuclei and abundant cytoplasm (Fig. 10-2). Hyperchromasia, increased mitotic figures, and necrosis are not characteristic of TCs; however, in some cases, nuclear atypia may be present. In some TCs, cells may exhibit a plasmacytoid appearance.

TYPICAL CARCINOID TUMOR, GROSS FEATURES

TCs are typically central but may be peripheral. They generally measure between 2 and 4 cm in diameter and are tan to yellow-red on cut section. The tumor may protrude into the airway and occasionally may obstruct the airway lumen. Hemorrhage and necrosis are not characteristic gross features of TCs (Figs. 10-3–10-5).

FIGURE 10-2 High-power image of Pap-stained cytology preparation of TC showing cells with round, uniform nuclei and small nucleoli, as well as conspicuous cytoplasm.

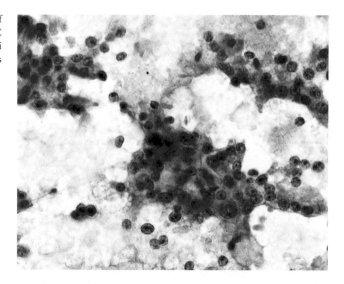

FIGURE 10-3 Gross cut section image of a central carcinoid tumor showing off-white to tan tumor, with no areas of necrosis or hemorrhage, occluding the bronchial airway.

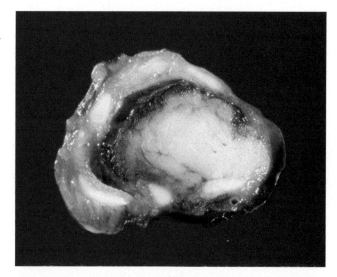

FIGURE 10-4 Gross image of a peripheral carcinoid tumor showing a well-circumscribed subpleural off-white tumor nodule that bulges on cut section, with no areas of hemorrhage or necrosis present.

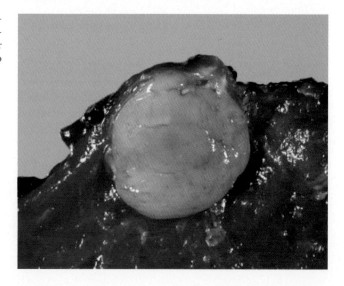

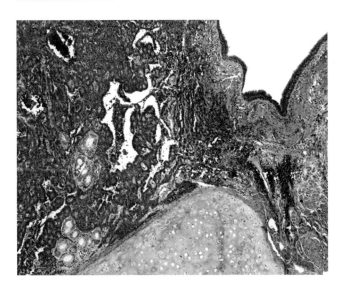

FIGURE 10-5 Low-power image of bronchial carcinoid tumor showing tumor bulging into the airway and abutting bronchial cartilage, with no necrosis present.

TYPICAL CARCINOID TUMOR, HISTOLOGY

TC is classically composed of a uniform population of polygonal cells with central nuclei with granular nuclear chromatin and moderately abundant associated eosinophilic cytoplasm. Nucleoli are generally absent but may be encountered in some cases. The cells are generally fairly uniform in appearance; however, nuclear atypia may be present and is not a criterion for diagnosing the lesion as an AC tumor (Fig. 10-6). Organoid (Fig. 10-7) and trabecular growth patterns (Fig. 10-8) are most frequently encountered and the background stroma is highly vascular. Other patterns that may be encountered are papillary growth, a pseudoglandular pattern (Fig. 10-9), and a follicular pattern (Fig. 10-10) in which the cells are arranged around eosinophilic material resembling colloid and prominent rosette formation (Fig. 10-11).[1,6] Variance in the cellular morphology may also occur and includes tumors with clear cells,[21] abundant oncocytic cytoplasm, acinic cell morphology, and tumors with intracytoplasmic melanin.[22,23] The stroma may similarly show unusual features such as calcification, ossification, or deposition of amyloid-like material (Fig. 10-12). Spindle cell morphology may be seen in peripheral tumors in particular (Fig. 10-13).[1,6]

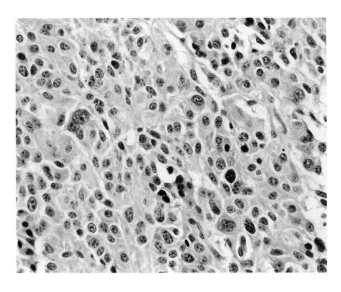

FIGURE 10-6 High-power image of TC showing nuclear atypia, which is not a criterion for the diagnosis of AC tumor. Note that there is an absence of necrosis and mitotic figures in this case.

FIGURE 10-7 High-power image of TC showing the classical appearance of TC, with a uniform population of polygonal cells containing finely granular nuclear chromatin and moderately abundant cytoplasm. The cells are arranged in an organoid pattern and lie within a vascular stroma.

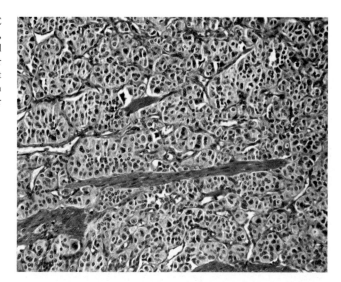

FIGURE 10-8 High-power image of TC showing trabecular pattern of tumor growth.

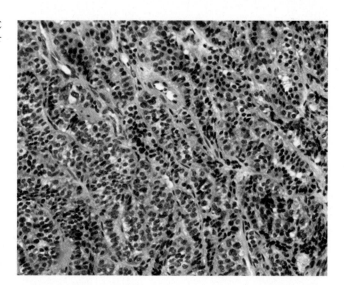

FIGURE 10-9 High-power image of TC containing a "pseudoglandular" growth pattern. Awareness of this pattern and presence of other neuroendocrine growth patterns should help avoid confusion with adenocarcinoma.

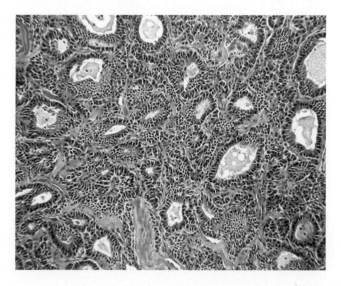

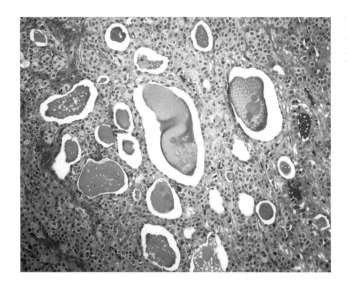

FIGURE 10-10 High-power image of TC containing so-called "follicular growth pattern" mimicking the appearance of thyroid follicles.

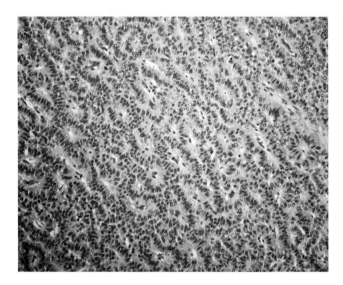

FIGURE 10-11 High-power image of TC with prominent rosette formation.

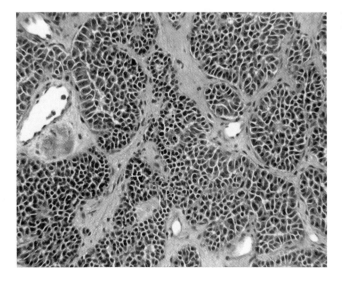

FIGURE 10-12 High-power image of TC with hyalinized collagenous stroma resembling amyloid.

FIGURE 10-13 High-power image of TC exhibiting spindle cell morphology. Such features are more frequently encountered in peripheral tumors.

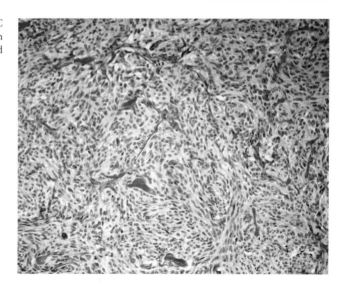

TYPICAL CARCINOID TUMOR, IMMUNOHISTOCHEMISTRY

TC will be positive for cytokeratin cocktails such as AE1/AE3 and CAM 5.2 in the majority of cases. Rare cases may be negative for keratins. TC is typically negative for both cytokeratin 7(CK7) and CK20 but a significant minority may be CK7 positive. Neuroendocrine markers such as synaptophysin, chromogranin, and CD56 (NCAM) are generally strongly positive (Figs. 10-14 and 10-15).[1,6] TTF-1 is typically negative in TC but may be positive in approximately a third of cases and is more commonly encountered in peripheral tumors.[24] In contrast to the higher grade neuroendocrine tumors, TTF-1 is considered supportive of a primary pulmonary origin in pulmonary carcinoids.[24,25] Of note, pulmonary carcinoid tumors have thus far been negative with PDX-1 and cdx-2, which typically stain nearly all pancreatic neuroendocrine tumors and ileal/appendiceal carcinoid tumors, respectively.[26] Napsin A, a proteinase involved in the maturation of surfactant protein B and found to have utility in supporting pulmonary origin for adenocarcinoma, has thus far been negative in pulmonary neuroendocrine carcinomas although further study on a larger number of cases is needed.[27] High-grade neuroendocrine carcinomas have recently been reported

FIGURE 10-14 High-power image of TC showing strong cytoplasmic immunopositivity with the neuroendocrine marker chromogranin.

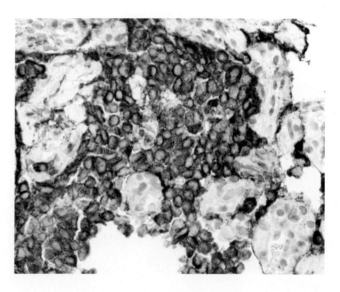

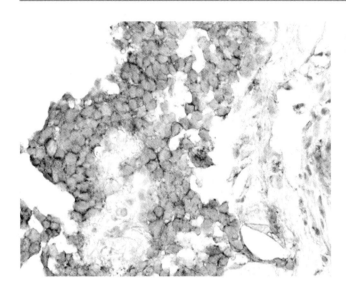

FIGURE 10-15 High-power image of TC showing tumor cell immunopositivity with CD56 (NCAM) in a membranous staining distribution.

to stain with PAX-5[28] as well as c-kit and bcl-2 in a high percentage of cases.[29] In contrast, these studies reported no staining of TC or AC with these markers with the exception of 1 case each of 16 TCs and 6 ACs being positive for bcl-2. [28,29]

Given that some series have reported that pulmonary carcinoid tumors are slightly more frequent in women, and the fact that some studies have reported a slightly elevated synchronous risk for breast cancer in patients with carcinoid tumors,[30] expression of estrogen and progesterone receptors is of interest. In a 2008 study by Sica et al. 23/42 (54%) of TCs and 6/7 (85%) of ACs were found to be positive for ER with expression ranging from focal to diffuse. PR expression was less frequent with only 26% and 29% of TCs and ACs, respectively, being positive.[31] This is in contrast to the study of Darvishian et al.[32] who, in a smaller study, did not demonstrate positive staining for ER in eight cases of carcinoid tumor and multiple tumorlets occurring in breast cancer patients.

As the presence of lymph node metastases is important in regard to overall survival, attempts have been made to correlate the presence or absence of particular markers with the likelihood of lymph node metastases. Pelosi et al.[33] reported that CD99 is present in the vast majority of TCs and ACs and the absence of this marker correlated with the occurrence of nodal metastases. In an earlier study, the same groups also reported that the presence of fascin immunoreactivity also correlated with the presence of nodal metastases.[34]

Molecular abnormalities in TC differ from those of both the high-grade neuroendocrine carcinomas (large cell neuroendocrine carcinoma [LCNEC] and small cell carcinoma [SCLC]), as well as those typically found in non–small cell lung carcinoma. Abnormalities of the MEN1 gene on chromosome 11 are commonly encountered, although TC does not frequently occur as part of Multiple Endocrine Neoplasia (MEN) syndromes (<5%).[35] TC, as well as AC, typically shows fewer mutations in genes such as p53 compared to high-grade neuroendocrine tumors. Abnormalities in p53 are seen in <5% of TCs and <1/3 of ACs but in the majority of LCNEC and SCLC. [36–38] Similarly, TCs and ACs do not show a significant rate of Rb inactivation and telomerase activity is seen in <10% of TCs, in contrast to >90% in the high-grade tumors.[39]

Chemotherapy and radiation therapy have generally had little success in treating carcinoid tumors. As such, the study of molecular aspects of these tumors with particular regard to potential targeted therapy is of interest. A 2009 study by Rickman et al.[40] examined the expression of the ErbB family (EGFR, Her2, Erb3, and Erb4) of receptor tyrosine kinases in pulmonary TC and AC. In this series, 45.8% of TCs and 28.6% of ACs exhibited positive staining for EGFR by immunohistochemistry. Molecular analysis, however, failed to reveal activating mutations within the EGFR kinase domain in any of the carcinoid tumors. The analysis did reveal a unique single nucleotide polymorphism in exon 20 (G to A substitution), which at present is of uncertain significance. The study also analyzed the tumors for k-ras mutations and found no mutations in either the TC or AC groups. In spite of the lack of activating EGFR kinase mutations in the tumors, the study subjected H727 carcinoid cell lines to erlotinib and noted a decrease in proliferative activity, suggesting this family of drugs may still have a potential therapeutic role that warrants further investigation.[40] All of the tumors in this study were negative for Erb2 (Her2), which is in keeping with a previous study by Wilkinson et al.[41] Additionally, the Rickman study demonstrated strong positive staining for ErbB3 and ErbB4. ErbB4 expression in non–small cell carcinomas has been correlated with a worse prognosis, but the significance in carcinoid tumors is uncertain at this point and requires further study.[40]

Evaluation of the efficacy of molecularly targeted agents in carcinoid tumors can be difficult as the number of cases in a given series is generally small. Agents that have shown some potential at the early clinical trial phase include those that particularly target angiogenesis such as vascular endothelial growth factor, platelet-derived growth factor, and mammalian target of rapamycin pathways. As such, bevucizumab, everoliums, and sunitinib have shown promising results in early trials but further study is needed.[8,9]

TYPICAL CARCINOID TUMOR, DIFFERENTIAL DIAGNOSIS

The differential diagnosis of TC is largely limited to distinguishing it from AC, LCNEC, and SCLC. As these tumors have similar immunohistochemical profiles, tumor morphology and the ability to evaluate cellular morphology, mitotic rate, and necrosis are the most reliable discriminating factors. Proliferation markers such as Ki-67, as would be expected, are expressed to a much lesser degree in TC and AC than the two higher grade tumors. Similarly, on average, AC has a higher degree of Ki-67 expression than TC, but there is much overlap between the two groups, and the discriminating value of this modality did not reach statistical significance in at least one study.[42–44]

Other entities to consider in the differential diagnosis of TC, depending on the tumor morphology, include adenoid cystic carcinoma and sclerosing pneumocytoma. These two entities are usually easily excluded by their lack of staining for neuroendocrine markers. Paraganglioma may enter the differential and, while positive for neuroendocrine markers, is typically negative for keratins, distinguishing it from carcinoid tumors. It should be noted that carcinoid tumors may rarely contain a population of S-100 positive sustentacular cells.[45]

Metastatic prostate carcinoma may occur as an endobronchial metastasis and closely mimic a neuroendocrine carcinoma morphologically. Metastatic prostate carcinoma is negative for neuroendocrine markers, and in spite of some reports of carcinoid tumors being positive for prostate specific antigen, a combination of negative NE markers and positive PSA and/or PAP is sufficient to prove a metastasis.[1,46]

Additional issues may arise on frozen section of carcinoid tumors. A recent study by Gupta et al.[47] demonstrated that carcinoid tumors were not infrequently misdiagnosed as squamous cell carcinoma, lymphoma, or metastatic breast cancer. Features determined as helpful in supporting a diagnosis of carcinoid at the time of frozen section included stromal hyalinization and "salt and pepper" chromatin, while the finding of irregular nuclear membranes or a mitotic rate >5 mitoses per 10 HPF favored an alternate diagnosis.[47]

TYPICAL CARCINOID TUMOR, HISTIOGENESIS

TCs are tumors of the amine precursor uptake and decarboxylation system and presumably arise from remnants of the neural crest.

References

1. Travis WD, Brambilla E, Muller-Hermelink K, et al. *Pathology and Genetics. Tumours of the Lung, Pleura, Thymus and Heart.* Lyon: IARC Press; 2004.
2. Aguayo SM, Miller YE, Waldron JA Jr, et al. Brief report: idiopathic diffuse hyperplasia of pulmonary neuroendocrine cells and airways disease. *N Engl J Med.* 1992;327(18):1285–1288.
3. Davies SJ, Gosney JR, Hansell DM, et al. Diffuse idiopathic pulmonary neuroendocrine cell hyperplasia: an under-recognised spectrum of disease. *Thorax.* 2007;62(3):248–252.
4. Gosney JR. Diffuse idiopathic pulmonary neuroendocrine cell hyperplasia as a precursor to pulmonary neuroendocrine tumors. *Chest.* 2004;125(5 suppl):108S.
5. Travis WD, Rush W, Flieder DB, et al. Survival analysis of 200 pulmonary neuroendocrine tumors with clarification of criteria for atypical carcinoid and its separation from typical carcinoid. *Am J Surg Pathol.* 1998;22(8):934–944.
6. Flieder DB. Neuroendocrine tumors of the lung: recent developments in histopathology. *Curr Opin Pulm Med.* 2002;8(4):275–280.
7. Garcia-Yuste M, Matilla JM, Cueto A, et al. Typical and atypical carcinoid tumours: analysis of the experience of the Spanish Multi-centric Study of Neuroendocrine Tumours of the Lung. *Eur J Cardiothorac Surg.* 2007;31(2):192–197.
8. Bertino EM, Confer PD, Colonna JE, et al. Pulmonary neuroendocrine/carcinoid tumors. A review article. *Cancer.* 2009;115:4434–4441.
9. Gustafsson BI, Kidd M, Chan A, et al. Bronchopulmonary neuroendocrine tumors. *Cancer.* 2008;113(1):5–21.
10. Lim E, Goldstraw P, Nicholson AG, et al. Proceedings of the IASLC international workshop on advances in pulmonary neuroendocrine tumors 2007. *J Thorac Oncol.* 2008;3(10):1194–1201.
11. Chong S, Lee KS, Kim BT, et al. Integrated PET/CT of pulmonary neuroendocrine tumors: diagnostic and prognostic implications. *Am J Roentgenol.* 2007;188(5):1223–1231.
12. Thomas CF, Jr., Tazelaar HD, Jett JR. Typical and atypical pulmonary carcinoids: outcome in patients presenting with regional lymph node involvement. *Chest.* 2001;119(4):1143–1150.
13. Wurtz A, Benhamed L, Conti M, et al. Results of systematic nodal dissection in typical and atypical carcinoid tumors of the lung. *J Thorac Oncol.* 2009;4(3):388–394.
14. Ferolla P, Daddi N, Urbani M, et al. Tumorlets, multicentric carcinoids, lymph-nodal metastases, and long-term behavior in bronchial carcinoids. *J Thorac Oncol.* 2009;4(3):383–387.
15. Srirajaskanthan R, Toumpanakis C, Karpathakis A, et al. Surgical management and palliative treatment in bronchial neuroendocrine tumours: a clinical study of 45 patients. *Lung Cancer.* 2009;65(1):68–73.
16. Lucchi M, Melfi F, Ribechini A, et al. Sleeve and wedge parenchyma-sparing bronchial resections in low-grade neoplasms of the bronchial airway. *J Thorac Cardiovasc Surg.* 2007;134(2):373–377.
17. Hage R, de la Riviere AB, Seldenrijk CA, et al. Update in pulmonary carcinoid tumors: a review article. *Ann Surg Oncol.* 2003;10(6):697–704.
18. Miller RR, Muller NL. Neuroendocrine cell hyperplasia and obliterative bronchiolitis in patients with peripheral carcinoid tumors. *Am J Surg Pathol.* 1995;19(6):653–658.
19. Aubry MC, Thomas CF Jr, Jett JR, et al. Significance of multiple carcinoid tumors and tumorlets in surgical lung specimens: analysis of 28 patients. *Chest.* 2007;131(6):1635–1643.
20. Travis WD, Giroux DJ, Chansky K, et al. The IASLC Lung Cancer Staging Project: proposals for the inclusion of broncho-pulmonary carcinoid tumors in the forthcoming (seventh) edition of the TNM Classification for Lung Cancer. *J Thorac Oncol.* 2008;3(11):1213–1223.
21. Gaffey MJ, Mills SE, Frierson HF Jr, et al. Pulmonary clear cell carcinoid tumor: another entity in the differential diagnosis of pulmonary clear cell neoplasia. *Am J Surg Pathol.* 1998;22(8):1020–1025.
22. Gal AA, Koss MN, Hochholzer L, et al. Pigmented pulmonary carcinoid tumor. An immunohistochemical and ultrastructural study. *Arch Pathol Lab Med.* 1993;117(8):832–836.
23. Goel A, Addis BJ. Pigmented atypical carcinoid of the lung. *Histopathology.* 2007;51(2):263–265.
24. Du EZ, Goldstraw P, Zacharias J, et al. TTF-1 expression is specific for lung primary in typical and atypical carcinoids: TTF-1-positive carcinoids are predominantly in peripheral location. *Hum Pathol.* 2004;35(7):825–831.

25. Saqi A, Alexis D, Remotti F, et al. Usefulness of CDX2 and TTF-1 in differentiating gastrointestinal from pulmonary carcinoids. *Am J Clin Pathol.* 2005;123(3):394–404.

26. Srivastava A, Hornick JL. Immunohistochemical staining for CDX-2, PDX-1, NESP-55, and TTF-1 can help distinguish gastrointestinal carcinoid tumors from pancreatic endocrine and pulmonary carcinoid tumors. *Am J Surg Pathol.* 2009;33(4):626–632.

27. Bishop JA, Sharma R, Illei PB. Napsin A and thyroid transcription factor-1 expression in carcinomas of the lung, breast, pancreas, colon, kidney, thyroid, and malignant mesothelioma. *Hum Pathol.* 2009 Sep 7.

28. Sica G, Vazquez MF, Altorki N, et al. PAX-5 expression in pulmonary neuroendocrine neoplasms: its usefulness in surgical and fine-needle aspiration biopsy specimens. *Am J Clin Pathol.* 2008;129(4):556–562.

29. LaPoint RJ, Bourne PA, Wang HL, et al. Coexpression of c-kit and bcl-2 in small cell carcinoma and large cell neuroendocrine carcinoma of the lung. *Appl Immunohistochem Mol Morphol.* 2007;15(4):401–406.

30. Cote ML, Wenzlaff AS, Philip PA, et al. Secondary cancers after a lung carcinoid primary: a population-based analysis. *Lung Cancer.* 2006;52(3):273–279.

31. Sica G, Wagner PL, Altorki N, et al. Immunohistochemical expression of estrogen and progesterone receptors in primary pulmonary neuroendocrine tumors. *Arch Pathol Lab Med.* 2008;132(12):1889–1895.

32. Darvishian F, Ginsberg MS, Klimstra DS, et al. Carcinoid tumorlets simulate pulmonary metastases in women with breast cancer. *Hum Pathol.* 2006;37(7):839–844.

33. Pelosi G, Leon ME, Veronesi G, et al. Decreased immunoreactivity of CD99 is an independent predictor of regional lymph node metastases in pulmonary carcinoid tumors. *J Thorac Oncol.* 2006;1(5):468–477.

34. Pelosi G, Pasini F, Fraggetta F, et al. Independent value of fascin immunoreactivity for predicting lymph node metastases in typical and atypical pulmonary carcinoids. *Lung Cancer.* 2003;42(2):203–213.

35. Debelenko LV, Brambilla E, Agarwal SK, et al. Identification of MEN1 gene mutations in sporadic carcinoid tumors of the lung. *Hum Mol Genet.* 1997;6(13):2285–2290.

36. Brambilla E, Negoescu A, Gazzeri S, et al. Apoptosis-related factors p53, Bcl2, and Bax in neuroendocrine lung tumors. *Am J Pathol.* 1996;149(6):1941–1952.

37. Kobayashi Y, Tokuchi Y, Hashimoto T, et al. Molecular markers for reinforcement of histological subclassification of neuroendocrine lung tumors. *Cancer Sci.* 2004;95(4):334–341.

38. Onuki N, Wistuba II, Travis WD, et al. Genetic changes in the spectrum of neuroendocrine lung tumors. *Cancer.* 1999;85(3):600–607.

39. Beasley MB, Lantuejoul S, Abbondanzo S, et al. The P16/cyclin D1/Rb pathway in neuroendocrine tumors of the lung. *Hum Pathol.* 2003;34(2):136–142.

40. Rickman OB, Vohra PK, Sanyal B, et al. Analysis of ErbB receptors in pulmonary carcinoid tumors. *Clin Cancer Res.* 2009;15(10):3315–3324.

41. Wilkinson N, Hasleton PS, Wilkes S, et al. Lack of C-erbB-2 protein expression in pulmonary carcinoid tumours. *J Clin Pathol.* 1991;44(4):343.

42. Arbiser ZK, Arbiser JL, Cohen C, et al. Neuroendocrine lung tumors: grade correlates with proliferation but not angiogenesis. *Mod Pathol.* 2001;14(12):1195–1199.

43. Costes V, Marty-Ane C, Picot MC, et al. Typical and atypical bronchopulmonary carcinoid tumors: a clinicopathologic and KI-67-labeling study. *Hum Pathol.* 1995;26(7):740–745.

44. Laitinen KL, Soini Y, Mattila J, et al. Atypical bronchopulmonary carcinoids show a tendency toward increased apoptotic and proliferative activity. *Cancer.* 2000;88(7):1590–1598.

45. Gosney JR, Denley H, Resl M. Sustentacular cells in pulmonary neuroendocrine tumours. *Histopathology.* 1999;34(3):211–215.

46. Copeland JN, Amin MB, Humphrey PA, et al. The morphologic spectrum of metastatic prostatic adenocarcinoma to the lung: special emphasis on histologic features overlapping with other pulmonary neoplasms. *Am J Clin Pathol.* 2002;117(4):552–557.

47. Gupta R, Dastane A, McKenna RJ Jr, et al. What can we learn from the errors in the frozen section diagnosis of pulmonary carcinoid tumors? An evidence-based approach. *Hum Pathol.* 2009;40(1):1–9.

Atypical Carcinoid Tumor

11

▶ Mary Beth Beasley

Atypical carcinoid tumor (AC) is a rare pulmonary neoplasm. Carcinoid tumors as a whole make up 1% to 2% of all pulmonary malignancies and AC is estimated to represent 11% to 24% of this number.[1] AC is defined in the 2004 World Health Organization (WHO) classification of pulmonary neoplasms as a carcinoid tumor with 2 to 10 mitoses per 10 HPF or necrosis. Most tumors will have both features, but it should be noted that occasionally a carcinoid will have necrosis without an elevated mitotic count and those tumors should be properly classified as AC. The current criteria were proposed in 1998 by Travis et al.[2,3] and were subsequently incorporated into the 1999 WHO classification. The evolution and continued debate regarding the appropriate criteria and nomenclature of these tumors are discussed in Chapter 12; however, one should note that, given the evolution of criteria for the classification of AC, older literature should be interpreted with caution given that some tumors previously classified as AC may be better classified as other neuroendocrine tumors given current guidelines.

The clinical characteristics of AC are similar to those of typical carcinoid tumors (TCs; see Chapter 10), although AC occurs in a slightly older age group and approximately 60% of patients with AC have a history of cigarette smoking. AC has a worse prognosis in comparison to TC, with a 5-year survival rate of 60% to 70% and a 10-year survival of 35% to 50%.[1,2,4,5] Lymph node metastases are present at the time of diagnosis in approximately 30% to 40% of patients.[1,2,4,6] The presence of nodal disease significantly effects prognosis in most studies, with one study reporting a 5-year survival of only 22% in patients with N2 disease.[1] Like TC, some cases of AC have been reported to arise in a background of diffuse idiopathic pulmonary neuroendocrine cell hyperplasia.[7]

ATYPICAL CARCINOID TUMORS, CYTOLOGY

Cytologically, ACs show features similar to those of TCs, including round, uniform nuclei and abundant cytoplasm, with additional cytologic features including necrosis and mitotic figures.

ATYPICAL CARCINOID TUMORS, GROSS FEATURES

ACs have the same gross appearance as TCs, typically measuring between 2 and 4 cm in diameter. The tumor may protrude into the airway, and occasionally may obstruct the airway lumen. ACs are usually tan to yellow-red on cut section; and in some cases, foci of hemorrhage, not characteristic of TCs, may be evident. Also, more ACs arise peripherally than do TCs (Fig. 11-1).

ATYPICAL CARCINOID TUMORS, HISTOLOGY

Like TC, AC is typically composed of a relatively uniform population of round to polygonal cells with finely granular chromatin and moderately abundant cytoplasm. AC most commonly has an organoid pattern of growth (Fig. 11-2), but an array of patterns similar to that in TC may also

FIGURE 11-1 Gross image of a peripheral AC showing gross features similar to those of the typical carcinoid tumor, with a well-circumscribed off-white to tan nodular lesion that bulges on cut section, with no areas of hemorrhage or necrosis.

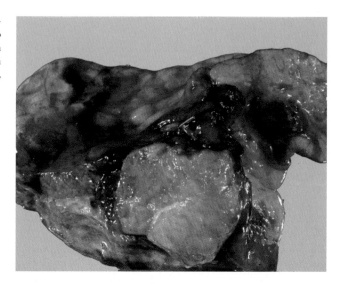

FIGURE 11-2 Atypical carcinoid exhibits neuroendocrine growth patterns similar to those encountered in typical carcinoid, exemplified here by an organoid pattern. Necrosis is obvious in this case.

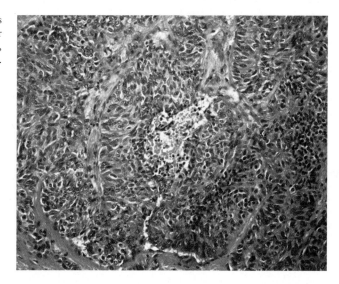

be encountered as well as areas of solid, less well-organized growth.[4] Nuclear pleomorphism is a point of interest. Pleomorphism is more commonly encountered in AC, but in the 1998 study by Travis et al.,[2,3] pleomorphism did not correlate with a worse prognosis by multivariate analysis and, therefore, is not currently included in the WHO definition as a factor discriminating TC from AC. As stated above, AC is distinguished from TC by the presence of necrosis or a mitotic count of 2 to 10 per 10 HPF. The necrosis is typically located within the center of the organoid tumor nests and may be focal or punctuate (Figs. 11-3–11-9). Occasional cases may have larger areas of infarct-like necrosis.[3,4] As these discriminating features may be present only focally, absence of these features on a core or transbronchial biopsy does not exclude an atypical carcinoid. As such, small biopsies should be designated "carcinoid tumor" with final classification left to a resected specimen. Tumors with a mitotic rate of 6 to 10 mitoses per 10 HPF have been shown to have a worse prognosis than those with 2 to 5 mitoses per 10 HPF.[4] Like TC, AC is treated surgically and typically shows minimal response to chemotherapy. Studies evaluating AC in regard to potential targeted therapies are discussed in Chapter 10.

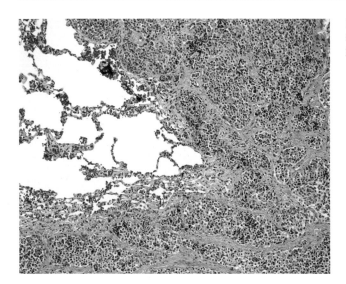

FIGURE 11-3 Medium-power image of AC showing tumor infiltrating lung parenchyma.

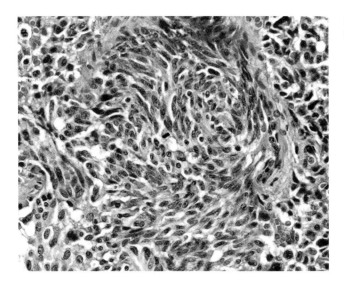

FIGURE 11-4 AC showing spindle cell features.

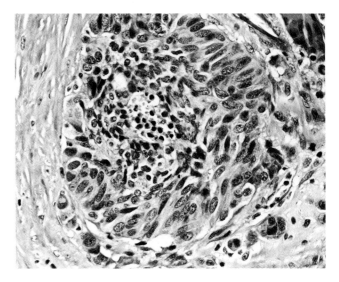

FIGURE 11-5 Atypical carcinoid is distinguished from typical carcinoid by a mitotic rate of 2 to 10 mitoses per 10 HPF or necrosis. Necrosis is often seen centrally within tumor nests and may be small punctuate foci, as seen here.

FIGURE 11-6 High-power image of AC showing scattered mitotic figures.

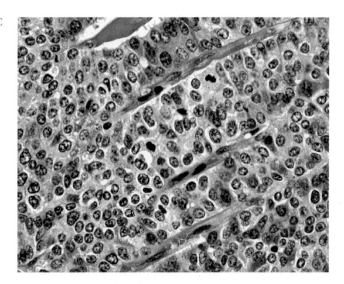

FIGURE 11-7 Aside from mitotic count and necrosis, typical carcinoid tumor cells are histologically similar to those of a typical carcinoid tumor and may show relatively uniform bland nuclei.

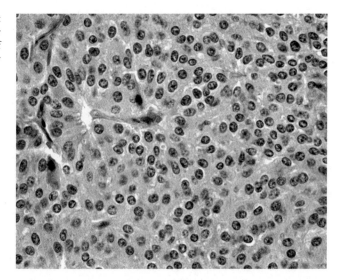

FIGURE 11-8 Atypia may be identified in ACs as in TCs and is not a criterion for their diagnoses.

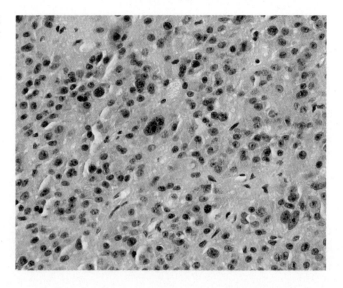

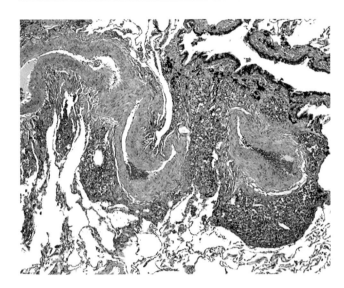

FIGURE 11-9 Medium-power image of AC showing involvement of peribronchiolar lymphatics with tumor.

ATYPICAL CARCINOID TUMORS, IMMUNOHISTOCHEMISTRY

Immunohistochemical staining patterns are essentially identical between TC and AC in regard to keratins and neuroendocrine markers (see Chapter 10). Like TC, TTF-1 is positive in AC in <50% of cases.[8] Proliferation markers have been studied in regard to separating the subtypes of neuroendocrine tumors. As stated in Chapter 10, TC and AC generally have a lower proliferation rate than the two high-grade carcinomas; however, significant overlap exists between TC and AC and between AC and the high-grade tumors. While proliferation rate has been shown to correlate with prognosis in at least one study,[9] another study did not find a statistically significant difference between proliferation rates in TC and AC.[10]

From a molecular standpoint, AC shows great similarity to TC (see also Chapter 10). Like TC, a significant number of ACs harbor mutations of the MEN1 locus at chromosome 11q13.[11] Additionally, AC shows relatively infrequent mutations of p53 and inactivation of Rb, although the percentage of tumors harboring such mutations is generally higher than that of TC and less than that of the two high-grade neuroendocrine tumors.[12–15]

ATYPICAL CARCINOID TUMOR, DIFFERENTIAL DIAGNOSIS

The differential diagnosis of AC includes TC as well as the two high-grade neuroendocrine tumors, large cell neuroendocrine carcinoma (LCNEC), and small cell lung carcinoma (SCLC) (Figs. 11-10 and 11-11). Immunohistochemical stains are of little utility in separating these entities, and the diagnosis rests on correct identification of the appropriate morphology and mitotic rate.

Occasionally, cases of metastatic breast cancer (Figs. 11-12–11-14) or metastatic prostate cancer may mimic AC or other NE tumors.[16,17] Appropriate immunohistochemical stains such as gross cystic disease fluid protein-15 (GCDFP-15) or mammoglobin for breast carcinoma and prostate-specific antigen or prostatic alkaline phosphatase are helpful in sorting out pulmonary NE tumors from metastases. It should be noted that a significant portion of AC will be positive for estrogen receptor and progesterone receptor and negative for TTF-1, and breast carcinomas may express neuroendocrine markers.[8,18]

FIGURE 11-10 High-power image of SCLC showing tumor cells with scant cytoplasm, relatively small nuclei with "salt and pepper" chromatin, nuclear molding, and abundant mitotic figures.

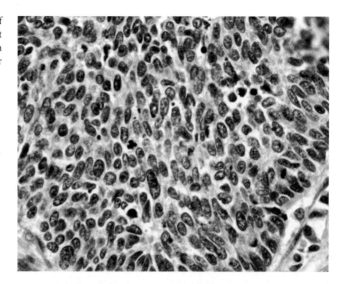

FIGURE 11-11 High-power image of LCNEC showing enlarged, hyperchromatic tumor cell nuclei, abundant cytoplasm, necrosis, rosette formation, and abundant mitotic figures.

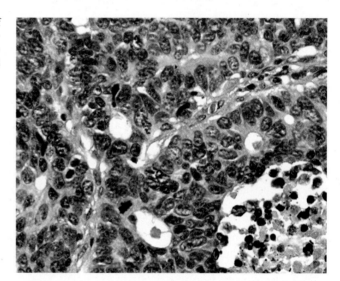

FIGURE 11-12 Metastatic breast cancer may mimic atypical carcinoid or other neuroendocrine carcinomas. This tumor has an organoid growth pattern, vascular background, and a suggestion of rosette formation.

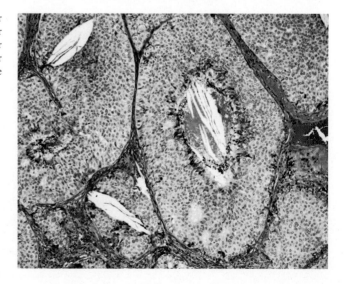

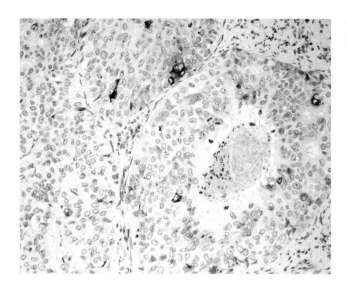

FIGURE 11-13 The tumor was positive for synaptophysin.

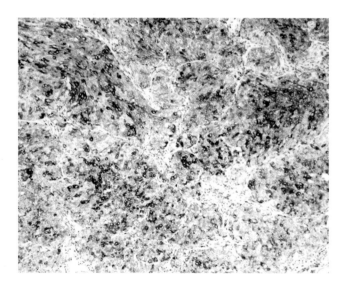

FIGURE 11-14 The tumor was also immunopositive with ER. The patient had a prior history of breast carcinoma 10 years previously, and the positive staining for GCDFP-15 provided the correct diagnosis. Review of the prior breast pathology revealed similar morphology and the original tumor was also synaptophysin positive.

ATYPICAL CARCINOID TUMOR, HISTIOGENESIS

As with TCs, ACs are tumors of the amine precursor uptake and decarboxylation system and presumably arise from remnants of the neural crest.

References

1. Lim E, Goldstraw P, Nicholson AG, et al. Proceedings of the IASLC international workshop on advances in pulmonary neuroendocrine tumors 2007. *J Thorac Oncol.* 2008;3(10):1194–1201.
2. Travis WD, Rush W, Flieder DB, et al. Survival analysis of 200 pulmonary neuroendocrine tumors with clarification of criteria for atypical carcinoid and its separation from typical carcinoid. *Am J Surg Pathol.* 1998;22(8):934–944.

3. Travis WD, Brambilla E, Muller-Hermelink K, et al. *Pathology and Genetics. Tumours of the Lung, Pleura, Thymus and Heart.* Lyon: IARC Press; 2004.
4. Beasley MB, Thunnissen FB, Brambilla E, et al. Pulmonary atypical carcinoid: predictors of survival in 106 cases. *Hum Pathol.* 2000;31(10):1255–1265.
5. Gustafsson BI, Kidd M, Chan A, et al. Bronchopulmonary neuroendocrine tumors. *Cancer.* 2008;113(1):5–21.
6. Wurtz A, Benhamed L, Conti M, et al. Results of systematic nodal dissection in typical and atypical carcinoid tumors of the lung. *J Thorac Oncol.* 2009;4(3):388–394.
7. Davies SJ, Gosney JR, Hansell DM, et al. Diffuse idiopathic pulmonary neuroendocrine cell hyperplasia: an under-recognised spectrum of disease. *Thorax.* 2007;62(3):248–252.
8. Du EZ, Goldstraw P, Zacharias J, et al. TTF-1 expression is specific for lung primary in typical and atypical carcinoids: TTF-1-positive carcinoids are predominantly in peripheral location. *Hum Pathol.* 2004;35(7):825–831.
9. Costes V, Marty-Ane C, Picot MC, et al. Typical and atypical bronchopulmonary carcinoid tumors: a clinicopathologic and KI-67-labeling study. *Hum Pathol.* 1995;26(7):740–745.
10. Arbiser ZK, Arbiser JL, Cohen C, et al. Neuroendocrine lung tumors: grade correlates with proliferation but not angiogenesis. *Mod Pathol.* 2001;14(12):1195–1199.
11. Debelenko LV, Brambilla E, Agarwal SK, et al. Identification of MEN1 gene mutations in sporadic carcinoid tumors of the lung. *Hum Mol Genet.* 1997;6(13):2285–2290.
12. Beasley MB, Lantuejoul S, Abbondanzo S, et al. The P16/cyclin D1/Rb pathway in neuroendocrine tumors of the lung. *Hum Pathol.* 2003;34(2):136–142.
13. Brambilla E, Negoescu A, Gazzeri S, et al. Apoptosis-related factors p53, Bcl2, and Bax in neuroendocrine lung tumors. *Am J Pathol.* 1996;149(6):1941–1952.
14. Onuki N, Wistuba II, Travis WD, et al. Genetic changes in the spectrum of neuroendocrine lung tumors. *Cancer.* 1999;85(3):600–607.
15. Kobayashi Y, Tokuchi Y, Hashimoto T, et al. Molecular markers for reinforcement of histological subclassification of neuroendocrine lung tumors. *Cancer Sci.* 2004;95(4):334–341.
16. Copeland JN, Amin MB, Humphrey PA, et al. The morphologic spectrum of metastatic prostatic adenocarcinoma to the lung: special emphasis on histologic features overlapping with other pulmonary neoplasms. *Am J Clin Pathol.* 2002;117(4):552–557.
17. Gupta R, Dastane A, McKenna RJ Jr, et al. What can we learn from the errors in the frozen section diagnosis of pulmonary carcinoid tumors? An evidence-based approach. *Hum Pathol.* 2009;40(1):1–9.
18. Sica G, Wagner PL, Altorki N, et al. Immunohistochemical expression of estrogen and progesterone receptors in primary pulmonary neuroendocrine tumors. *Arch Pathol Lab Med.* 2008;132(12):1889–1895.

Update on Classification of Neuroendocrine Carcinomas

12

▶ Mary Beth Beasley

Pulmonary neuroendocrine (NE) carcinomas are generally considered to encompass a spectrum of tumors including the low-grade typical carcinoid (TC) (Fig. 12-1), the intermediate-grade atypical carcinoid (AC) (Fig. 12-2), and the two high-grade carcinomas: large cell neuroendocrine carcinoma (LCNEC) (Fig. 12-3) and small cell lung carcinoma (SCLC) (Fig. 12-4). These tumors have overt neuroendocrine morphology from a histologic standpoint and generally show evidence of neuroendocrine differentiation either immunohistochemically or ultrastructurally (neuroendocrine granules).

The 2004 World Health Organization (WHO) classification of pulmonary tumors does not actually classify the NE carcinomas as a group, although they are typically thought of as representing a continuum.[1] Currently, the WHO classification categorizes the two carcinoid subtypes as a group, while LCNEC is a subtype of large cell carcinoma and SCLC is a separate category. LCNEC and SCLC both additionally have a "combined" subtype as both of these tumors may be combined with other non–small cell lung carcinomas (NSCLCs), such as adenocarcinoma or squamous cell carcinoma, or they may be combined with each other.

Aside from these four tumors, other pulmonary tumors may also exhibit evidence of neuroendocrine differentiation by immunohistochemical methods. Such tumors include pulmonary blastoma, desmoplastic small round cell tumor, paraganglioma, and primitive neuroectodermal tumor (Figs. 12-5 and 12-6).[1] Most notably, NSCLC otherwise lacking morphologic features typically associated with neuroendocrine differentiation may exhibit positive staining with neuroendocrine markers such as chromogranin, synaptophysin, or CD56. These tumors are referred to as "NSCLCs with neuroendocrine differentiation." The reported frequency of this finding is variable but is up to 20% to 30% in some series. The significance of this finding has been the subject of several studies, and while results have been somewhat variable, most series indicate this finding is not of clinical or prognostic significance.[2–8] Further complicating the picture is the existence of a group of large cell carcinomas that have overt neuroendocrine morphology from a histologic standpoint yet lack evidence of neuroendocrine differentiation by immunohistochemical or ultrastructural grounds. Such tumors have been termed "large cell carcinomas with neuroendocrine morphology" and the clinical significance of this category is unclear.[6,9] The existence of tumors with neuroendocrine morphology yet lacking evidence of neuroendocrine differentiation by immunohistochemical or ultrastructural grounds, and vice versa, has, however, raised the valid point as to whether neuroendocrine tumors should be defined by morphologic or immunohistochemical grounds, or a combination thereof (Figs. 12-7–12-9).[10]

The classification of NE carcinomas of the lung has evolved over the years and remains the subject of much debate. Much of the current controversy centers on the continued utilization of the "carcinoid" nomenclature for TC and AC, the criteria for AC, and whether a true distinction exists between LCNEC and SCLC. Other issues have evolved from increasing immunophenotypic, clinical, and molecular information. Reproducibility of diagnoses using the current classification

FIGURE 12-1 High-power image of TC showing characteristic organoid morphology, a uniform cell population, and by definition fewer than 2 mitoses per 10 HPF and lacking necrosis.

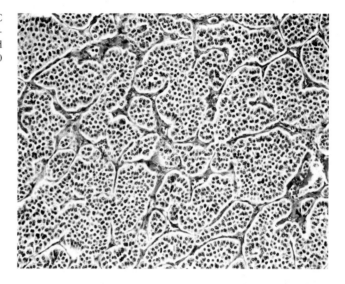

FIGURE 12-2 High-power image of AC showing organoid growth pattern with central punctuate areas of necrosis and mitotic figures.

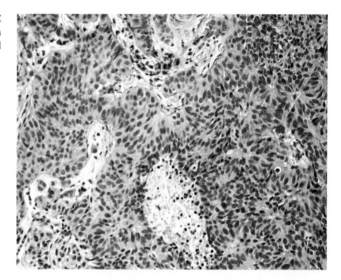

FIGURE 12-3 High-power image of LCNEC showing organoid growth and rosette formation. Central necrosis and numerous mitotic figures are present.

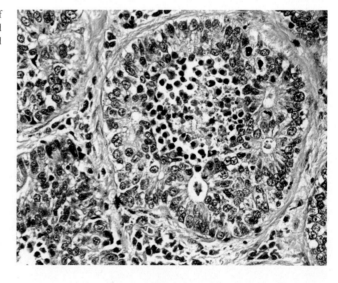

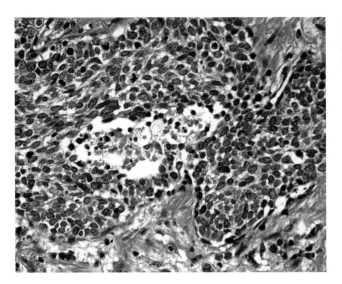

FIGURE 12-4 High-power image of small cell carcinoma is characterized by cells with hyperchromatic nuclei, scant cytoplasm, and numerous mitotic figures.

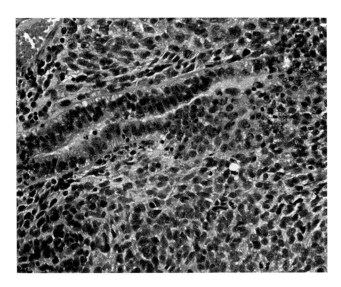

FIGURE 12-5 High-power image of pulmonary blastoma showing a combination of epithelial component resembling fetal adenocarcinoma and mesenchymal component containing primitive-appearing malignant spindle cells in a myxoid stroma.

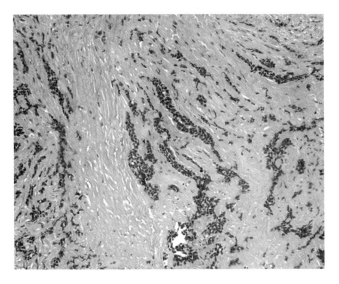

FIGURE 12-6 Medium-power image of desmoplastic small round cell tumor showing strands and cords of small round blue cells, with little cytoplasm and nuclear molding, lying within a densely fibrotic stroma.

FIGURE 12-7 High-power image of large cell carcinoma with histologic features characteristic of LCNEC, including peripheral palisading and vague rosette formation. Immunostains for neuroendocrine markers were negative. This is an example of a carcinoma best termed large cell carcinoma with neuroendocrine morphology.

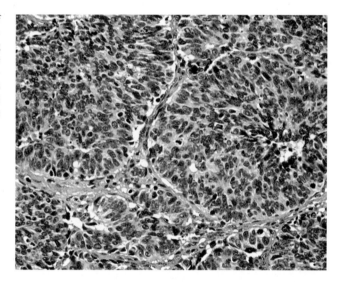

FIGURE 12-8 Medium-power image of a large cell carcinoma that shows no rosette formation, necrosis, or peripheral palisading suggestive of LCNEC.

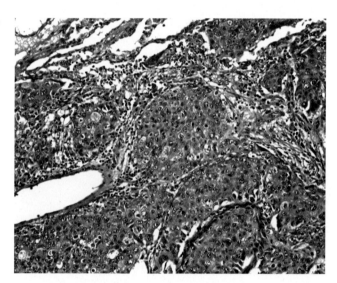

FIGURE 12-9 Immmunostains performed on the case shown in Figure 12-6 included neuroendocrine markers, and synaptophysin positivity was observed in tumor cells. How to best categorize this tumor remains controversial.

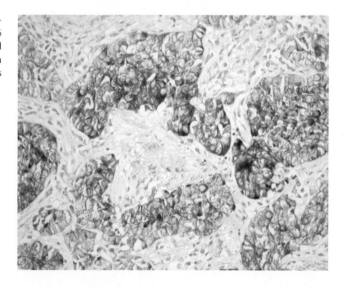

scheme is also problematic. While agreement is generally good for TC and SCLC, it is less so for AC and LCNEC, even among experienced pulmonary pathologists.[11]

Criticisms of the current WHO scheme also include the fact that the criteria are applicable primarily to large specimens, whereas the majority of lung carcinomas are diagnosed on small biopsies or cytology specimens, where one may not have sufficient tumor to count mitoses in 10 high power fields (HPF) and evaluation of the growth pattern may be difficult. Currently, it is usually not possible to reliably separate TC from AC on a small biopsy, and it is extremely difficult to make a definitive diagnosis of LCNEC. While sample size and other issues inherent with small biopsies will remain a factor, further evaluation to make the classification more applicable to small biopsies is under investigation.

This chapter addresses some of the more common issues and controversies surrounding this group of tumors at the present time, acknowledging that further study is needed to clarify many of these concerns and, most importantly, to provide clinical relevance to the classification of this group of neoplasms. Detailed pathologic information for each tumor will not be repeated here, and the reader is referred to the respective chapters on each tumor for this information. A summary of the current pulmonary neuroendocrine tumors is presented in Table 12-1, and the current WHO definitions of the major pulmonary neuroendocrine tumors are presented in Table 12-2. The continued debate and need for coordinated study of these tumors have prompted the International Association for the Study of Lung Cancer to form an international registry of pulmonary neuroendocrine tumors for detailed study of many of these issues.[4]

EVOLVING ISSUES WITH CARCINOID TUMOR

The primary issues surrounding carcinoid tumors involve the preferred nomenclature for these tumors and the definition of AC. The concept of a tumor with prognostic and morphologic features "in between" those of TC and SCLC has long been recognized. The first attempt to define AC was made by Arrigoni et al.[12] in 1972. Arrigoni proposed that AC be defined as a carcinoid tumor with (a) 1 mitotic figure per 1 to 2 HPF; (b) necrosis; (c) pleomorphism, hyperchromatism, and an abnormal nuclear cytoplasmic ratio; and (d) areas of increased cellularity and disorganization. Arrigoni et al.[12] did not specify whether one, multiple, or all of the criteria should be met and many of the criteria are subjective.[12] The entity of LCNEC was not proposed until 1991,[13]

Table 12-1	Neuroendocrine tumors of the lung

I. Tumors with neuroendocrine morphology
   Carcinoid
      TC
      AC
      LCNEC
      Combined LCNEC
      SCLC
      Combined SCLC
II. NSCLC with neuroendocrine differentiation
III. Other tumors with neuroendocrine features/differentiation
   Pulmonary blastoma
   Primitive neuroectodermal tumor
   Desmoplastic small round cell tumor
   Paraganglioma
   Carcinomas with rhabdoid phenotype

Table 12-2	Current WHO definitions of NE carcinomas[1]

TC
  A carcinoid tumor with fewer than 2 mitoses per 2 mm², lacking necrosis, and 0.5 cm or larger
AC
  A carcinoid tumor with 2–10 mitoses per 2 mm² or necrosis
LCNEC
  A tumor with a neuroendocrine morphology (organoid, palisading, rosettes, trabeculae), a high mitotic rate (11 or greater per 2 mm²), cytologic features of an NCSLC (large cell size, low nuclear to cytoplasmic ratio, vesicular, coarse or fine chromatin, frequent nucleoli), and positive immunohistochemical staining for one of more neuroendocrine markers (other than neuron-specific enolase) and/or neuroendocrine granules by electron microscopy.
SCLC
  A tumor with small cell size (generally less than the diameter of three resting lymphocytes), scant cytoplasm, finely granular nuclear chromatin, absent or faint nucleoli, a high mitotic rate (11 or greater per 2 mm²), and frequent necrosis, often in large zones.

Source: *Pathology and Genetics. Tumors of the Lung, pleura, thymus and Heart.* Lyon: IARC Press;2004.

and the current criteria for TC and AC were not proposed until 1998,[14] with criteria for both entities incorporated into the 1999 and 2004 WHO classification schemes.[1] In the interim, several other authors proposed various classification schemes for ACs using similar criteria to those of Arrigoni et al. and proposals for differing terminology also emerged. Such schemes include those of Paladugu et al.[15] who proposed the term "Kulchitsky cell carcinoma" with grade I corresponding to TC and grade II to AC. Mark and Ramirez[16] proposed "peripheral small cell carcinoma resembling carcinoid tumor" with subclassification into low and high grades, and Warren et al.[17] proposed three subsets of "well-differentiated NE carcinoma" for what would correspond to different grades of carcinoid tumors. These classification schemes clearly include some tumors that would be categorized as LCNEC using the current WHO criteria. While the current definitions of TC and AC appear relatively straightforward on the surface, criticisms remain. Critics are in favor of eliminating the "carcinoid" nomenclature and replacing it with subtypes/grades of "NE carcinoma," which is felt to better reflect the biologic potential of the tumors, while proponents of the "carcinoid" scheme argue that retention of the traditional nomenclature reduces potential confusion associated with a nomenclature shift. Critics of the current WHO scheme further argue that the current definition of AC places too much emphasis on a single criterion, namely mitotic activity. Indeed, one major pulmonary pathology textbook currently recommends the use of the criteria of El-Naggar et al.[18,19] In this scheme, neuroendocrine tumors are classified as "grade 1", "grade 2," and "grade 3" NE carcinomas. In this classification, grade 2 is essentially equivalent to AC, and criteria are a mitotic rate of 5 or more per 10 HPF, discernable nuclear pleomorphism, at least focal necrosis, and at least focal loss of organoid growth pattern. It is recommended that at least two of these criteria should be present to make this diagnosis.[19] Continued study of these tumors in a systematic fashion will hopefully provide clarification of this area, but it should be noted that consistent use of existing criteria should be employed to facilitate uniform study of this group of tumors.

Tumor location in regard to TC is another area of renewed interest. Historically, carcinoid tumors were typically separated into "central" and "peripheral" subtypes. The WHO currently does not recognize a distinction based on tumor location. However, given that peripheral TCs are more frequently multifocal or associated with multiple tumorlets/neuroendocrine hyperplasia,[20] are more frequently TTF-1 positive,[21] and more frequently exhibit a spindle cell morphology,[1,20] the issue has been raised as to whether peripheral tumors are distinct from central tumors.

Finally, in spite of TCs having a good prognosis in most cases, a small percentage of TCs will behave in an aggressive fashion.[4,14] Further evaluation of this subset of tumors is necessary in order to elucidate any biological difference between these malignant tumors and their malignant but indolent counterparts and to determine optimal treatment of these tumors.

DO NEUROENDOCRINE CARCINOMAS REPRESENT A CONTINUUM?

The concept of NE carcinomas as a continuum from low grade to high grade has also been questioned. A link between carcinoid tumors and SCLC was initially suggested by the work of Bensch et al.[22] who documented the presence of neurosecretory granules in both tumors. It has been traditionally thought that all NE carcinomas arise from the neuroendocrine Kulchitsky cells in the bronchial mucosa, although direct evidence to support this is lacking.[10] While TC, AC, LCNEC, and SCLC are generally thought of as representing a continuum, in the 2004 WHO classification, carcinoid tumors, SCLC, and LCNEC are categorized separately, with LCNEC regarded as a subtype of large cell carcinoma.[1] Indeed, TC and AC have major clinical, epidemiologic, and genetic differences from LCNEC and SCLC. As such, it would appear that carcinoid tumors and the two high-grade tumors represent biologically separate entities. LCNEC and SCLC are typically seen in an older age group and have a clear cut association with smoking in comparison to the carcinoid tumors. Additionally, the two high-grade tumors are seen more frequently in males while TC and AC have an equal sex incidence with some reports indicating a slightly higher incidence in females.[1,23–26] TC and AC may be associated with DIPNECH, which has not been reported with LCNEC or SCLC, and these entities do not otherwise have a known precursor lesion.[27–31] Further, there is no evidence that the carcinoid tumors progress to high-grade carcinomas. LCNEC and SCLC have not been reported in association with MEN1 syndrome.[25,26] Differences in immunohistochemical staining also exist, such as more frequent staining with TTF-1 and PAX-5 in the high-grade tumors in comparison to the carcinoids.[21,32,33] Such findings highlight that there are clear differences between the carcinoid tumors and the two high-grade tumors. Molecular studies, as discussed in the previous chapters, also highlight differences among these tumors. The finding of MEN-1 abnormalities in TC and AC but not in the high-grade tumors suggests a different pathway of development.[34,35] Depending on one's perspective, the molecular findings such as the increasing frequency of p53, telomerase, and Rb abnormalities from TC to SCLC might illustrate evidence of disparate qualities between the carcinoid tumors and the high-grade tumors, or they may provide evidence of an accumulation of abnormalities in keeping with the concept of a continuum.[36–39]

It is also of interest that TC and AC do not occur in combination with other histologic types of lung cancer such as adenocarcinoma or squamous cell carcinoma, as may be seen in LCNEC and SCLC.[1,4] This finding has led to the hypothesis that SCLC, LCNEC, and combined forms of these tumors arise from a common precursor cell that differs from TC/AC. Given the rarity of combined tumors, there is currently no extensive data on the genetic abnormalities of these combined tumors. Fellegara et al.[40] utilized microdissection techniques to analyze the separate components of a combined adenocarcinoma/SCLC/LCNEC and found loss of heterozygosity involving the same allele in 9 of 30 informative microsatellite markers in all components and 13 of 30 markers in 2 components.[40] While only a single case, similar findings were reported in a series of cases by Huang et al.[41] but again only one of their combined cases was a combined NE carcinoma. However, such findings suggest the possibility of a monoclonal origin from a pluripotent epithelial stem cell.

Another interesting aspect regarding the concept of NE carcinomas as a continuum is the relative wide gap between the mitotic rates of AC and the high-grade tumors. Currently, neuroendocrine tumors with a mitotic rate of >10 mitoses per 10 HPF are classified as LCNEC or SCLC depending on the cellular features.[1] However, the majority of LCNEC and SCLC will have a mitotic rate of 50 per 10 HPF, and tumors with a lower mitotic rate of 11 to 30 mitoses per 10 HPF are surprisingly infrequent. In the original paper proposing criteria for LCNEC, the number of tumors with mitotic rates in this range was too few to statistically evaluate as an independent group, and thus they were included in LCNEC.[13] Other literature evaluating this group of tumors is largely lacking. A paper by Huang et al.[42] in 2002 somewhat attempted to address this group of tumors by creating an additional category of neuroendocrine tumors that the authors termed "poorly differentiated NE carcinoma." Conceptually, the authors presented this tumor as a "high-grade AC" in between what they term "moderately differentiated NE carcinoma" (i.e., AC) and "undifferentiated NE carcinomas" (i.e., LCNEC and SCLC). In the abstract, the authors present their "poorly differentiated" category as being defined as having >10 mitoses per 10 HPF and the "undifferentiated category" as having >30 mitoses per 10 HPF. However, the materials and methods section reports a mitotic count range of between 34 and 98 mitoses (mean 64) for the "poorly differentiated" tumors, a mean of 77 with no range given for "undifferentiated LCNEC," and a range of 42 to 115 mitoses for "undifferentiated small cell NE carcinoma."[42] Thus, the significance of tumors with a mitotic count between 11 and 30 mitoses per 10 HPF was not evaluated in this paper and remains an area in need of further investigation.

DO SMALL CELL CARCINOMA AND LARGE CELL NEUROENDOCRINE CARCINOMA WARRANT SEPARATE DESIGNATIONS?

SCLC and LCNEC are both high-grade tumors with a dismal prognosis. The overall survival for LCNEC ranges from 15% to 57% with differences being attributable to the stage.[4,24,25] Stage for stage, LCNEC has a worse 5-year survival rate than other NSCLC but does not have a statistically significant survival difference in comparison to SCLC.[43] The primary issue with LCNEC is that it is currently unclear whether LCNEC responds to chemotherapy in the same manner as SCLC or whether a more optimal treatment exists. Some studies have demonstrated that LCNEC does show a similar clinical response to cisplatin-based chemotherapy as SCLC.[44–47] These are studies of only a small number of patients, which is not unexpected given the rarity of LCNEC, and a coordinated effort to better define the optimal treatment for these tumors is warranted.

On a molecular level, SCLC and LCNEC do have numerous similarities but some differences do exist. A study by Peng et al.[48] evaluating a large number of genomic alterations in SCLC and LCNEC using an array-based technique found that losses at 3p26–22, 4q21, 4q24, and 4q31 were detected at significant levels in SCLC, whereas gains at 2q31, 2q32.2, and 2q33 and loss at 6p21.3 were significantly correlated with LCNEC. A statistically significant difference in allelic loss of 5q33 between SCLC and LCNEC was reported by Hiroshima et al.[49] and Ullmann et al.[50] reported gains of 3q occurred more frequently in SCLC while gains of 6p were more frequent in LCNEC. Additionally, they reported that deletions of 10q, 16q, and 17p were less frequently observed in LCNEC compared to SCLC.[50] Interestingly, D'Adda et al.[51] utilized microdissection techniques to evaluate the components of combined SCLC/LCNEC separately and compared the results to those of pure SCLC or LCNEC. The authors found that in the combined tumors, both components shared a common pattern of alterations of 17p13.1, 3p14.2–3p21.2, 5q21, and 9p21. The authors noted that these alterations are generally involved in early carcinogenesis and hypothesized that the findings suggested a close relationship between the two components and might suggest a common origin. The authors did find differences between the two components although none reached statistical significance. Another interesting finding in this study was that genetic alterations were noted in both components of the combined tumors that have not been highly reported in either tumor in the "pure" form. The authors suggested that the findings implied that the two components in the combined tumors potentially had more commonality with each other than they did with their "pure" counterparts and further suggested that combined SCLC/LCNEC may represent a possible "transition" from in the spectrum between LCNEC and SCLC.[51]

References

1. Travis WB, Brambilla E, Müller-Hermelink HK, et al, eds. *World Health Organization Classification of Tumours. Pathology and Genetics of Tumours of the Lung, Pleura, Thymus and Heart.* Lyon: IARC Press; 2004.

2. Howe MC, Chapman A, Kerr K, et al. Neuroendocrine differentiation in non-small cell lung cancer and its relation to prognosis and therapy. *Histopathology.* 2005;46(2):195–201.

3. Ionescu DN, Treaba D, Gilks CB, et al. Nonsmall cell lung carcinoma with neuroendocrine differentiation—an entity of no clinical or prognostic significance. *Am J Surg Pathol.* 2007;31(1):26–32.

4. Lim E, Goldstraw P, Nicholson AG, et al. Proceedings of the IASLC international workshop on advances in pulmonary neuroendocrine tumors 2007. *J Thorac Oncol.* 2008;3(10):1194–1201.

5. Pelosi G, Pasini F, Sonzogni A, et al. Prognostic implications of neuroendocrine differentiation and hormone production in patients with Stage I nonsmall cell lung carcinoma. *Cancer.* 2003;97(10):2487–2497.

6. Peng WX, Sano T, Oyama T, et al. Large cell neuroendocrine carcinoma of the lung: a comparison with large cell carcinoma with neuroendocrine morphology and small cell carcinoma. *Lung Cancer.* 2005;47(2):225–233.

7. Sorhaug S, Steinshamn S, Haaverstad R, et al. Expression of neuroendocrine markers in non-small cell lung cancer. *APMIS.* 2007;115(2):152–163.

8. Sterlacci W, Fiegl M, Hilbe W, et al. Clinical relevance of neuroendocrine differentiation in non-small cell lung cancer assessed by immunohistochemistry: a retrospective study on 405 surgically resected cases. *Virchows Arch.* 2009;455(2):125–132.

9. Zacharias J, Nicholson AG, Ladas GP, et al. Large cell neuroendocrine carcinoma and large cell carcinomas with neuroendocrine morphology of the lung: prognosis after complete resection and systematic nodal dissection. *Ann Thorac Surg.* 2003;75(2):348–352.

10. Warren WH, Hammar SP. The dispersed neuroendocrine system, its bronchopulmonary elements, and neuroendocrine tumors presumed to be derived from them: myths, mistaken notions, and misunderstandings. *Semin Thorac Cardiovasc Surg.* 2006;18(3):178–182.

11. Travis WD, Gal AA, Colby TV, et al. Reproducibility of neuroendocrine lung tumor classification. *Hum Pathol.* 1998;29(3):272–279.

12. Arrigoni MG, Woolner LB, Bernatz PE. Atypical carcinoid tumors of the lung. *J Thorac Cardiovasc Surg.* 1972;64(3):413–421.

13. Travis WD, Linnoila RI, Tsokos MG, et al. Neuroendocrine tumors of the lung with proposed criteria for large-cell neuroendocrine carcinoma. An ultrastructural, immunohistochemical, and flow cytometric study of 35 cases. *Am J Surg Pathol.* 1991;15(6):529–553.

14. Travis WD, Rush W, Flieder DB, et al. Survival analysis of 200 pulmonary neuroendocrine tumors with clarification of criteria for atypical carcinoid and its separation from typical carcinoid. *Am J Surg Pathol.* 1998;22(8):934–944.

15. Paladugu RR, Benfield JR, Pak HY, et al. Bronchopulmonary Kulchitzky cell carcinomas. A new classification scheme for typical and atypical carcinoids. *Cancer.* 1985;55(6):1303–1311.

16. Mark EJ, Ramirez JF. Peripheral small-cell carcinoma of the lung resembling carcinoid tumor. A clinical and pathologic study of 14 cases. *Arch Pathol Lab Med.* 1985;109(3):263–269.

17. Warren WH, Memoli VA, Gould VE. Well differentiated and small cell neuroendocrine carcinomas of the lung. Two related but distinct clinicopathologic entities. *Virchows Arch B Cell Pathol Incl Mol Pathol.* 1988;55(5):299–310.

18. el-Naggar AK, Ballance W, Karim FW, et al. Typical and atypical bronchopulmonary carcinoids. A clinicopathologic and flow cytometric study. *Am J Clin Pathol.* 1991;95(6):828–834.

19. Wick MR, Leslie K, Ritter J, et al. Neuroendocrine neoplasms of the lung. In: Leslie KO, Wick MR, editors. *Practical pulmonary pathology. A diagnostic approach.* Philadelphia, PA: Churchill Livingston; 2005:423–463.

20. Miller RR, Muller NL. Neuroendocrine cell hyperplasia and obliterative bronchiolitis in patients with peripheral carcinoid tumors. *Am J Surg Pathol.* 1995;19(6):653–658.

21. Du EZ, Goldstraw P, Zacharias J, et al. TTF-1 expression is specific for lung primary in typical and atypical carcinoids: TTF-1-positive carcinoids are predominantly in peripheral location. *Hum Pathol.* 2004;35(7):825–831.

22. Bensch KG, Corrin B, Pariente R, et al. Oat-cell carcinoma of the lung. Its origin and relationship to bronchial carcinoid. *Cancer*. 1968;22(6):1163–1172.

23. Nicholson SA, Beasley MB, Brambilla E, et al. Small cell lung carcinoma (SCLC): a clinicopathologic study of 100 cases with surgical specimens. *Am J Surg Pathol*. 2002;26(9):1184–1197.

24. Travis WD. Lung tumours with neuroendocrine differentiation. *Eur J Cancer*. 2009;45(suppl 1): 251–266.

25. Gustafsson BI, Kidd M, Chan A, et al. Bronchopulmonary neuroendocrine tumors. *Cancer*. 2008; 113(1):5–21.

26. Bertino EM, Confer PD, Colonna JE, et al. Pulmonary neuroendocrine/carcinoid tumors. A review article. *Cancer*. 2009;115:4434–4441.

27. Adams H, Brack T, Kestenholz P, et al. Diffuse idiopathic neuroendocrine cell hyperplasia causing severe airway obstruction in a patient with a carcinoid tumor. *Respiration*. 2006;73(5):690–693.

28. Aguayo SM, Miller YE, Waldron JA Jr, et al. Brief report: idiopathic diffuse hyperplasia of pulmonary neuroendocrine cells and airways disease. *N Engl J Med*. 1992;327(18):1285–1288.

29. Davies SJ, Gosney JR, Hansell DM, et al. Diffuse idiopathic pulmonary neuroendocrine cell hyperplasia: an under-recognised spectrum of disease. *Thorax*. 2007;62(3):248–252.

30. Ge Y, Eltorky MA, Ernst RD, et al. Diffuse idiopathic pulmonary neuroendocrine cell hyperplasia. *Ann Diagn Pathol*. 2007;11(2):122–126.

31. Gosney JR. Diffuse idiopathic pulmonary neuroendocrine cell hyperplasia as a precursor to pulmonary neuroendocrine tumors. *Chest*. 2004;125(5 suppl):108S.

32. Rossi G, Marchioni A, Milani M, et al. TTF-1, cytokeratin 7, 34betaE12, and CD56/NCAM immunostaining in the subclassification of large cell carcinomas of the lung. *Am J Clin Pathol*. 2004;122(6):884–893.

33. Sica G, Vazquez MF, Altorki N, et al. PAX-5 expression in pulmonary neuroendocrine neoplasms: its usefulness in surgical and fine-needle aspiration biopsy specimens. *Am J Clin Pathol*. 2008;129(4): 556–562.

34. Debelenko LV, Swalwell JI, Kelley MJ, et al. MEN1 gene mutation analysis of high-grade neuroendocrine lung carcinoma. *Genes Chromosomes Cancer*. 2000;28(1):58–65.

35. Debelenko LV, Brambilla E, Agarwal SK, et al. Identification of MEN1 gene mutations in sporadic carcinoid tumors of the lung. *Hum Mol Genet*. 1997;6(13):2285–2290.

36. Beasley MB, Lantuejoul S, Abbondanzo S, et al. The P16/cyclin D1/Rb pathway in neuroendocrine tumors of the lung. *Hum Pathol*. 2003;34(2):136–142.

37. Brambilla E, Negoescu A, Gazzeri S, et al. Apoptosis-related factors p53, Bcl2, and Bax in neuroendocrine lung tumors. *Am J Pathol*. 1996;149(6):1941–1952.

38. Onuki N, Wistuba II, Travis WD, et al. Genetic changes in the spectrum of neuroendocrine lung tumors. *Cancer*. 1999;85(3):600–607.

39. Zaffaroni N, De PD, Villa R, et al. Differential expression of telomerase activity in neuroendocrine lung tumours: correlation with gene product immunophenotyping. *J Pathol*. 2003;201(1): 127–133.

40. Fellegara G, D'Adda T, Pilato F, et al. Genetics of a combined lung small cell carcinoma and large cell neuroendocrine carcinoma with adenocarcinoma. *Virchows Arch*. 2008;453:107–115.

41. Huang J, Behrens C, Wistuba II, et al. Clonality of combined tumors. *Arch Pathol Lab Med*. 2002;126(4):437–441.

42. Huang Q, Muzitansky A, Mark EJ. Pulmonary neuroendocrine carcinomas. A review of 234 cases and a statistical analysis of 50 cases treated at one institution using a simple clinicopathologic classification. *Arch Pathol Lab Med*. 2002;126(5):545–553.

43. Takei H, Asamura H, Maeshima A, et al. Large cell neuroendocrine carcinoma of the lung: a clinicopathologic study of eighty-seven cases. *J Thorac Cardiovasc Surg*. 2002;124(2):285–292.

44. Rossi G, Cavazza A, Marchioni A, et al. Role of chemotherapy and the receptor tyrosine kinases KIT, PDGFRalpha, PDGFRbeta, and Met in large-cell neuroendocrine carcinoma of the lung. *J Clin Oncol*. 2005;23(34):8774–8785.

45. Iyoda A, Hiroshima K, Moriya Y, et al. Postoperative recurrence and the role of adjuvant chemotherapy in patients with pulmonary large-cell neuroendocrine carcinoma. *J Thorac Cardiovasc Surg*. 2009;138(2):446–453.

46. Iyoda A, Hiroshima K, Moriya Y, et al. Prospective study of adjuvant chemotherapy for pulmonary large cell neuroendocrine carcinoma. *Ann Thorac Surg*. 2006;82(5):1802–1807.

47. Yamazaki S, Sekine I, Matsuno Y, et al. Clinical responses of large cell neuroendocrine carcinoma of the lung to cisplatin-based chemotherapy. *Lung Cancer.* 2005;49(2):217–223.

48. Peng WX, Shibata T, Katoh H, et al. Array-based comparative genomic hybridization analysis of high-grade neuroendocrine tumors of the lung. *Cancer Sci.* 2005;96(10):661–667.

49. Hiroshima K, Iyoda A, Shida T, et al. Distinction of pulmonary large cell neuroendocrine carcinoma from small cell lung carcinoma: a morphological, immunohistochemical, and molecular analysis. *Mod Pathol.* 2006;19(10):1358–1368.

50. Ullmann R, Petzmann S, Sharma A, et al. Chromosomal aberrations in a series of large-cell neuroendocrine carcinomas: unexpected divergence from small-cell carcinoma of the lung. *Hum Pathol.* 2001;32(10):1059–1063.

51. D'Adda T, Pelosi G, Lagrasta C, et al. Genetic alterations in combined neuroendocrine neoplasms of the lung. *Mod Pathol.* 2008.

13

Sarcomatoid (Sarcomatous) Carcinoma

▶ Sanja Dacic

Sarcomatoid carcinomas are rare and make up only 0.3% to 1.3% of all lung malignancies.[1] These tumors are defined by 2004 WHO criteria as a poorly differentiated non–small cell lung carcinomas (NCSLCs) that contain a component of sarcoma or sarcoma-like (spindle or giant cells or both) differentiation. Although the diagnosis may be suspected on transbronchial biopsy or fine needle aspiration, surgical resection is necessary for definitive classification and diagnosis.

SARCOMATOID CARCINOMA, CYTOLOGY

Cytologically, sarcomatoid carcinomas exhibit spindle cell elements. Malignant epithelial, giant cell, or heterologous (e.g., malignant cartilaginous, osseous, or rhabdomyomatous) elements may be present as well (Fig. 13-1).

SARCOMATOID CARCINOMA, GROSS FEATURES

Sarcomatoid carcinomas can arise in the central or peripheral lung, usually as a large mass between 3 and 11 cm. Grossly, the cut surface is gray-white with areas of necrosis and hemorrhage (Fig. 13-2).

SARCOMATOID CARCINOMA, HISTOLOGY

Five subgroups of sarcomatoid carcinomas are recognized including pleomorphic carcinomas, spindle cell carcinomas, giant cell carcinoma, carcinosarcoma, and pulmonary blastoma. Three of these entities are discussed below. Giant cell carcinoma and pulmonary blastoma are discussed separately in Chapters 14 and 15.

Pleomorphic carcinoma consists of a poorly differentiated squamous cell carcinoma, adenocarcinoma, or large cell carcinoma admixed with spindle or giant cells constituting ≥10% of the tumor (Fig. 13-3). Spindle cells may have epithelioid or mesenchymal appearance. The stroma may be fibrous or myxoid. Malignant giant cells are polygonal, are uninucleated or multinucleated, and have dense eosinophilic cytoplasm and pleomorphic nuclei. Emperiopolesis is common (Fig. 13-4). Large vessel invasion associated with necrosis is usually present.[2–6]

Carcinosarcoma is a malignant tumor consisting of a mixture of carcinoma and sarcoma containing differentiated sarcomatous elements, such as malignant cartilage, bone, or skeletal muscle (Fig. 13-5). Squamous cell carcinoma is the most common carcinomatous component (45%–70%), followed by adenocarcinoma (20%–31%) and large cell carcinoma (10%). An undifferentiated spindle cell sarcoma component is most frequently present, followed by rhabdomyosarcoma, osteosarcoma, or chondrosarcoma. More than one differentiated sarcomatous component may be present. Sarcomatous component is often the predominant component, and the foci of carcinoma are often small.[7,8]

Spindle cell carcinoma is defined as an NSCLC consisting of only spindle-shaped tumor cells which are identical to the spindle cell component of pleomorphic carcinomas (Fig. 13-6).

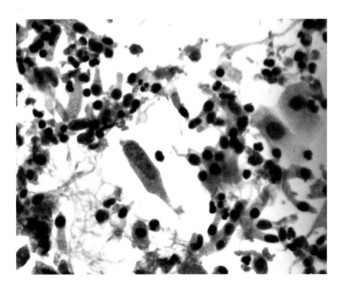

FIGURE 13-1 High-power image of Pap-stained cytology preparation of sarcomatoid carcinoma showing an enlarged, hyperchromatic malignant spindle tumor cell within a background of bronchial mucosal cells.

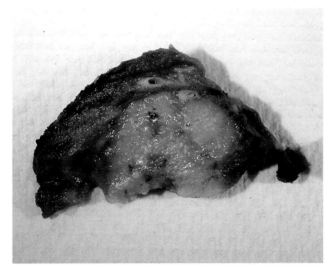

FIGURE 13-2 Gross image of a wedge resection specimen containing sarcomatoid carcinoma, specifically in this case chondrosarcoma, showing a peripheral well-circumscribed tumor with a glistening, off-white cut surface and focal small areas of hemorrhage.

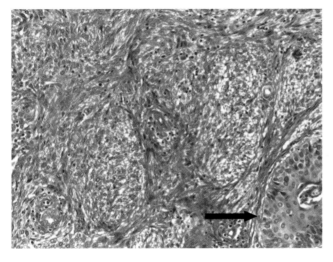

FIGURE 13-3 Medium-power image of pleomorphic carcinoma composed of a conventional squamous cell carcinoma (*arrow*) admixed with more than 10% of malignant spindle cells.

FIGURE 13-4 High-power image of sarcomatoid carcinoma exhibiting emperiopolesis.

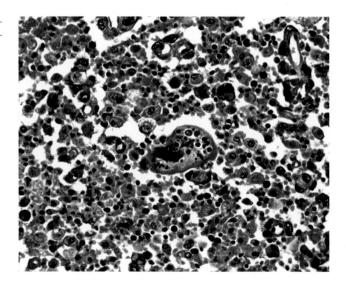

FIGURE 13-5 Medium-power image of carcinosarcoma exhibiting a mixture of a conventional squamous cell carcinoma (*arrow*) as well as true sarcomatous components including chondrosarcoma (**A**) and rhabdomyosarcoma (**B**).

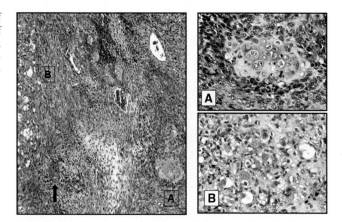

FIGURE 13-6 Medium-power image of spindle carcinoma composed of spindle-shaped cells with irregular nuclear contours and hyperchromasia (inset) and admixed with scattered and focally prominent lymphoplasmacytic inflammatory infiltrates. Specific patterns of adenocarcinoma, squamous cell, large cell, or giant cell carcinoma are not present.

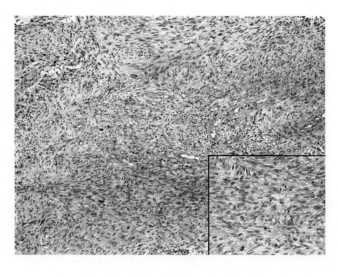

Irregular fascicles of obviously malignant spindle cells with nuclear hyperchromasia and prominent nucleoli are seen. Adenocarcinoma, giant cell, squamous cell, or large cell carcinoma are not seen.[5,8,9]

SARCOMATOID CARCINOMA, IMMUNOHISTOCHEMISTRY

According to WHO criteria, immunohistochemistry is not necessary if sarcomatoid tumor demonstrates a component of conventional NSCLC on routine light microscopy.[1] Sarcomatoid carcinomas often co-express cytokeratin, vimentin, CEA, and SMA. In some cases, multiple cytokeratins and EMA are necessary to demonstrate epithelial differentiation in the sarcomatous component. When cytokeratin stains are negative, it may be very difficult to differentiate these tumors from primary or metastatic sarcomas. Chondrosarcoma will stain with S100 protein and rhabdomyosarcoma with muscle markers. Strong cytokeratin positivity is most helpful in making the diagnosis of sarcomatoid carcinomas, but depending on the tumor's morphology, cytokeratin-positive sarcomas may remain in the differential diagnosis (Figs. 13-7–13-10).[5]

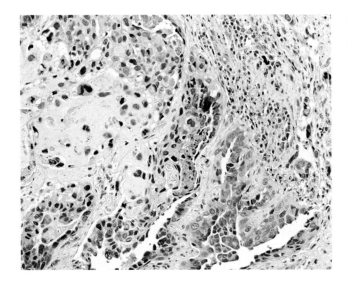

FIGURE 13-7 High-power image of carcinosarcoma showing both epithelial and chondrosarcomatous elements.

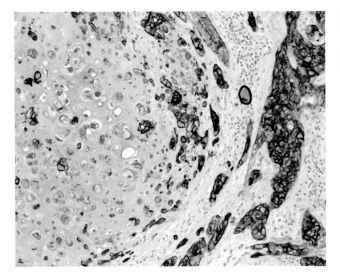

FIGURE 13-8 High-power image of the tumor shown in Figure 13-6 exhibiting immunopositivity with pankeratin within both epithelial and mesenchymal tumor components.

FIGURE 13-9 High-power image of the same area of tumor as shown in Figure 13-6 exhibiting tumor cell immunopositivity with vimentin within the chondrosarcomatous component, but not within the epithelial component.

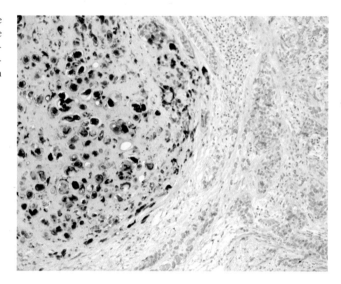

FIGURE 13-10 High-power image of the same area as shown in Figure 13-6 exhibiting tumor cell immunopositivity with monoclonal CEA within the epithelial component, but not within the chondrosarcomatous component.

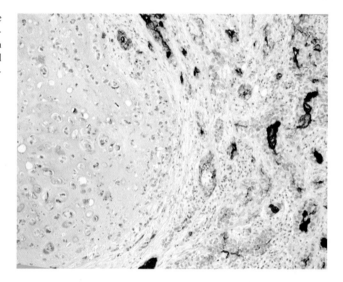

SARCOMATOID CARCINOMA, DIFFERENTIAL DIAGNOSIS

Table 13-1 summarizes immunohistochemical profiles of sarcomatoid neoplasms of the lung and pleura. Pleomorphic carcinomas may be difficult to differentiate from reactive process, sarcomas, and mesotheliomas.[5,10–12] Adequate sampling of a case usually allows identification of the carcinomatous component. Features of spindle cell carcinoma that may lead to misinterpretation as a benign process include vascular invasion with associated infarction, necrosis with cavitation and surrounding fibrohistiocytic reaction, secondary infection and inflammation, and interstitial growth by the neoplastic cells.[13] Separation of spindle cell carcinomas from cytokeratin-positive sarcomas, particularly synovial sarcoma, may be difficult; however, both variants of synovial sarcoma (monophasic and biphasic) have characteristic morphology. The spindle cells arranged in fascicles have uniform, tapering nuclei and pale poorly defined cytoplasm in a variably collagenous, often hyaline in appearance, stoma. Stromal mast cells and a hemangiopericytoma-like vascular pattern are common findings. Cytokeratin and EMA tend to be focally positive. EMA

Table 13-1	Summary of immunohistochemical profiles of spindle proliferations of the lung and pleura			
Antibody	Sarcomatoid Mesothelioma	Sarcomatoid Carcinoma	Synovial Sarcoma	Solitary Fibrous Tumor
Keratin	+	+	+	−
Calretinin	±	−	−	−
TTF	−	±	−	−
WT-1	±	±	−	−
CEA	±	+	−	−
EMA	−	±	+	−
Desmin	±	±	±	±
Actin	±	±	±	±
S100	±	−	±	±
CD34	−	−	−	+
BCL-2	−	−	±	+
Vimentin	+	±	+	+

is more sensitive and stains more cells than keratin. Demonstration of the reproducible tumor translocation t(X;18) (p11.2;q11.2) by FISH is very helpful.

SARCOMATOID CARCINOMA, HISTOGENESIS

The histogenesis of sarcomatoid carcinomas has engendered much controversy over the years, with numerous studies using ultrastructural, immunohistochemical, and, more recently, molecular studies in an attempt to provide a comprehensive explanation. The monoclonal theory proposed a common origin of mesenchymal and epithelial components from a single totipotent stem cell. Molecular studies have established that the epithelial and sarcomatoid components of pleomorphic carcinomas and carcinosarcomas have identical molecular profiles, including equivalent patterns of acquired allelic loss, p53 mutational profile, and X chromosome inactivation.[14-16] It is generally agreed that sarcomatoid carcinoma has a poorer prognosis than stage-matched conventional NSCLC.[17,18] This may be in part related to the high rate of *KRAS* mutations observed in these tumors.[17]

References

1. Travis WB, Brambilla E, Müller-Hermelink HK, et al., eds. *World Health Organization Classification of Tumours. Pathology and Genetics of Tumours of the Lung, Pleura, Thymus and Heart.* Lyon: IARC Press; 2004.
2. Fishback NF, Travis WD, Moran CA, et al. Pleomorphic (spindle/giant cell) carcinoma of the lung. A clinicopathologic correlation of 78 cases. *Cancer.* 1994;73:2936–2945.
3. Mochizuki T, Ishii G, Nagai K, et al. Pleomorphic carcinoma of the lung: clinicopathologic characteristics of 70 cases. *Am J Surg Pathol.* 2008;32:1727–1735.
4. Nappi O, Wick MR. Sarcomatoid neoplasms of the respiratory tract. *Semin Diagn Pathol.* 1993;10:137–147.

5. Pelosi G, Sonzogni A, De Pas T, et al. Pulmonary sarcomatoid carcinomas: a practical overview. *Int J Surg Pathol.* 2009; Jan 14; [Epub ahead of print].

6. Wick MR, Ritter JH, Humphrey PA. Sarcomatoid carcinomas of the lung: a clinicopathologic review. *Am J Clin Pathol.* 1997;108:40–53.

7. Koss MN, Hochholzer L, Frommelt RA. Carcinosarcomas of the lung: a clinicopathologic study of 66 patients. *Am J Surg Pathol.* 1999;23:1514–1526.

8. Nappi O, Glasner SD, Swanson PE, et al. Biphasic and monophasic sarcomatoid carcinomas of the lung. A reappraisal of 'carcinosarcomas' and 'spindle-cell carcinomas'. *Am J Clin Pathol.* 1994;102:331–340.

9. Wick MR, Ritter JH, Nappi O. Inflammatory sarcomatoid carcinoma of the lung: report of three cases and clinicopathologic comparison with inflammatory pseudotumors in adult patients. *Hum Pathol.* 1995;26:1014–1021.

10. Cagle PT, Truong LD, Roggli VL, et al. Immunohistochemical differentiation of sarcomatoid mesotheliomas from other spindle cell neoplasms. *Am J Clin Pathol.* 1989;92:566–571.

11. Husain AN, Colby TV, Ordonez NG, et al. Guidelines for pathologic diagnosis of malignant mesothelioma: a consensus statement from the International Mesothelioma Interest Group. *Arch Pathol Lab Med.* 2009;133:1317–1331.

12. Takeshima Y, Amatya VJ, Kushitani K, et al. Value of immunohistochemistry in the differential diagnosis of pleural sarcomatoid mesothelioma from lung sarcomatoid carcinoma. *Histopathology.* 2009;54: 667–676.

13. Colby TV. Malignancies in the lung and pleura mimicking benign processes. *Semin Diagn Pathol.* 1995;12:30–44.

14. Dacic S, Finkelstein SD, Sasatomi E, et al. Molecular pathogenesis of pulmonary carcinosarcoma as determined by microdissection-based allelotyping. *Am J Surg Pathol.* 2002;26:510–516.

15. Holst VA, Finkelstein S, Colby TV, et al. p53 and K-ras mutational genotyping in pulmonary carcinosarcoma, spindle cell carcinoma, and pulmonary blastoma: implications for histogenesis. *Am J Surg Pathol.* 1997;21:801–811.

16. Pelosi G, Scarpa A, Manzotti M, et al. K-ras gene mutational analysis supports a monoclonal origin of biphasic pleomorphic carcinoma of the lung. *Mod Pathol.* 2004;17:538–546.

17. Italiano A, Cortot AB, Ilie M, et al. EGFR and KRAS status of primary sarcomatoid carcinomas of the lung: Implications for anti-EGFR treatment of a rare lung malignancy. *Int J Cancer.* 2009; Jun 2; [Epub ahead of print].

18. Ito K, Oizumi S, Fukumoto S, et al. Clinical characteristics of pleomorphic carcinoma of the lung. *Lung Cancer.* 2009; Jul 3; [Epub ahead of print].

Giant Cell Carcinoma

14

▶ Sanja Dacic

G iant cell carcinoma is an extremely rare variant of non–small cell carcinoma composed of bizarre, pleomorphic, very large mononucleated or multinucleated tumor giant cells identical to the giant cells found in pleomorphic carcinoma (see Chapter 13). Adenocarcinoma, squamous cell carcinoma, and large cell carcinoma are not features of giant cell carcinoma.[1]

GIANT CELL CARCINOMA, CYTOLOGY

Giant cell carcinoma is a rare tumor and not typically diagnosed by cytology; however, aspiration may show a mixture of inflammatory cells and tumor cells, with occasional giant tumor cells identified.

GIANT CELL CARCINOMA, GROSS FEATURES

Giant cell carcinomas tend to form well-circumscribed masses that on cut section are tan-yellow to gray and show areas of necrosis and hemorrhage.

GIANT CELL CARCINOMA, HISTOLOGY

The tumor cells in giant cell carcinoma are discohesive and associated with a marked inflammatory infiltrate, usually composed of neutrophils. Tumor cells have abundant eosinophilic cytoplasm often showing leukocyte emperiopolesis (neutrophils penetrating the cytoplasm of the tumor giant cells), phagocytosed anthracotic pigment, or hyaline globules (Figs. 14-1–14-3). Nuclei are hyperchromatic to vesicular and contain prominent nucleoli. Pleomorphic giant cells are identified throughout the tumor and are typically very large and often bizarre multinucleated or multilobated cells (Figs. 14-4–14-6).[2–5]

GIANT CELL CARCINOMA, IMMUNOHISTOCHEMISTRY

The tumor cells often co-express cytokeratin, vimentin, CEA, and smooth muscle markers. TTF-1 may be positive in some cases.[4,5]

GIANT CELL CARCINOMA, DIFFERENTIAL DIAGNOSIS

The differential diagnosis includes other types of NSCLC with giant cells, primary and metastatic sarcomas (pleomorphic rhabdomyosarcoma), adrenocortical carcinoma, choriocarcinoma, and other pleomorphic malignant tumors. Beta-HCG can be seen in lung carcinomas and therefore should not be used as a marker of metastatic choriocarcinoma. The giant cells of giant cell carcinoma should not be confused with osteoclast-type multinucleated giant cells, which are non-neoplastic cells that may be found in any subtype of sarcomatoid lung carcinomas. While giant cells may be identified in lung cancers after radiation therapy, the diagnostic criteria of giant cell carcinoma are not present.

FIGURE 14-1 Medium-power image of pulmonary giant cell tumor showing a well-circumscribed tumor with abundant giant cells and associated inflammatory cells.

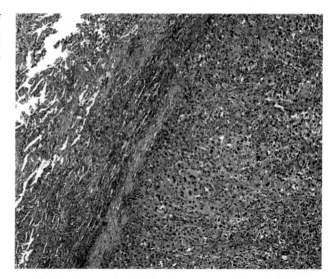

FIGURE 14-2 High-power image of giant cell carcinoma showing discohesive malignant giant cells that are polygonal, uninucleated or multinucleated, with dense eosinophilic cytoplasm. A marked neutrophilic inflammatory infiltrate is present.

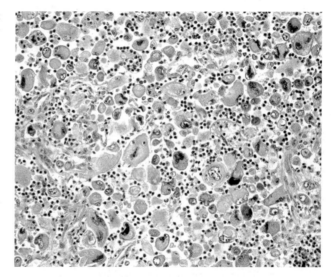

FIGURE 14-3 Giant cells with leukocyte emperiopolesis are a characteristic feature of giant cell carcinoma.

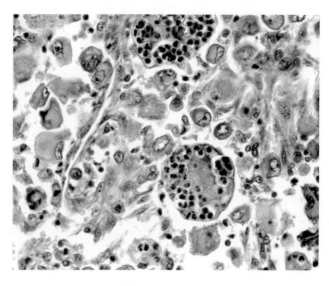

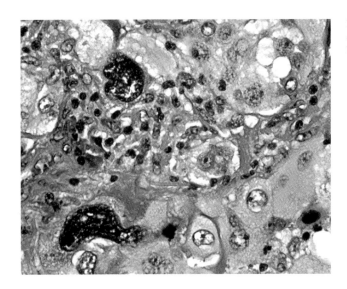

FIGURE 14-4 High-power image of giant cell carcinoma highlighting the large, bizarre hyperchromatic nuclei.

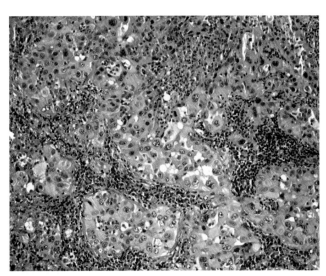

FIGURE 14-5 High-power image of giant cell carcinoma highlighting an area with an abundant inflammatory cell infiltrate surrounding nests of tumor cells.

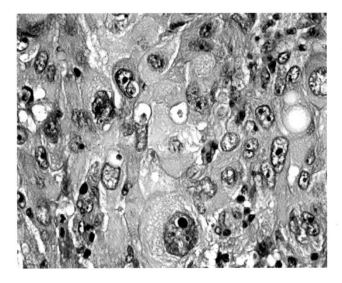

FIGURE 14-6 High-power image of giant cell carcinoma showing abundant eosinophilic cytoplasm within tumor cells.

GIANT CELL CARCINOMA, HISTIOGENESIS

Giant cell carcinomas arise from primitive cells, presumably of pulmonary epithelial origin.

References

1. Travis WB, Brambilla E, Müller-Hermelink HK, et al., eds. *World Health Organization Classification of Tumours. Pathology and Genetics of Tumours of the Lung, Pleura, Thymus and Heart.* Lyon: IARC Press; 2004.
2. Addis BJ, Dewar A, Thurlow NP. Giant cell carcinoma of the lung—immunohistochemical and ultra-structural evidence of dedifferentiation. *J Pathol.* 1988;155:231–240.
3. Attanoos RL, Papagiannis A, Suttinont P, et al. Pulmonary giant cell carcinoma: pathological entity or morphological phenotype? *Histopathology.* 1998;32:225–231.
4. Pelosi G, Sonzogni A, De Pas T, et al. Pulmonary sarcomatoid carcinomas: a practical overview. *Int J Surg Pathol.* 2009; Jan 14; [Epub ahead of print].
5. Rossi G, Cavazza A, Sturm N, et al. Pulmonary carcinomas with pleomorphic, sarcomatoid, or sarcomatous elements: a clinicopathologic and immunohistochemical study of 75 cases. *Am J Surg Pathol.* 2003;27:311–324.

Pulmonary Blastoma

15

▶ Sanja Dacic

Pulmonary blastoma is a rare biphasic tumor composed of primitive malignant glands resembling well-differentiated fetal adenocarcinoma and immature, embryonic-type sarcomatous stroma.[1]

PULMONARY BLASTOMA, CYTOLOGY

Pulmonary blastomas are rare tumors that are not typically diagnosed cytologically. Cytologic features include malignant glandular cells or malignant mesenchymal spindle cells, or both.

PULMONARY BLASTOMA, GROSS FEATURES

Pulmonary blastomas typically are large, well-circumscribed masses that have a tan to tan-yellow fleshy cut surface (Figs. 15-1 and 15-2). They often have satellite lesions and associated pleural effusions.

PULMONARY BLASTOMA, HISTOPATHOLOGY

The glycogen-rich tubules and primitive stroma resemble fetal lung between 10 and 16 weeks gestation ("pseudoglandular stage"). The tubules are lined by pseudostratified, nonciliated columnar cells with clear or lightly eosinophilic cytoplasm. Subnuclear or supranuclear vacuoles containing glycogen are producing an endometrioid appearance (Figs. 15-3–15-8). A small amount of mucin within the glandular lumens may be present, but intracellular mucin is unusual. Similar to fetal adenocarcinomas, morular structures composed of squamous nests can be seen. Stomal cells have blastema-like configuration and have a similar appearance to Wilms tumor of the kidney. Stromal cells may be round, oval, or spindlelike. Foci of differentiated sarcomatous elements such as rhabdomyosarcoma, osteosarcoma, or chondrosarcoma may be found.[2,3]

PULMONARY BLASTOMA, IMMUNOHISTOCHEMISTRY

The epithelial component, including glands and morules, is diffusely positive for epithelial markers such as cytokeratin 7, AE1/AE3, EMA, CEA, and TTF-1. Neuroendocrine markers such as chromogranin A and synaptophysin, Clara cell antigen, and polypeptide hormones (calcitonin, ACTH, serotonin, L-enkephalin) are focally positive. The sarcomatous stroma is diffusely immunoreactive for vimentin and muscle- specific actin. Focal cytokeratin AE1/AE3 positivity may be present. Desmin, myoglobin, and S100 protein can be expressed if specific muscle or cartilage mesenchymal differentiation is present.[4–6]

PULMONARY BLASTOMA, DIFFERENTIAL DIAGNOSIS

Pulmonary blastomas should be distinguished from fetal adenocarcinomas, pleuropulmonary blastomas, and primary or metastatic sarcomas. Morphology together with immunohistochemistry and molecular studies should differentiate between these tumors. If areas of predominantly

FIGURE 15-1 Gross image of pulmonary blastoma showing a well-circumscribed, tan fleshy tumor mass.

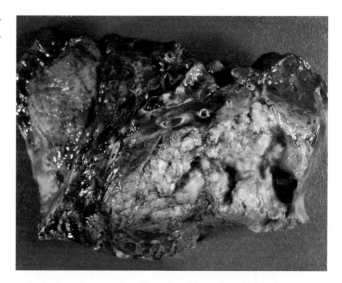

FIGURE 15-2 Closer gross image of pulmonary blastoma highlighting the fleshy character of the tumor on cut section.

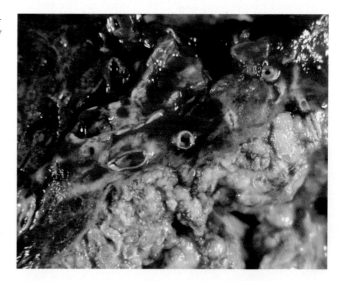

FIGURE 15-3 Low-power image of pulmonary blastoma showing a cellular mass with surrounding fibrous stroma within which nests and cords of tumor cell are arranged.

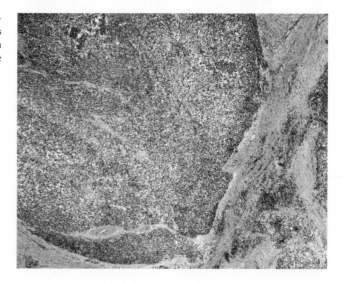

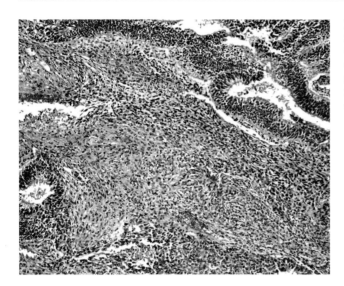

FIGURE 15-4 Pulmonary blastoma resembles "pseudoglandular stage" of the fetal lung between 10 and 16 weeks of gestation. It is composed of malignant glands resembling well-differentiated fetal adenocarcinoma and sarcomatous embryonic-type stroma.

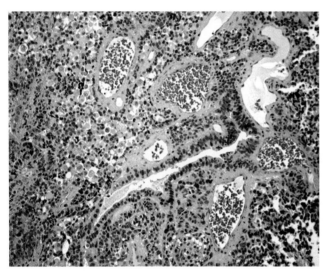

FIGURE 15-5 High-power image of pulmonary blastoma with a sarcomatous component composed predominantly of blastema-like, loosely arranged round to oval tumor cells.

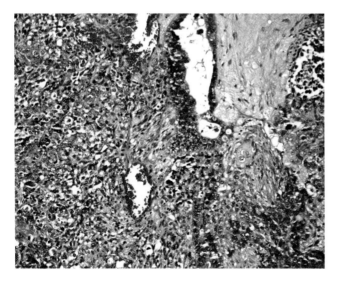

FIGURE 15-6 High-power image of pulmonary blastoma showing sarcomatous component with an area of myxoid change.

FIGURE 15-7 High-power image of pulmonary blastoma showing abundant subnuclear vacuolization of the epithelial component, and a sarcomatous component made up predominantly of spindle cells.

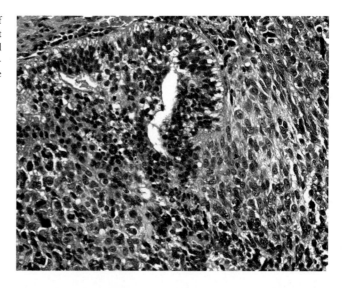

FIGURE 15-8 PAS staining highlights nonciliated columnar cells with subnuclear and supranuclear glycogen.

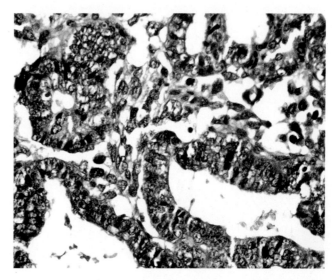

FIGURE 15-9 Medium-power image of lung containing pulmonary blastoma showing an area of predominantly epithelioid component, which could potentially be misdiagnosed as primary or metastatic adenocarcinoma.

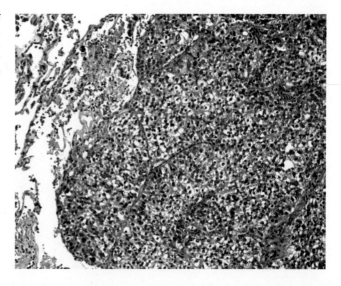

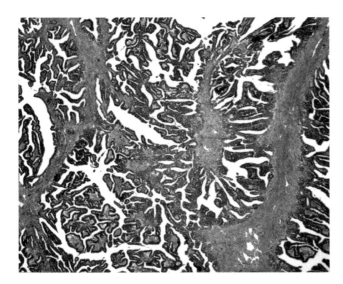

FIGURE 15-10 Medium-power image of well-differentiated fetal adenocarcinoma showing a villiform pattern of gland arrangement reminiscent of fetal lung or endometrium.

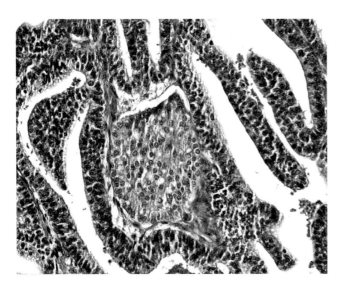

FIGURE 15-11 High-power image of well-differentiated fetal adenocarcinoma showing a rounded squamoid morule made up of polygonal cells containing eosinophilic cytoplasm. Surrounding glandular component shows glycogen-rich cytoplasm with basally arranged nuclei.

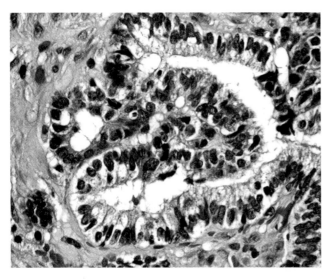

FIGURE 15-12 High-power image of well-differentiated fetal adenocarcinoma exhibiting subnuclear and supranuclear vacuolization within the glandular component.

mesenchymal component or epithelial component are biopsied, then the tumor may be potentially misdiagnosed as primary or metastatic sarcoma or adenocarcinoma, respectively (Fig. 15-9). The distinction between pulmonary blastoma and fetal adenocarcinoma is important as pulmonary blastoma generally has a much worse prognosis than fetal adenocarcinoma (Figs. 15-10–15-12).

PULMONARY BLASTOMA, HISTIOGENESIS

Pulmonary blastomas presumably arise from a primitive precursor cell. Genotyping has shown that both the epithelial and spindle cell components arise from a single clone.

References

1. Travis WB, Brambilla E, Müller-Hermelink HK, et al., eds. *World Health Organization Classification of Tumours. Pathology and Genetics of Tumours of the Lung, Pleura, Thymus and Heart.* Lyon: IARC Press; 2004.
2. Koss MN, Hochholzer L, O'Leary T. Pulmonary blastomas. *Cancer.* 1991;67:2368–2381.
3. Priest JR, McDermott MB, et al. Pleuropulmonary blastoma: a clinicopathologic study of 50 cases. *Cancer.* 1997;80:147–161.
4. Nakatani Y, Miyagi Y, Takemura T, et al. Aberrant nuclear/cytoplasmic localization and gene mutation of beta-catenin in classic pulmonary blastoma: beta-catenin immunostaining is useful for distinguishing between classic pulmonary blastoma and a blastomatoid variant of carcinosarcoma. *Am J Surg Pathol.* 2004;28:921–927.
5. Rossi G, Cavazza A, Sturm N, et al. Pulmonary carcinomas with pleomorphic, sarcomatoid, or sarcomatous elements: a clinicopathologic and immunohistochemical study of 75 cases. *Am J Surg Pathol.* 2003;27:311–324.
6. Yousem SA, Wick MR, Randhawa P, et al. Pulmonary blastoma. An immunohistochemical analysis with comparison with fetal lung in its pseudoglandular stage. *Am J Clin Pathol.* 1990;93:167–175.

Salivary Gland–like Carcinomas

16

Primary salivary gland tumors of the lung are extremely rare, usually slow-growing, low-grade neoplasms that make up only 0.1% to 0.2% of all lung cancers.[1] They originate from the submucosal glands of the tracheobronchial tree, and therefore, clinical signs and symptoms are related to endobronchial growth of these tumors. They have similar morphology and genetic abnormalities as their salivary gland counterparts. Patients with salivary gland lung tumors are often younger than other bronchogenic carcinoma patients and up to 40% of patients are nonsmokers. Only small case series about presentation, diagnosis, and management of these tumors have been reported in literature. The recommended treatment is complete surgical resection. The most important differential diagnosis is with a late metastasis from a head and neck salivary gland tumor. Since there are no morphologic criteria to distinguish between these two possibilities, a detailed clinical history should be obtained. Most frequently reported tumors include mucoepidermoid carcinoma (MEC), adenoid cystic carcinoma (ADC), and epithelial-myoepithelial carcinoma.[2–10] Other salivary gland–like tumors have been rarely identified as primary lung tumors, including acinic cell carcinoma, pleomorphic adenoma, pneumocytic adenomyoepithelioma, and polymorphous low-grade adenocarcinomas.[11–17]

MUCOEPIDERMOID CARCINOMA

Pulmonary MECs are rare malignant neoplasms, making up fewer than 1% of primary lung neoplasms. Based on morphologic and cytologic features, tumors are divided into low- and high-grade subtypes. The prognosis of MUC depends on the tumor grade, clinical stage, and completeness of surgical resection. Low-grade tumors have excellent prognosis, whereas high-grade tumors tend to behave similarly to non–small cell lung carcinomas.

Mucoepidermoid Carcinoma, Cytology
MEC is not typically diagnosed cytologically; however, cytology may show bland glandular cells, squamoid cells, and goblet cells.

Mucoepidermoid Carcinoma, Gross Features
MECs usually present as sessile, polypoid, or pedunculated masses. They are generally centrally located, arising in the large airways and ranging in size from approximately 0.5 to 6 cm (Fig. 16-1).[7] High-grade lesions frequently show infiltrative growth patterns. The cut surface is gray-white-tan in color, frequently with cystic change and a mucoid appearance.

Mucoepidermoid Carcinoma, Histology
MEC is composed of three cell types including mucus-secreting, squamous, and intermediate cells. The relative proportion of each component is one of the criteria for histologic grading. Necrosis, nuclear pleomorphism, mitoses, and solid or nested growth patterns for the intermediate or squamous cells are commonly used criteria. Low-grade tumors predominantly show cystic changes admixed with solid areas (Figs. 16-2–16-4). Cystic areas are lined by cytologically bland columnar, goblet, cuboidal, clear or oncocytic-appearing mucin-producing cells. High-grade

FIGURE 16-1 A small sessile off-white mucoepidermoid carcinoma bulges slightly into the lumen at the 6 o'clock position. It is covered with bronchial mucosa and is not ulcerated.

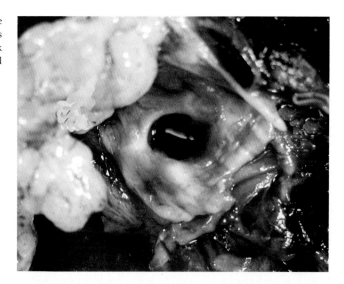

FIGURE 16-2 Low-power image of a pedunculated bronchial MEC showing bronchial wall on the left and a pedunculated tumor mass with obvious cystic spaces protruding into the bronchial lumen.

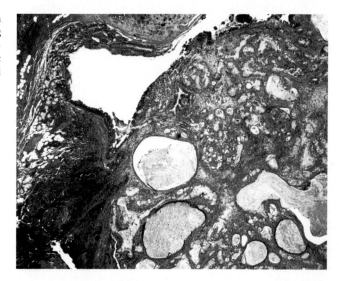

FIGURE 16-3 Higher power image shows predominantly goblet cells and intermediate cells in this low-grade MEC.

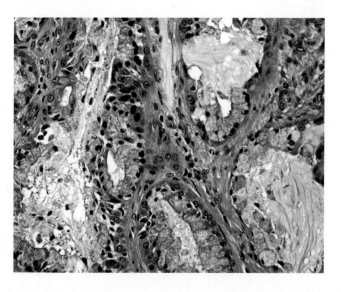

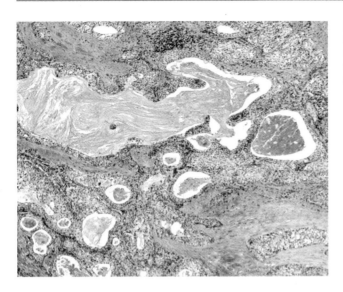

FIGURE 16-4 Low-grade MEC predominantly composed of cystic spaces filled with colloid-like mucus and lined by cytologically bland columnar to cuboidal cells.

tumors show predominance of solid areas (Figs. 16-5–16-7). Keratin pearls are not seen. The stroma is usually edematous, with hyalinization, calcification, ossification, and granulomatous reactions, adjacent to areas of mucus extravasation.

Mucoepidermoid Carcinoma, Immunohistochemistry

The heterogeneity of the immunohistochemical profile does not correlate with the tumor grade. All three cell types of MEC are strongly positive for AE1 and cytokeratin 7 and weakly positive for cytokeratin AE3, CK18, and CK8/18/19.[18,19] The intermediate cells are strongly positive for monoclonal cytokeratins CK34bE12, but luminal cells are negative. Cytokeratin 5/6 is positive in areas with squamous differentiation. TTF-1 is negative. Cytokeratin 10, cytokeratin 20, α-smooth muscle actin, HHF35, GFAP, and S100 are all negative. The most characteristic chromosomal abnormality is the t(11; 19)(q21;p13), which involves two genes: *m*ucoepidermoid *c*arcinoma *t*ranslocated *1* (*MECT1*) gene and a *m*ammalian *m*astermind-*l*ike *2* (*MAML2*) located on chromosomes 19p13 and 11q21, respectively.[20–22] Similar to primary salivary gland MEC, bronchopulmonary MEC with MAML2 gene rearrangement more frequently occurred in younger patients with histologically low-grade tumors.

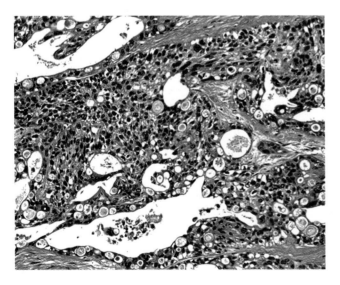

FIGURE 16-5 High-grade MEC with predominance of solid areas showing cytologic atypia.

FIGURE 16-6 Medium-power image of high-grade MEC showing markedly atypical squamoid cells without squamous pearls or single cell keratinization.

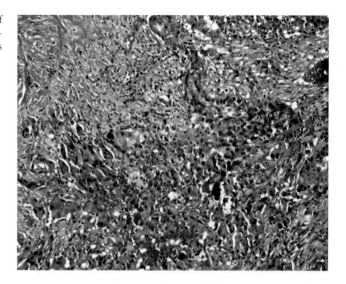

FIGURE 16-7 Medium-power image of high-grade MEC showing tumor necrosis with associated atypical squamoid cells.

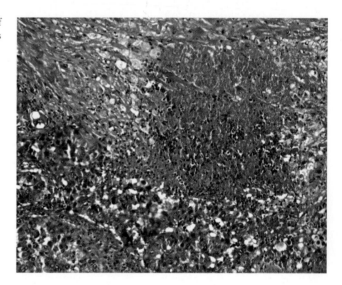

Mucoepidermoid Carcinoma, Differential Diagnosis

Primary lung neoplasms, including squamous cell, adenosquamous, and adenocarcinoma constitute the major differential diagnosis for bronchopulmonary MEC. Lack of TTF-1 expression in MEC may be useful in differentiating MEC from primary lung adenocarcinoma. MAML2 gene rearrangement is not detected in primary lung squamous, adenosquamous, and adenocarcinomas and may represent an important diagnostic marker (Figs. 16-8 and 16-9).[20]

Mucoepidermoid Carcinoma, Histiogenesis

MECs presumably arise from primitive tracheobronchial mucous gland cells.

ADENOID CYSTIC CARCINOMA

ACC is the second most common malignant tumor found in the trachea and main bronchi after the squamous cell carcinoma. ACCs affect adults in their fourth and fifth decades without sex predilection.[7] The majority of tumors are endobronchial and therefore symptoms are related to

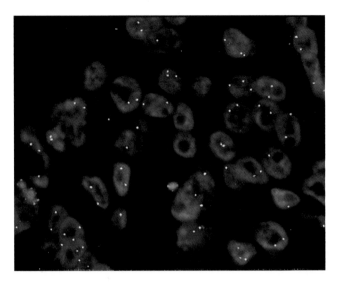

FIGURE 16-8 FISH analysis of bronchopulmonary MEC with the BAC probes RP11-16K (*orange*) and RP11-676L3 (*green*) for MAML2 gene. Cells negative for rearrangement show hybridization signals from both BAC probes located in proximity to one another resulting in a yellow signal.

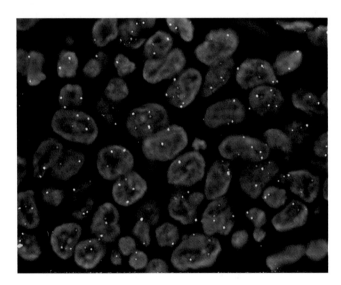

FIGURE 16-9 FISH analysis of bronchopulmonary MEC with the BAC probes RP11-16K (*orange*) and RP11-676L3 (*green*) for MAML2 gene. Cells with MAML2 gene rearrangement show one pair of signals (green and orange) in juxtaposition and one green and one orange signal separated.

bronchial obstruction.[6] In contrast to other types of salivary gland tumors of the lung, ACCs tend to present at a higher stage.

Adenoid Cystic Carcinoma, Cytology

ACC is not typically diagnosed cytologically; however, cytology may show uniform-appearing small cells, round to oval uniform nuclei, a high nuclear-cytoplasm ratio, and hyaline eosinophilic or myxoid stromal fragments.

Adenoid Cystic Carcinoma, Gross Features

Pulmonary ADCs measure approximately 2 cm, typically ranging from 1 to 4 cm.[7] ACC usually forms a soft and tan polypoid endobronchial submucosal lesion. It is frequently well circumscribed, but infiltrative margins into peribronchial soft tissue and lung parenchyma may be observed in some cases (Fig. 16-10).

Adenoid Cystic Carcinoma, Histology

The growth pattern of ACC is similar to its salivary gland counterpart. The most frequent growth patterns include cribriform, tubular, and solid. Cribriform growth pattern shows cyst-like areas surrounded by tumor cells and filled with basophilic, Alcian blue–positive glycosaminoglycans.

FIGURE 16-10 This pulmonary ADC has spread circumferentially throughout the bronchial wall and encroaches upon the bronchial lumen.

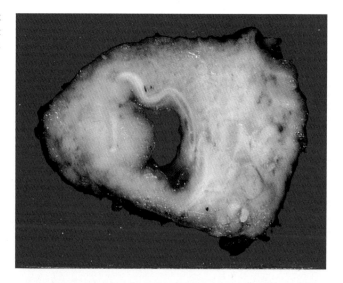

FIGURE 16-11 Medium-power image of pulmonary ADC showing cylindrical mucinous matrix with surrounding small oval cells with little cytoplasm.

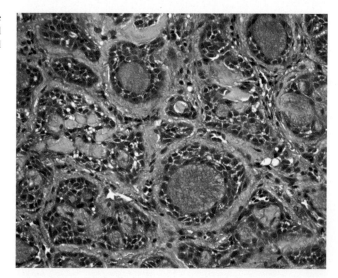

FIGURE 16-12 High-power image of pulmonary ADC showing cribriform pattern distribution of cells with relatively uniform tumor cells with little cytoplasm.

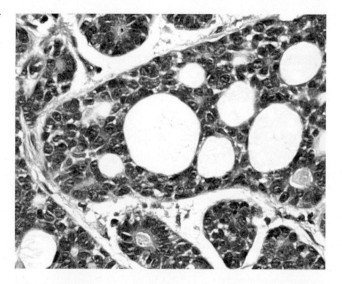

The islands of tumor cells are separated by an excessive, eosinophilic basement membrane–like material of variable thickness. The tumor cells are small with scant cytoplasm and dark hyperchromatic, oval to angulated nuclei (Figs. 16-11 and 16-12). Mitoses are scant. A prominent perineural, bronchial cartilage and bronchial mucosal invasion are seen in about 40% of cases.

Adenoid Cystic Carcinoma, Immunohistochemistry

The immunoprofile of ACC is that of ductal and myoepithelial tumor. The ductal cells usually show more intense staining for wide-spectrum and low molecular weight cytokeratins than myoepithelial cells. The myoepithelial tumor cells are also positive for vimentin, smooth-muscle actin, calponin, S100 protein, and p63.[23]

Adenoid Cystic Carcinoma, Differential Diagnosis

The diagnosis of ACC can be challenging on a small biopsy specimen. The most difficult differential diagnosis is of a primary lung adenocarcinoma. Immunohistochemical studies may help to differentiate between these two possibilities. Expression of myoepithelial markers such as actin, calponin, and p63 would favor the diagnosis of ACC.

Adenoid Cystic Carcinoma, Histiogenesis

ACC presumably arises from a primitive tracheobronchial gland cell.

References

1. Travis WB, Brambilla E, Müller-Hermelink HK, et al., eds. *World Health Organization Classification of Tumours. Pathology and Genetics of Tumours of the Lung, Pleura, Thymus and Heart.* Lyon: IARC Press; 2004.
2. Doganay L, Bilgi S, Ozdil A, et al. Epithelial-myoepithelial carcinoma of the lung. A case report and review of the literature. *Arch Pathol Lab Med* 2003;127:e177–e180.
3. Fulford LG, Kamata Y, Okudera K, et al. Epithelial-myoepithelial carcinomas of the bronchus. *Am J Surg Pathol.* 2001;25:1508–1514.
4. Martins C, Fonseca I, Roque L, et al. Malignant salivary gland neoplasms: a cytogenetic study of 19 cases. *Eur J Cancer.* 1996;32B:128–132.
5. Maziak DE, Todd TR, Keshavjee SH, et al. Adenoid cystic carcinoma of the airway: thirty-two-year experience. *J Thoracic Cardiovasc Surg.* 1996;112:1522–1531.
6. Molina JR, Aubry MC, Lewis JE, et al. Primary salivary gland-type lung cancer: spectrum of clinical presentation, histopathologic and prognostic factors. *Cancer.* 2007;110:2253–2259.
7. Moran CA. Primary salivary gland-type tumors of the lung. *Semin Diagn Pathol.* 1995;12:106–122.
8. Nguyen CV, Suster S, Moran CA. Pulmonary epithelial-myoepithelial carcinoma: a clinicopathologic and immunohistochemical study of 5 cases. *Human Pathol.* 2009;40:366–373.
9. Wilson RW, Moran CA. Epithelial-myoepithelial carcinoma of the lung: immunohistochemical and ultrastructural observations and review of the literature. *Human Pathol.* 1997;28:631–635.
10. Yousem SA, Hochholzer L. Mucoepidermoid tumors of the lung. *Cancer.* 1987;60:1346–1352.
11. Chang T, Husain AN, Colby T, et al. Pneumocytic adenomyoepithelioma: a distinctive lung tumor with epithelial, myoepithelial, and pneumocytic differentiation. *Am J Surg Pathol.* 2007;31:562–568.
12. Cho KD, Jung JH, Cho DG, et al. Primary polymorphous low-grade adenocarcinoma of lung treated by sleeve bronchial resection: a case report. *J Korean Med Sci.* 2007;22:373–376.
13. Fechner RE, Bentinck BR, Askew JB Jr. Acinic cell tumor of the lung. A histologic and ultrastructural study. *Cancer.* 1972;29:501–508.
14. Fitchett J, Luckraz H, Gibbs A, et al. A rare case of primary pleomorphic adenoma in main bronchus. *Ann Thorac Surg.* 2008;86:1025–1026.
15. Hara M, Sato Y, Kitase M, et al. CT and MR findings of a pleomorphic adenoma in the peripheral lung. *Rad Med.* 2001;19:111–114.

16. Moran CA, Suster S, Koss MN. Acinic cell carcinoma of the lung ("Fechner tumor"). A clinicopathologic, immunohistochemical, and ultrastructural study of five cases. *Am J Surg Pathol.* 1992;16:1039–1050.

17. Sakamoto H, Uda H, Tanaka T, et al. Pleomorphic adenoma in the periphery of the lung. Report of a case and review of the literature. *Arch Pathol Lab Med.* 1991;115:393–396.

18. Sanchez-Mora N, Parra-Blanco V, Cebollero-Presmanes M, et al. Mucoepidermoid tumors of the bronchus. Ultrastructural and immunohistochemical study. Histogenic correlations. *Histol Histopathol.* 2007;22:9–13.

19. Shilo K, Foss RD, Franks TJ, et al. Pulmonary mucoepidermoid carcinoma with prominent tumor-associated lymphoid proliferation. *Am J Surg Pathol.* 2005;29:407–411.

20. Achcar Rde O, Nikiforova MN, Dacic S, et al. Mammalian mastermind like 2 11q21 gene rearrangement in bronchopulmonary mucoepidermoid carcinoma. *Hum Pathol.* 2009;40:854–860.

21. Tonon G, Gehlhaus KS, Yonescu R, et al. Multiple reciprocal translocations in salivary gland mucoepidermoid carcinomas. *Cancer Genet Cytogenet.* 2004;152:15–22.

22. Tonon G, Modi S, Wu L, et al. t(11;19)(q21;p13) translocation in mucoepidermoid carcinoma creates a novel fusion product that disrupts a Notch signaling pathway. [erratum appears in Nat Genet. 2003 Mar;33(3):430.] *Nat Genet.* 2003;33:208–213.

23. Aubry M-C, Heinrich MC, Molina J, et al. Primary adenoid cystic carcinoma of the lung: absence of KIT mutations. *Cancer.* 2007;110:2507–2510.

Metastatic Tumors to the Lung

▶ Timothy Craig Allen

Metastatic tumors to the lungs are the most common lung neoplasm, and the lungs are the recipient of more metastatic neoplasms than any other organ.[1-4] Cancers from essentially any site in the body can metastasize to the lung.[5-7] The lungs are the only organ for which the entire blood and lymphatic supply flow, and their dense capillary network is often the first encountered by circulating tumor cells entering the venous blood supply from the ductus lymphaticus.[1,8] The lungs are the site of metastases in 20% to 54% of cases in patients with extrapulmonary primary malignant neoplasms, and in 15% to 25%, the lung is the only site of metastasis.[3,9-11] Common sites of metastatic tumors to the lung include lung, gastrointestinal tract, breast, pancreas, kidney, melanoma, thyroid, liver, and prostate.[1-3,6,12,13] Lymphatic spread of tumor is commonly found with metastases from the stomach, breast, ovary, prostate, and lung; and hematogenous spread of tumor is often identified with metastases from the breast, kidney, colon, and testes.[2] According to the International Registry of Lung Metastases, 44% of metastases are carcinomas, 42% sarcomas, 7% germ cell tumors, and 6% melanomas. Colorectal carcinoma comprised 33% of metastatic tumors to the lung, with 20% breast, 19% renal, 12% head and neck, 7% uterus, and 3% lung.[14-16] In many cases there is a clinical history of an extrapulmonary primary tumor, and situations involving nonpulmonary occult primary tumors are relatively uncommon; however, 3% to 7% of patients with lung cancer also have another, independent, nonpulmonary primary tumor.[3,14,17] In many cases, histology alone is enough to reliably diagnose the primary tumor, especially in cases where the primary is known.[3,18] The major problem in diagnosing a metastatic tumor to the lung occurs in the setting of a solitary nodule, an atypical presentation such as a cavitating tumor or a central tumor, or a poorly differentiated tumor with ambiguous histological and immunohistochemical features. In some cases, it is impossible to distinguish whether a lung tumor is primary or metastatic.[1,3,6,7,13,14,18-20]

Clinically, patients with metastases to the lungs often do not exhibit pulmonary symptoms; however, patients with endobronchial tumor may have cough and hemoptysis as well as obstructive symptoms such as dyspnea and wheezing. Chest pain may be present if there is pleural involvement with tumor.[1,3,6,13,21] Radiologically, chest x-ray, high-resolution CT scan, and PET imaging are often employed in the evaluation of patients with suspected lung metastases.[1,3,22,23] While CT scan has generally replaced chest x-ray alone for the preoperative evaluation of patients with suspected metastases to the lung, PET scans and, more recently, PET/CT imaging are more frequently being used in addition to CT scan for evaluation of these patients, with results reportedly superior to CT scan alone.[22,24] Along with the clinical and radiologic correlative findings, the gross and microscopic features assist in determining which, if any, immunostains or group immunostains may be valuable in further differentiating the tumor metastatic to the lung.

METASTATIC TUMORS TO THE LUNG, GROSS FEATURES

Grossly, metastatic neoplasms metastatic to the lungs typically involve the lower lobes bilaterally with multiple, often peripheral, well-circumscribed tumor nodules that range from many small military tumor nodules to large "cannonball" masses that may be confluent (Figs. 17-1and 17-2). Solitary pulmonary nodules may also be a manifestation of metastatic disease to the lungs and

FIGURE 17-1 Gross image of lung containing numerous "cannonball" metastatic tumor nodules in a patient with a history of renal cell carcinoma.

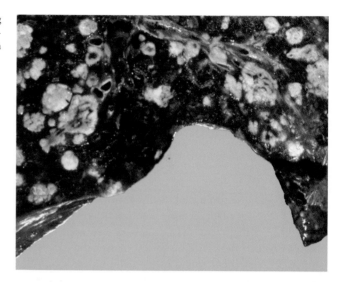

FIGURE 17-2 Gross image of lung containing numerous small tumor nodules in a miliary distribution in a patient with a history of ovarian carcinoma.

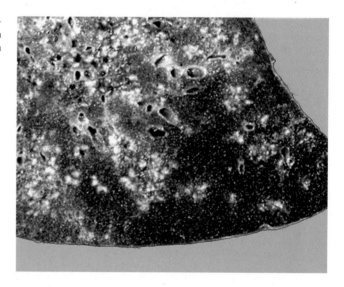

occur in 3% to 9% of cases of metastatic tumor to the lung (Fig. 17-3).[1,3,6,13,23,25,26] The specific gross presentation varies with the type of metastasis; however, melanomas, germ cell tumors, and ovarian carcinomas often present with a miliary pattern, and renal cell carcinomas and sarcomas usually present with a "cannonball" pattern of metastasis. Tumor involving the lung and having a thick, rind-like layer of tumor over the lung surface may represent pleural diffuse malignant mesothelioma, metastatic tumor to the pleura with lung involvement, or primary pulmonary pseudomesotheliomatous carcinoma (Fig. 17-4). Mucin-producing adenocarcinoma metastases, such as ovarian, breast, or gastrointestinal tract metastases, may show a yellow-tan glistening mucoid cut surface, with or without areas of necrosis or hemorrhage (Fig. 17-5). A similar glistening mucoid cut surface may be seen with myxoid sarcomas, often arising primarily in the retroperitoneum or the extremities. Renal cell carcinomas, liposarcomas, adrenal cortical tumors, and sex cord stromal tumors that are metastatic to the lung often show a yellow or golden appearance, indicative of glycogen or lipid, on cut surface. Tumors that appear red or red-brown on cut section may contain diffuse hemorrhage or areas of hemorrhagic necrosis, suggestive of angiosarcoma, gastrointestinal stromal tumor, or choriocarcinoma, among others. Metastatic sarcomas and metastatic lymphomas may present a gray, "fish-flesh" appearance on cut section. Metastatic melanomas may show variable areas of black coloration (Fig. 17-6). A hard, bony or firm

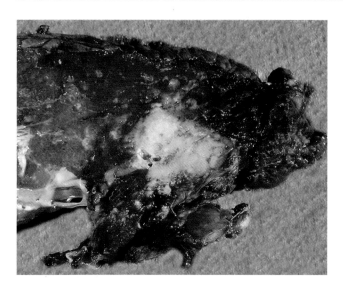

FIGURE 17-3 Gross image of lung containing a somewhat multinodular firm off-white to tan irregularly marginated tumor mass in a patient with a history of breast carcinoma. The gross image is also consistent with a lung primary neoplasm.

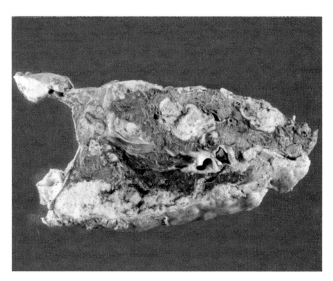

FIGURE 17-4 Gross image of "pseudomesotheliomatous carcinoma" in a patient with a history of colon carcinoma. The gross presentation is consistent with metastatic tumor to the pleura with invasion of the lung, with primary pulmonary pseudomesotheliomatous carcinoma arising in the lung and spreading in a rind-like manner along the pleura, and with pleural diffuse malignant mesothelioma arising in the pleura and spreading into the lung parenchyma. As histologic patterns may vary, clinical and radiologic correlations are very important in determining an appropriate immunostaining panel to assist in accurate diagnosis.

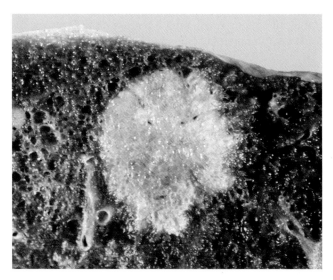

FIGURE 17-5 Gross image of lung containing a tumor mass with a glistening, mucoid cut surface in a patient with a history of mucinous ovarian adenocarcinoma.

FIGURE 17-6 Gross image of lung containing a tumor mass with areas of dark brown to black coloration in a patient with a history of melanoma.

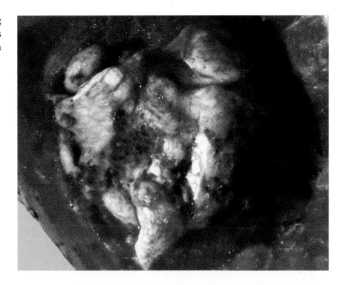

FIGURE 17-7 Gross image of the lung containing an irregularly marginated, gray-tan tumor mass with areas of hemorrhage and a "gritty" cut surface in a patient with a history of carcinosarcoma.

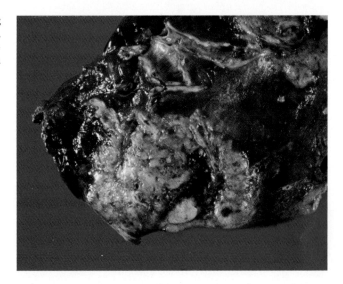

gritty consistency identified on cut section suggests bone- or cartilage-producing tumors such as chondrosarcoma and osteosarcoma. Other tumors that may exhibit a gritty consistency on cut section include teratoma, carcinosarcoma, and psammoma body–producing tumors such as papillary thyroid carcinoma and ovarian carcinoma (Fig. 17-7).[1–4,6,12,13,23,25,27,28]

METASTATIC TUMORS TO THE LUNG, HISTOLOGY

Histologically and cytologically, metastatic tumors to the lungs may mimic the histologic and cytologic features of their primary tumors; however, these histologic and cytologic features may not be specific. When it is unknown whether a lesion represents a primary lung tumor or a metastasis, features such as multifocality of tumor, pushing rounded tumor margin, lack of central fibrosis or elastotic scarring, prominent and diffuse lymphatic involvement, dirty necrosis, and a prominent lymphocytic component within the tumor are nonspecific features suggestive of metastasis.[6] Some metastases have histologic features that give little guidance as to primary site of the tumor. Such is often the case with poorly differentiated or undifferentiated non–small cell carcinomas in the lung. There is also little histologic guidance found with squamous cell carcinomas metastatic to the lung; their histologic characteristics significantly overlap and may be essentially identical regardless of primary site of tumor, be the primary site lung, cervix, skin, or head and neck, or another potential primary site (Fig. 17-8).

Adenocarcinomatous histologic features such as acinar, cribriform, and papillary patterns are not specific enough to significantly aid in determining a metastatic tumor's primary site. Nonetheless, some histologic characteristics may provide guidance as to metastatic tumor origin. Common tumors metastatic to the lung may have histologic features that suggest primary site. Colon adenocarcinomas metastatic to the lung often show tumor with prominently pseudostratified nuclei lining acinar or cribriform pattern spaces, along with sometimes prominent areas of dirty necrosis (Figs. 17-9 and 17-10). While colon adenocarcinoma as well as other tumors such as pancreatic adenocarcinoma that metastasize to the lung may exhibit prominent mucin production, the histologic feature is relatively nonspecific and of more limited benefit in determining the primary site of the metastasis. Mucinous carcinoma with characteristic pools of mucin with epithelial neoplastic cells "floating" in the mucin frequently arises from pancreatic, gastrointestinal, and beast primary sites (Figs. 17-11 and 17-12). The histologic features of solid

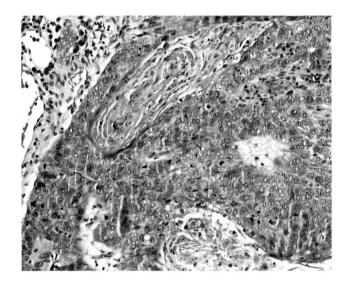

FIGURE 17-8 Medium-power image of metastatic squamous cell carcinoma to the lung in a patient with a history of squamous cell carcinoma of the oropharynx. The histologic features, including keratin pearl formation seen here, are nonspecific and not in and of themselves helpful in identifying the primary site of tumor.

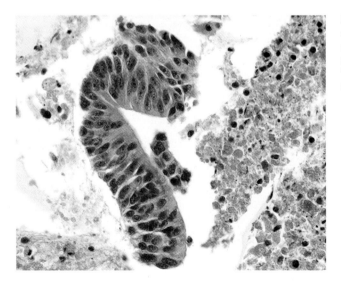

FIGURE 17-9 High-power image of a cell block section from a fine needle aspiration of a lung mass in a patient with a history of colon carcinoma showing "dirty necrosis" and tumor cells showing nuclear pseudostratification.

FIGURE 17-10 Medium-power image of a resection of a solitary lung nodule in a nonsmoking patient showing adenocarcinoma with prominent nuclear pseudostratification. Based on the histologic findings, colonoscopy was performed and colon adenocarcinoma was identified.

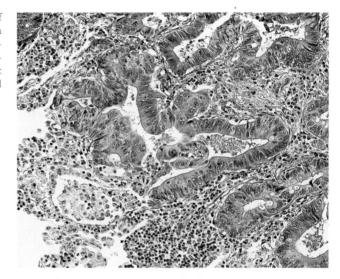

FIGURE 17-11 Medium-power image of lung showing mucinous adenocarcinoma, with nests of relatively uniform tumor cells "floating" in a lake of mucin in a patient with a history of mucinous adenocarcinoma of the breast.

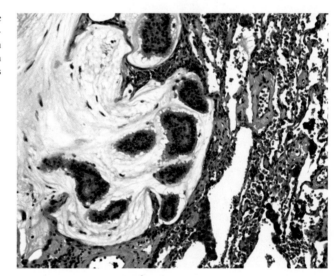

FIGURE 17-12 High-power image of the case shown in Figure 17-11 highlighting the uniformity of the tumor cell nuclei.

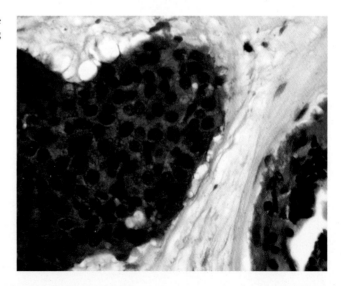

or trabecular patterns of adenocarcinoma with areas of comedonecrosis and relatively uniform nuclear pleomorphism within tumor cells suggest metastatic breast carcinoma, especially if the patient is a woman (Fig. 17-13). Metastatic prostate cancer to the lung should be considered in men where histologic features of the lung tumor show relatively uniform glandular spaces and relatively uniform tumor cells exhibiting prominent nucleoli. Papillary architecture with areas of colloid production grooved nuclei, and nuclear pseudoinclusions suggest metastatic papillary thyroid carcinoma to the lung (Figs. 17-14 and 17-15). Remember in these cases the metastatic thyroid carcinoma TTF-1 immunopositivity is not helpful in distinguishing the tumor as being a primary lung neoplasm.

While tumor cells containing large, red nucleoli may suggest metastatic melanoma to the lung, metastatic melanoma is characterized by its ability to display various histologic patterns. As such, a high index of suspicion must be maintained and melanoma should frequently be considered in the differential diagnosis of metastatic lung disease (Figs. 17-16–17-18). Nonetheless, other nonadenocarcinomatous tumors metastatic to the lung may exhibit histologic features that

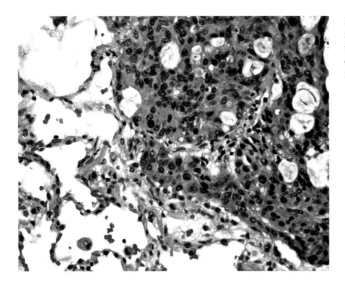

FIGURE 17-13 Medium-power image of metastatic invasive ductal carcinoma to the lung showing tumor cells with abundant cytoplasm and relatively uniform nuclei.

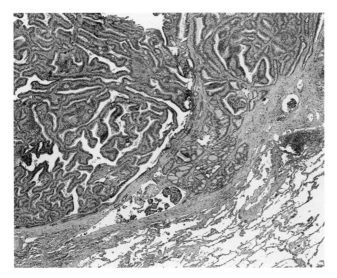

FIGURE 17-14 Low-power image of metastatic papillary thyroid carcinoma showing a tumor mass with prominent papillary structures in a patient with a history of papillary thyroid carcinoma.

FIGURE 17-15 High-power image of the case shown in Figure 17-14 showing nuclear pseudoinclusion at the top of the image.

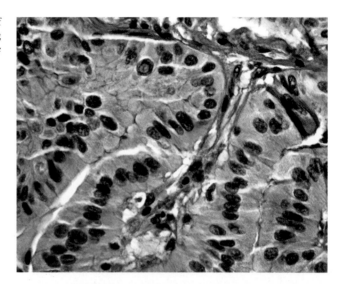

FIGURE 17-16 High-power image of melanoma metastatic to the lung showing histologic features often identified in melanoma, including prominent, often red, nucleoli and melanin pigment.

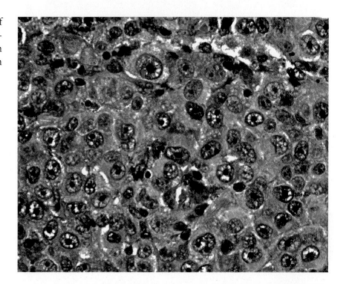

FIGURE 17-17 High-power image of melanoma metastatic to the lung showing histologic features reminiscent of primary pulmonary poorly differentiated adenocarcinoma or large cell carcinoma.

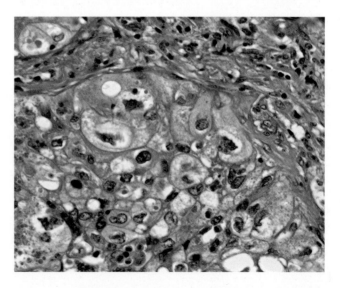

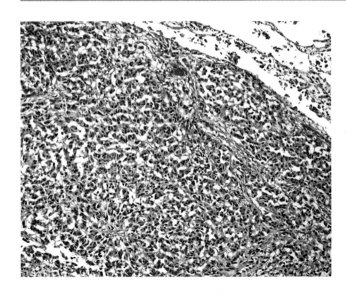

FIGURE 17-18 Medium-power image of melanoma metastatic to the lung showing a generally trabecular pattern of tumor growth.

provide clues to primary site of tumor. Histologic features of generally uniform nuclei containing prominent nucleoli and abundant clear cytoplasm suggest renal cell carcinoma, particularly when tumor cells are arranged in nests and exhibiting prominent blood vessels (Fig. 17-19). Sarcomas metastatic to the lung may show liposarcomatous or leiomyosarcomatous histologic features, suggesting primary origin from retroperitoneum and uterus or gastrointestinal tract, respectively. Histologic features of synovial sarcoma, while occasionally representing a primary lung tumor, often represent metastatic tumor from a synovial sarcoma arising in an extremity. Mixed or biphasic tumors in the lung, showing a mixture of malignant spindled cells with areas of often high-grade, undifferentiated epithelioid cells, may be either primary or metastatic. Primary biphasic lung neoplasms include, among others, carcinosarcoma and pulmonary blastoma. Metastatic biphasic lung neoplasms include, among others, carcinosarcomas of breast or gastrointestinal origin, synovial sarcoma, uterine adenosarcoma, and biphasic diffuse malignant mesothelioma. Biphasic diffuse malignant mesothelioma cases show a wide variety of sarcomatous and epithelial histologic features (Fig. 17-20). Immunostains are of benefit in differentiating between these various differential diagnoses.[1,3,13,14,29–41]

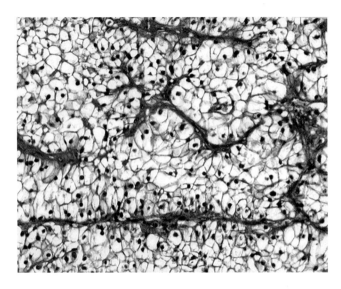

FIGURE 17-19 Medium-power image of renal cell carcinoma metastatic to the lung showing tumor cells arranged in nests with characteristic clear to pink cytoplasm and relatively uniform nuclei, and associated vascular structures.

FIGURE 17-20 Medium-power image of metastatic biphasic diffuse malignant mesothelioma to the lung that arose in the peritoneum. There is both a glandular component and a spindle cell component present.

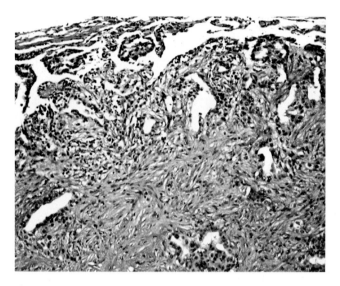

METASTATIC TUMORS TO THE LUNG, IMMUNOHISTOCHEMISTRY

Immunohistochemical staining, cytogenetic analysis, and molecular studies performed on cytologic or histologic material are often used to assist in characterizing lung tumors as primary or metastatic and to further characterize the potential primary sites of the metastases.[1–3,13,19,39,42–45] Immunohistochemistry is often vital in making a correct diagnosis in these cases. It is important that the pathologist considers each case carefully in determining which immunostains to perform, because (a) as there are no entirely specific tumor markers, the use of a panel of a few carefully selected immunohistochemical markers is often necessary; (b) limited tissue is often available for immunostains, as tissue is frequently procured by cytologic or small biopsy methods; (c) negative immunostains are generally unhelpful in excluding differential diagnoses; and (d) the use of a large panel of immunostains without appropriate care in selecting them on a case by case basis may result in confusing, overlapping results that, rather than assisting the pathologist in making the correct diagnosis, merely increase confusion and uncertainty about the diagnosis, for which the frequently performed but somewhat desperate addition of even more immunostains is unlikely to eliminate.[2,3,5,39,42–45]

Especially in cases of poorly differentiated tumors, determination of the tumor's lineage may require the inclusion of immunohistochemical stains. Epithelial immunohistochemical markers include pankeratin marker AE1/AE3 and low molecular weight keratin marker CAM5.2. Care must be taken in the use of keratin stains in the diagnosis of poorly differentiated tumors, as some carcinomas such as hepatocellular carcinoma and adrenal cortical carcinoma may be keratin negative, keratin immunopositivity does not distinguish carcinoma from mesothelioma, and keratin immunopositivity may be identified in some sarcomas and occasionally in melanoma.[3,6,13,42,43,46] Renal cell carcinoma metastatic to the lung may show immunopositivity with CD10, vimentin, and renal cell carcinoma marker; however, lack of specificity requires that one be cautious in his or her interpretation. Prostate-specific antigen and prostatic acid phosphatase are helpful in diagnosing metastatic prostate cancer to the lung. Gross cystic disease fluid protein 15 (GCDFP 15), also termed BRST-2, may be of benefit in determining whether a lung cancer is of breast origin; however, it is not an extremely sensitive marker, so lack of immunopositivity does not exclude a breast primary. Mammaglobin may also be of some benefit in diagnosing metastatic breast cancer to the lung; however, it is less specific than GCDFP 15.[46] Estrogen and progesterone receptor markers may be found in primary carcinomas other than breast carcinoma, including primary lung carcinoma, and are of no benefit in helping to differentiate a lung cancer as a breast metastasis. Nonmucinous ovarian adenocarcinomas metastatic to the lung often show immuno-positivity with CK7 and monoclonal CEA, and mucinous ovarian adenocarcinomas may also be CK20 immunopositive.[42,46,47] Urothelial cancers metastatic to the lung may show thrombomodulin immunopositivity; however, thrombomodulin may be identified in a number of other tumors and its immunopositivity must be interpreted cautiously. While uroplakins are fairly specific, they are not sensitive enough to be of great benefit in diagnosing metastatic urothelial cancer to the lung.

Identification of melanoma immunohistochemically generally involves the use of S100 and a more specific melanoma marker such as HMB-45 or MelanA/MART1. Care must be taken in interpreting these markers; however, as many spindle cell melanomas are immunonegative with, and perivascular epithelioid tumors (PEComas) immunopositive with, the more specific immunostains.[3,6,14,48,49] Leukocyte common antigen (CD45) is very helpful in determining whether a lung tumor with features of a small blue round cell tumor, either primary or metastatic, is of hematopoietic origin. It is not uncommonly employed in some cases of small cell lung cancer to exclude the diagnosis of lymphoma when the histology is not completely diagnostic. If CD45 immunopositivity is present, further workup of the lesion immunohistochemically in order to bet-ter classify the hematopoietic neoplasm is usually necessary.[3,6,13,14,46] Occasionally, immunostains are necessary to assist in diagnosing germ cell tumors metastatic to the lung. Alpha fetoprotein immunostain is helpful in diagnosing yolk sac tumors; however, staining may be patchy. Alpha fetoprotein is also often identified in hepatocellular carcinomas. Another immunostain typically positive in germ cell tumors, placental alkaline phosphatase, is generally positive in embryonal carcinomas, yolk sac tumors, and seminomas and may be identified in some choriocarcinomas. Placental alkaline phosphatase is not specific for germ cell tumors; however, it may be identified in numerous malignant tumors.[3,13,42,43,46,50] The immunohistochemical identification of mesenchy-mal tumors is problematic and often one of exclusion, because vimentin, an immunohistochemi-cal stain generally positive in mesenchymal tumors, is not infrequently identified in carcinomas. Vimentin immunopositivity may also be exhibited in mesotheliomas and melanomas.[3,6,13,43] Clini-cal and radiologic history is often helpful when metastatic diffuse malignant mesothelioma to the lung is a consideration. Often, the differential diagnosis includes mesothelioma versus primary pulmonary adenocarcinoma with pleural involvement. In these cases, a panel of immunostains is necessary to assist the pathologist in making the proper diagnosis. Although panels vary, immu-nostains generally positive in mesothelioma include calretinin (nuclear and cytoplasmic stain-ing), WT-1, thrombomodulin HBME-1, D2-40, mesothelin, and CK5/6 (Figs. 17-21 and 17-22). None of these immunostains, including calretinin, is specific for mesothelioma. Immunostains

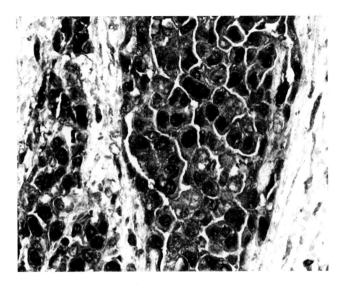

FIGURE 17-21 High-power image of calretinin staining of diffuse malignant mesothelioma, showing cytoplasmic and also strong nuclear staining of the tumor cells.

FIGURE 17-22 High-power image of
HBME-1 staining of diffuse malignant
mesothelioma, showing membranous
tumor cell staining.

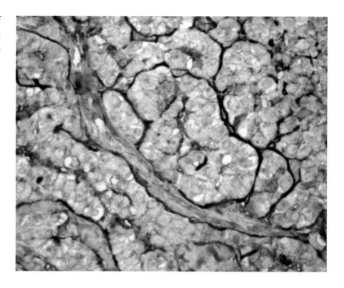

often used in these panels that are typically positive in adenocarcinoma include MOC-31, Ber-EP4, B72.3, TTF-1, Leu-M1, and CEA. Given the prognostic and legal implications of the diagnosis of diffuse malignant mesothelioma, care must be taken in interpreting these immunostain panels. Differentiation between some epithelial diffuse malignant mesotheliomas and primary pulmonary squamous cell carcinoma may also be problematic.[3,6,51–54]

Even if the tumor lineage is clear, diagnosis of the primary site of a tumor metastatic to the lung may require immunostains. Differentiating adenocarcinoma arising from the lung from adenocarcinoma arising from the colon is often a concern, and the use of a panel of immunostains including CK7, CK20, TTF-1, and CDX-2 assists in making the proper diagnosis. Primary lung adenocarcinomas are generally CK7 and TTF-1 immunopositive; whereas, primary colon adenocarcinomas are typically CK20 and CDX-2 immunopositive. Immunostain with TTF-1 is typically positive in small cell carcinomas, large cell neuroendocrine carcinomas, and adenocarcinomas and is typically negative in squamous cell carcinomas and large cell carcinomas. Note, however, that small cell carcinoma TTF-1 immunopositivity is not conclusive of a lung primary, as small cell carcinomas from other sites, such as cervix, bladder, and prostate, may also exhibit TTF-1 positivity (Fig. 17-23).[34]

FIGURE 17-23 High-power image of lung
adenocarcinoma showing strong nuclear
tumor cell immunopositivity with TTF-1.

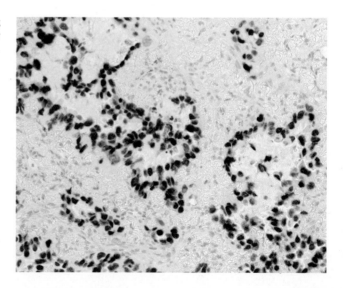

Recently, studies have examined the use of a molecular approach to differentiating primary lung neoplasms and neoplasms metastatic to the lung. Using gene expression profiling, the levels of expression of hundreds or even thousands of genes can be determined simultaneously via the use of microarrays. Real-time polymerase chain reaction testing is also being examined as a diagnostic method in the workup of tumors of unknown origin. These studies are still generally used as research tools; however, in the future, such technology might allow for accurate and timely determination of a tumor's type and site of origin.[20,55–62]

References

1. Dail D, Cagle PT, Marchevsky AM, et al. Metastases to the lung. In: Travis WD, Brambilla, E, Muller-Hermelink, HK, Harris CC, eds. *World Health Organization Classification of Tumours: Tumours of the Lung, Pleura, Thymus and Heart*. Lyon: IARC Press; 2004:122–124.
2. Laga AC, Allen TC, Bedrossian C, et al. Metastatic carcinoma. In: Cagle PT, ed. *Color Atlas and Text of Pulmonary Pathology*. 2nd ed. Philadelphia, PA: Lippincott Williams & Wilkins; 2008:74–76.
3. Dail D. Metastases to and from the lung. In: Tomashefski JF CP, Farver CF, Fraire AE, eds. *Dail and Hammar's Pulmonary Pathology*. 3rd ed. New York, NY: Springer; 2008:735–766.
4. Varadhachary GR, Abbruzzese JL, Lenzi R. Diagnostic strategies for unknown primary cancer. *Cancer*. 2004;100:1776–1785.
5. Allen TC, Cagle, PT. Metastases to the lung. In: Allen TC, Cagle PT, eds. *Frozen Section Library: Lung*. New York, NY: Springer; 2009:61–84.
6. Jones KD. Malignant epithelial neoplasms. In: Cagle PT, Allen TC, Beasley MB, eds. *Diagnostic Pulmonary Pathology*. 2nd ed. New York, NY: Informa; 2008:611–626.
7. Al-Brahim N, Ross C, Carter B, et al. The value of postmortem examination in cases of metastasis of unknown origin-20-year retrospective data from a tertiary care center. *Ann Diagn Pathol*. 2005;9:77–80.
8. Zetter BR. The cellular basis of site-specific tumor metastasis. *N Engl J Med*. 1990;322:605–612.
9. Crow J, Slavin G, Kreel L. Pulmonary metastasis: a pathologic and radiologic study. *Cancer*. 1981;47:2595–2602.
10. Farrell JT. Pulmonary metastasis: a pathologic, clinical, roetgenologic study based on 78 cases seen at necropsy. *Radiology*. 1935;24:444–451.
11. Johnson RM, Lindskog GE. 100 cases of tumor metastatic to lung and mediastinum. Treatment and results. *JAMA*. 1967;202:94–98.
12. Anton RC, Schwartz MR, Kessler ML, et al. Metastatic carcinoma of the prostate mimicking primary carcinoid tumor of the lung and mediastinum. *Pathol Res Pract*. 1998;194:753–758.
13. Cagle PT. Differential diagnosis between pulmonary and metastatic carcinomas. In: Brambilla C, Brambilla E, eds. *Lung Tumors: Fundamental Biology and Clinical Management*. New York, NY: Marcel Dekker; 1999:127–137.
14. Castro CY, Chhieng DC. Cytology and surgical pathology of neoplasms of the lung. In: Chhieng DC, Siegal GP, eds. *Updates in Diagnostic Pathology*. New York, NY: Springer; 2005:70–90.
15. Pastorino U, McCormack PM, Ginsberg RJ. A new staging proposal for pulmonary metastases. The results of analysis of 5206 cases of resected pulmonary metastases. *Chest Surg Clin N Am*. 1998;8:197–202.
16. Friedel G, Pastorino U, Ginsberg RJ, et al. Results of lung metastasectomy from breast cancer: prognostic criteria on the basis of 467 cases of the International Registry of Lung Metastases. *Eur J Cardiothorac Surg*. 2002;22:335–344.
17. Yesner R, Carter D. Pathology of carcinoma of the lung. Changing patterns. *Clin Chest Med*. 1982;3:257–289.
18. Muller KM, Respondek M. Pulmonary metastases: pathological anatomy. *Lung*. 1990;168(suppl):1137–1144.
19. Dacic S. Molecular diagnostics of pulmonary neoplasms. In: Cagle PT, Allen TC, Beasley MB, eds. *Diagnostic Pulmonary Pathology*. 2nd ed. New York, NY: Informa; 2008:745–753.
20. Ma XJ, Patel R, Wang X, et al. Molecular classification of human cancers using a 92-gene real-time quantitative polymerase chain reaction assay. *Arch Pathol Lab Med*. 2006;130:465–473.

21. Whitesell PL, Peters SG. Pulmonary manifestations of extrathoracic malignant lesions. *Mayo Clin Proc.* 1993;68:483–491.

22. Timmerman RD, Bizekis CS, Pass HI, et al. Local surgical, ablative, and radiation treatment of metastases. *CA Cancer J Clin.* 2009;59:145–170.

23. Seo JB, Im JG, Goo JM, et al. Atypical pulmonary metastases: spectrum of radiologic findings. *Radiographics.* 2001;21:403–417.

24. Reinhardt MJ, Wiethoelter N, Matthies A, et al. PET recognition of pulmonary metastases on PET/CT imaging: impact of attenuation-corrected and non-attenuation-corrected PET images. *Eur J Nucl Med Mol Imaging.* 2006;33:134–139.

25. Davidson RS, Nwogu CE, Brentjens MJ, et al. The surgical management of pulmonary metastasis: current concepts. *Surg Oncol.* 2001;10:35–42.

26. Toomes H, Delphendahl A, Manke HG, et al. The coin lesion of the lung. A review of 955 resected coin lesions. *Cancer.* 1983;51:534–537.

27. Kohler HF, Neves RI, Brechtbuhl ER, et al. Cutaneous angiosarcoma of the head and neck: report of 23 cases from a single institution. *Otolaryngol Head Neck Surg.* 2008;139:519–524.

28. Lin JF, Slomovitz BM. Uterine sarcoma 2008. *Curr Oncol Rep.* 2008;10:512–518.

29. Miller AJ, Mihm MC Jr. Melanoma. *N Engl J Med.* 2006;355:51–65.

30. Yoney A, Eren B, Eskici S, et al. Retrospective analysis of 105 cases with uterine sarcoma. *Bull Cancer.* 2008;95:E10–E17.

31. Diemel KD, Klippe HJ, Branseheid D. Pulmonary metastasetomy for osteosarcoma: is it justified? *Recent Results Cancer Res.* 2009;179:183–208.

32. Ettinger DS, Agulnik M, Cristea M, et al. Occult primary. *J Natl Compr Canc Netw.* 2008;6:1026–1060.

33. Galer CE, Kies MS. Evaluation and management of the unknown primary carcinoma of the head and neck. *J Natl Compr Canc Netw.* 2008;6:1068–1075.

34. Kaufmann O, Dietel M. Expression of thyroid transcription factor-1 in pulmonary and extrapulmonary small cell carcinomas and other neuroendocrine carcinomas of various primary sites. *Histopathology.* 2000;36:415–420.

35. Gomez-Roca C, Raynaud CM, Penault-Llorca F, et al. Differential expression of biomarkers in primary non-small cell lung cancer and metastatic sites. *J Thorac Oncol.* 2009.

36. Vollmer RT. Primary lung cancer vs. metastatic breast cancer: a probabilistic approach. *Am J Clin Pathol.* 2009;132:391–395.

37. Briccoli A, Rocca M, Salone M, et al. High grade osteosarcoma of the extremities metastatic to the lung: Long-term results in 323 patients treated combining surgery and chemotherapy, 1985–2005. *Surg Oncol.* 2009.

38. Apostolou G, Biteli M, Chatzipantelis P. Cytopathological diagnosis of metastatic pleomorphic liposarcoma in the lung: a report of a case correlated with the histopathology of the primary tumour. *Diagn Cytopathol.* 2009;37:667–670.

39. Herbst J, Jenders R, McKenna R, et al. Evidence-based criteria to help distinguish metastatic breast cancer from primary lung adenocarcinoma on thoracic frozen section. *Am J Clin Pathol.* 2009;131: 122–128.

40. Mercer RR, Lucas NC, Simmons AN, et al. Molecular discrimination of multiple primary versus metastatic squamous cell cancers of the head/neck and lung. *Exp Mol Pathol.* 2009;86:1–9.

41. Seward SM, Richardson DL, Leon ME, et al. Metastatic squamous cell carcinoma of the vulva to the lung confirmed with allelotyping. *Int J Gynecol Pathol.* 2009;28:497–501.

42. Jagirdar J. Application of immunohistochemistry to the diagnosis of primary and metastatic carcinoma to the lung. *Arch Pathol Lab Med.* 2008;132:384–396.

43. Vege DS, Soman CS, Joshi UA, et al. Undifferentiated tumors: an immunohistochemical analysis on biopsies. *J Surg Oncol.* 1994;57:273–276.

44. Gupta R, McKenna R Jr, Marchevsky AM. Lessons learned from mistakes and deferrals in the frozen section diagnosis of bronchioloalveolar carcinoma and well-differentiated pulmonary adenocarcinoma: an evidence-based pathology approach. *Am J Clin Pathol.* 2008;130:11–20; quiz 146.

45. Gupta R, Dastane A, McKenna RJ Jr, et al. What can we learn from the errors in the frozen section diagnosis of pulmonary carcinoid tumors? An evidence-based approach. *Hum Pathol.* 2009;40:1–9.

46. Bahrami A, Truong LD, Ro JY. Undifferentiated tumor: true identity by immunohistochemistry. *Arch Pathol Lab Med.* 2008;132:326–348.

47. Cathro HP, Stoler MH. Expression of cytokeratins 7 and 20 in ovarian neoplasia. *Am J Clin Pathol.* 2002;117:944–951.

48. Clarkson KS, Sturdgess IC, Molyneux AJ. The usefulness of tyrosinase in the immunohistochemical assessment of melanocytic lesions: a comparison of the novel T311 antibody (anti-tyrosinase) with S-100, HMB45, and A103 (anti-melan-A). *J Clin Pathol.* 2001;54:196–200.

49. Jungbluth AA, Iversen K, Coplan K, et al. Expression of melanocyte-associated markers gp-100 and Melan-A/MART-1 in angiomyolipomas. An immunohistochemical and rt-PCR analysis. *Virchows Arch.* 1999;434:429–435.

50. Emerson RE, Ulbright TM. The use of immunohistochemistry in the differential diagnosis of tumors of the testis and paratestis. *Semin Diagn Pathol.* 2005;22:33–50.

51. Marchevsky AM. Application of immunohistochemistry to the diagnosis of malignant mesothelioma. *Arch Pathol Lab Med.* 2008;132:397–401.

52. Ordonez NG. Immunohistochemical diagnosis of epithelioid mesothelioma: an update. *Arch Pathol Lab Med.* 2005;129:1407–1414.

53. Ordonez NG. D2-40 and podoplanin are highly specific and sensitive immunohistochemical markers of epithelioid malignant mesothelioma. *Hum Pathol.* 2005;36:372–380.

54. Ordonez NG. The diagnostic utility of immunohistochemistry in distinguishing between mesothelioma and renal cell carcinoma: a comparative study. *Hum Pathol.* 2004;35:697–710.

55. Bhattacharjee A, Richards WG, Staunton J, et al. Classification of human lung carcinomas by mRNA expression profiling reveals distinct adenocarcinoma subclasses. *Proc Natl Acad Sci USA.* 2001;98:13790–13795.

56. Dennis JL, Vass JK, Wit EC, et al. Identification from public data of molecular markers of adenocarcinoma characteristic of the site of origin. *Cancer Res.* 2002;62:5999–6005.

57. Bloom G, Yang IV, Boulware D, et al. Multi-platform, multi-site, microarray-based human tumor classification. *Am J Pathol.* 2004;164:9–16.

58. Varadhachary GR, Talantov D, Raber MN, et al. Molecular profiling of carcinoma of unknown primary and correlation with clinical evaluation. *J Clin Oncol.* 2008;26:4442–4448.

59. Waldman SA, Terzic A. A study of microRNAs in silico and in vivo: diagnostic and therapeutic applications in cancer. *FEBS J.* 2009;276:2157–2164.

60. Tothill RW, Kowalczyk A, Rischin D, et al. An expression-based site of origin diagnostic method designed for clinical application to cancer of unknown origin. *Cancer Res.* 2005;65:4031–4040.

61. Santos ES, Perez CA, Raez LE. How is gene-expression profiling going to challenge the future management of lung cancer? *Future Oncol.* 2009;5:827–8235.

62. Horlings HM, van Laar RK, Kerst JM, et al. Gene expression profiling to identify the histogenetic origin of metastatic adenocarcinomas of unknown primary. *J Clin Oncol.* 2008;26:4435–4441.

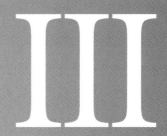
Imaging

Current Imaging Techniques for the Diagnosis and Staging of Lung Cancer

18

▶ Philip T. Cagle
▶ Ronald E. Fisher

INTRODUCTION

Radiology and nuclear medicine play a vital role in the diagnosis, staging, and treatment of lung cancer and typically provide the basis for obtaining specimens for the surgical pathologist. Computerized tomography (CT), magnetic resonance imaging (MRI), and positron emission tomography (PET) have been in use for decades as imaging techniques for many purposes, including detection and evaluation of primary lung tumors and metastases.[1–4] The frequent use of CT and high resolution CT (HRCT) in the diagnosis of chest diseases, including interstitial lung diseases, has resulted in the increased detection of incidental lung nodules, including clinically unsuspected lung cancers which, in turn, has led to renewed interest in the possibilities of lung cancer screening.[5] Currently, several imaging techniques are popular for the diagnosis and staging of primary lung cancers and their metastases. These include PET/CT co-registration for diagnosis, staging, planning therapy and evaluating response to therapy,[1–4,6–11] and endobronchial ultrasound (EBUS)-guided transbronchial needle aspiration and transesophageal endoscopic ultrasound (EUS)-guided fine needle aspiration primarily for diagnosing mediastinal lymph node metastases.[12–20]

CT AND MRI

CT and MRI have been in routine clinical use for anatomic imaging for decades and the images they produce should be very familiar to surgical pathologists. CT scanners, using x-rays, and MRI scanners, using radio frequency, produce multiple two-dimensional cross-sectional images or "slices" of tissue that can be reconstructed in three dimensions. Both may be enhanced by the use of contrast agents. MRI provides images in any plane. Although earlier CT scanners could only provide images in an axial or near-axial plane (computed axial tomography or CAT scanners), current multidetector CT (MDCT) scanners generate data that subsequently can be reconstructed in any plane. There are advantages and disadvantages to both techniques, but CT is preferred for solid thoracic tumors such as lung cancer in most situations.[1,2]

PET AND PET/CT

PET is a nuclear medicine technique in which a radioactively labeled compound or radiotracer is injected into the patient.[3,4,6–11] Fluorine-18-fluorodeoxyglucose (FDG) is the radiotracer most often used to detect cancers. A positron-emitting radionuclide with a short half-life (fluorine-18 has a half-life slightly <2 hours) is incorporated into a metabolically active compound (glucose) to produce the radiotracer FDG. The FDG is injected into the patient's bloodstream and concentrates in normal body tissues, inflammatory lesions, and tumors in proportion to the cells' glucose metabolic rate that use glucose at a high rate, including brain and liver, and in some inflammatory lesions. Most cancers have an increased rate of glucose metabolism due to their high reproductive rates and their inefficient use of glucose—poorly differentiated tumors cannot undergo aerobic metabolism even if sufficient oxygen is present. As a result, most cancers have to transport a large amount of glucose across their cell membranes in order to generate a sufficient amount of ATP. Once in the cell, FDG is phosphorylated to FDG-6-phosphate by hexokinase. FDG-6-phosphate, however, cannot be metabolized further because an oxygen atom has been replaced with fluorine. And because mammalian cells lack significant levels of the phosphatase needed to remove the phosphate group, the molecule is trapped inside cells. The more glucose (and thus FDG) a cell transports in, the more FDG is trapped inside it and the "hotter" it will appear on an FDG PET scan. Most cancers are hot on PET, with poorly differentiated, high-grade tumors being extremely hot (Fig. 18-1).[3,4,6–11]

After injection of the FDG, there is a wait period of about an hour for the radiotracer to become concentrated in the body tissues. The patient is placed in a scanner that records the tissue concentration of the radiotracer as it decays. As the radiotracer decays, it emits a positron. The emitted positron encounters an electron resulting in electron-positron annihilation with production of gamma rays or annihilation photons that are detected by the scanner. Computer analysis is then used to reconstruct images of the tracer concentration in three-dimensional space. Metabolically active tissues, including most lung cancers, are expected to display greater concentrations of FDG, often measured as standardized uptake value (SUV).[3,4,6–11]

Today, PET scan is used in combination with CT scan which allows areas of metabolic activity detected by the PET scan to be correlated with the corresponding anatomic structures via CT scan. Today, PET scanners integrated with MDCT scans allow more exact integration (image registration) of the PET and CT images since the two procedures can be performed in immediate sequence in one session, without the patient changing the position.[3,4,6–11]

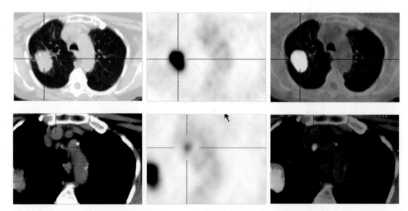

FIGURE 18-1 PET-CT: Adenocarcinoma. A 71-year-old woman with a lung mass on CXR and CT. Biopsy = primary pulmonary adenocarcinoma. PET is performed for staging. **Top images**: *Left*: CT axial slice shows right upper lobe mass. *Middle*: PET axial slice at the same level shows marked uptake (SUV = 15). *Right*: PET image in color superimposed on the gray-scale CT image shows that the marked uptake corresponds precisely to the mass. **Bottom images**: *Left*: CT axial slice shows two small right upper paratracheal lymph nodes. *Middle*:PET axial slice at the same level shows mild, but significant, focal uptake near the nodes (SUV = 3.5). The arrow at top is incidental. *Right*: PET image in color superimposed on the gray-scale CT image shows that the uptake corresponds precisely to one of the lymph nodes. Mediastinoscopy subsequently showed this to be a small metastasis.

EUS AND EBUS

Staging of lung cancer patients often involves sampling of mediastinal lymph nodes for examination by the surgical pathologist. Mediastinoscopy is a surgical procedure performed under general anesthesia that has been used for sampling of mediastinal lymph nodes for decades. For the past few decades, fine needle aspiration of mediastinal lymph nodes through the wall of the esophagus using an endoscope or through the wall of the bronchus using a bronchoscope has provided several advantages over mediastinoscopy.[12–20] These procedures have been further enhanced by using ultrasound to identify target tissues rather than performing aspirations blindly (Figs. 18-2 and 18-3). Advantages of EUS and EBUS over mediastinoscopy include (a) surgery with general anesthesia and use of an operating room is not required, (b) additional lymph node stations that are inaccessible to mediastinoscopy can be reached (including hilar and postcarinal nodes), and (c) these procedures can be repeated if needed whereas repeat mediastinoscopy is often difficult.[12–20]

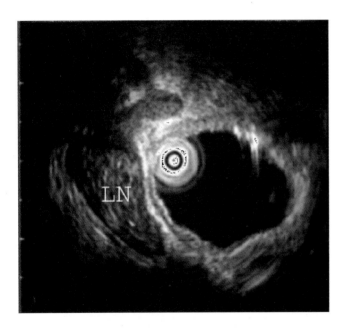

FIGURE 18-2 EBUS image of a lymph node (LN) adjacent to the airway wall. The airway wall layers are also clearly visible. (Reprinted from Herth FJ, Lunn W, Eberhardt R, et al. Transbronchial versus transesophageal ultrasound-guided aspiration of enlarged mediastinal lymph nodes. *Am J Respir Crit Care Med.* 2005 May 15;171(10):1164–1167, with permission.)

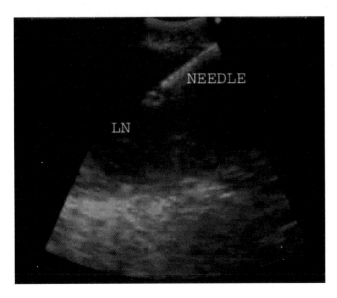

FIGURE 18-3 Image of a transesophageal EUS-guided needle puncture of a lymph node. The LN and the needle passing into it are clearly visible. (Reprinted from Herth FJ, Lunn W, Eberhardt R, et al. Transbronchial versus transesophageal ultrasound-guided aspiration of enlarged mediastinal lymph nodes. *Am J Respir Crit Care Med.* 2005 May 15;171(10):1164–1167, with permission.)

Transesophageal EUS typically employs an endosonoscope which is an endoscope with an ultrasound transducer in its tip. Fine needle aspiration of suspicious lymph nodes can be performed under real-time ultrasound guidance. For EBUS, an ultrasound probe is introduced through the bronchoscope and the positions of the target lymph nodes are identified prior to fine needle aspiration. The pathologist may be asked to perform a rapid cytology check onsite to confirm the quality of the specimen. Rates of successfully sampling the desired lymph nodes and of obtaining a specific diagnosis are reported to exceed 90% when both methods are combined. [12–20]

References

1. Truong MT, Munden RF, Movsas B. Imaging to optimally stage lung cancer: conventional modalities and PET/CT. *J Am Coll Radiol.* 2004;1(12):957–964.
2. Hicks RJ, Lau E, Alam NZ, et al. Imaging in the diagnosis and treatment of non-small cell lung cancer. *Respirology.* 2007;12(2):165–172.
3. Freudenberg LS, Rosenbaum SJ, Beyer T, et al. PET versus PET/CT dual-modality imaging in evaluation of lung cancer. *Radiol Clin North Am.* 2007;45(4):639–644.
4. Von Schulthess GK, Hany TF. Imaging and PET-PET/CT imaging. *J Radiol.* 2008;89(3 pt 2): 438–447.
5. Chirieac LR, Flieder DB. High-resolution computed tomography screening for lung cancer: unexpected findings and new controversies regarding adenocarcinogenesis. *Arch Pathol Lab Med.* 2010;134(1):41–48.
6. Rankin S. PET/CT for staging and monitoring non small cell lung cancer. *Cancer Imaging.* 2008;8(Spec No A):S27–S31.
7. Groth SS, Whitson BA, Maddaus MA. Radiographic staging of mediastinal lymph nodes in non-small cell lung cancer patients. *Thorac Surg Clin.* 2008;18(4):349–361.
8. De Wever W, Stroobants S, Coolen J, et al. Integrated PET/CT in the staging of nonsmall cell lung cancer: technical aspects and clinical integration. *Eur Respir J.* 2009;33(1):201–212.
9. Hellwig D, Baum RP, Kirsch C. FDG-PET, PET/CT and conventional nuclear medicine procedures in the evaluation of lung cancer: a systematic review. *Nuklearmedizin.* 2009;48(2):59–69.
10. Poeppel TD, Krause BJ, Heusner TA, et al. PET/CT for the staging and follow-up of patients with malignancies. *Eur J Radiol.* 2009;70(3):382–392.
11. Kligerman S, Digumarthy S. Staging of non-small cell lung cancer using integrated PET/CT. *Am J Roentgenol.* 2009;193(5):1203–1211.
12. Herth FJ, Lunn W, Eberhardt R, et al. Transbronchial versus transesophageal ultrasound-guided aspiration of enlarged mediastinal lymph nodes. *Am J Respir Crit Care Med.* 2005;171(10): 1164–1167.
13. Micames CG, McCrory DC, Pavey DA, et al. Endoscopic ultrasound-guided fine-needle aspiration for non-small cell lung cancer staging: a systematic review and metaanalysis. *Chest.* 2007;131(2): 539–548.
14. Vilmann P, Puri R. The complete 'medical' mediastinoscopy (EUS-FNA + EBUS-TBNA). *Minerva Med.* 2007;98(4):331–338.
15. Eloubeidi MA. Endoscopic ultrasound-guided fine-needle aspiration in the staging and diagnosis of patients with lung cancer. *Semin Thorac Cardiovasc Surg.* 2007(Fall);19(3):206–211.
16. Yasufuku K, Nakajima T, Fujiwara T, et al. Role of endobronchial ultrasound-guided transbronchial needle aspiration in the management of lung cancer. *Gen Thorac Cardiovasc Surg.* 2008;56(6): 268–276.
17. Navani N, Janes SM, Spiro SG. Lung cancer staging with minimally invasive endoscopic techniques. *JAMA.* 2008;299(21):2509.
18. Navani N, Spiro SG, Janes SM. Mediastinal staging of NSCLC with endoscopic and endobronchial ultrasound. *Nat Rev Clin Oncol.* 2009;6(5):278–286.
19. Anantham D, Koh MS, Ernst A. Endobronchial ultrasound. *Respir Med.* 2009;103(10):1406–1414.
20. Talebian M, von Bartheld MB, Braun J, et al. EUS-FNA in the preoperative staging of non-small cell lung cancer. *Lung Cancer.* 2009; [Epub ahead of print].

Correlation of Imaging with Pathology of Lung Cancer

19

▶ Ronald E. Fisher

▶ Philip T. Cagle

INTRODUCTION

Current imaging techniques correlate very well with the pathology for purposes of diagnosis and staging of lung cancer, although there are limitations including false positives, and confirmation by pathology is still desirable or necessary in many situations. This chapter provides a brief overview of the correlation of imaging with the pathology of lung cancer.[1–21]

LUNG CANCER DIAGNOSIS AND STAGING

CT and PET have long been successfully used for lung cancer diagnosis and staging. A meta-analysis published in 2006 reported that the sensitivity and specificity of PET in diagnosing single pulmonary nodules and masses is 96% and 78%, respectively, and the sensitivity and specificity of PET in mediastinal lymph node staging is 83% and 92%, respectively.[3] Use of PET/CT scans permits identification of unsuspected lung carcinoma metastases in 20% of patients missed by more traditional imaging techniques (Fig. 19-1).[1]

However, a number of studies conclude that PET/CT scan is not ready to replace surgical biopsies, including mediastinoscopy, for the diagnosis and staging of lung cancer patients. In one recent study, pathologic examination altered CT-determined stage in two thirds of patients and PET-determined stage in half of patients.[7] In a study of 200 patients undergoing PET/CT followed by staging mediastinoscopy and, if appropriate, resection, PET/CT correctly staged 49.5% of patients, under-staged 29.5%, and over-staged 21%.[15] It has been suggested that PET/CT has improved sensitivity of staging at the expense of less specificity due to an increase in false positives.[6] Resolving issues related to false positives and false negatives on PET or PET/CT scans is needed to avoid unnecessary costs and surgeries.[5,6,11,16,20,21] The pathologic correlates of false-positive PET scans are discussed further below.

ESTIMATING TUMOR SIZE

Most lung cancers present as masses or nodules on CT scans. Determination of tumor size and gross tumor volume is a component of lung cancer staging and radiotherapy. Estimating tumor size and gross tumor volume from imaging studies, including CT, PET, and PET/CT, has limitations in terms of interobserver differences and correlation with pathology. Peritumoral reaction, atelectasis, obstructive pneumonia, and opacities due to chest structures may hinder the interpretation. When possible, confirmation of tumor size by pathologic examination is desirable.[7,9]

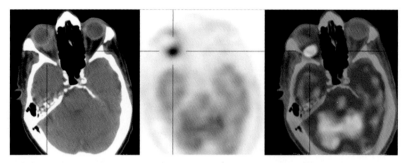

FIGURE 19-1 PET-CT: Squamous cell carcinoma metastasis, in a 75-year-old man with SOB, productive cough admitted for pneumonia, rule out malignancy. PET-CT showed marked uptake in right lower lobe consolidation (not shown), subsequently found to be primary squamous cell carcinoma. PET-CT also revealed an unexpected malignancy in right retrobulbar region. The patient mentioned blurry vision in the right eye on admission history. *Left:* CT axial slice shows small mass posterior to the right eyeball. *Middle:* PET axial slice at the same level shows marked tracer uptake in the mass (SUV = 10). *Right:* PET-CT fused images localize the uptake precisely to the mass. Retrobulbar masses in patients with a known primary malignancy are virtually always metastases. PET-CT also showed a metastasis in the liver and in the left adrenal gland (not shown).

LUNG CANCER SCREENING

Screening for lung cancer with CT scans has resulted in detection of more "early" carcinomas but has not yet yielded improved long-term survival.[11,17,20,21] Based on these observations, it has been suggested that some lung cancers may be relatively "stable" and slow growing and are perhaps not precursors to more aggressive, advanced lung cancers.[21]

BRONCHIOLOALVEOLAR CARCINOMA AND INVASIVE ADENOCARCINOMA

Pure bronchioloalveolar carcinoma classically presents as a nodular ground-glass opacity on CT scan, consistent with its lepidic growth pattern.[2,8] The presence of associated solid areas indicates an invasive component. Localized ground-glass opacities with solid areas are consistent with mixed pattern adenocarcinomas consisting of an invasive component (solid area) and a bronchioloalveolar component (ground-glass opacity). Bronchioloalveolar carcinomas classically have a low standard uptake value (SUV) on PET scan, consistent with their biologic behavior (Fig. 19-2).

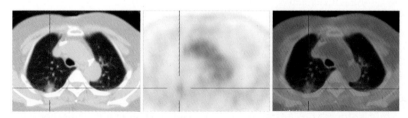

FIGURE 19-2 PET-CT: Bronchioloalveolar carcinoma. Pt is a 62-year-old woman with a 2-month history of cough and small nodular infiltrate on CT. *Left:* CT axial slice shows ground-glass nodular density in right upper lobe. *Middle:* PET axial slice at the same level shows detectable, but very mild, tracer uptake (SUV = 1.9). *Right:* PET image in color superimposed on gray-scale CT image shows that the PET uptake corresponds to the CT nodular density. Note that the low degree of PET uptake favors a benign inflammatory process, such as pneumonitis, but also occurs with bronchoalveolar carcinoma.

FALSE POSITIVES AND FALSE NEGATIVES ON PET AND PET/CT SCAN

Elevated FDG concentrations and increased SUVs on PET scans can be seen in a variety of benign conditions and inflammatory lesions. These include mycobacterial infections, fungal infections, bacterial infections, sarcoidosis, sarcoid-like reaction to tumors, radiation pneumonitis, postsurgical conditions, benign neoplasms, coal worker's pneumoconiosis, and cryptogenic organizing pneumonia.[4,5,10,12,13,14,18] PET scans of mediastinal lymph nodes may show increased FDG concentrations and SUVs with benign conditions including reactive follicular hyperplasia, reactive sinus histiocytosis, fibrotic micronodules, and, occasionally, granulomas.[18] Bronchioloalveolar carcinomas, carcinoid tumors, and low-grade lymphomas may have false-negative PET scans due to the low metabolic activity of these types of cancer; nodules and lymph nodes smaller than 1 cm can also be falsely negative.[4]

References

1. MacManus MP, Hicks RJ, Matthews JP, et al. High rate of detection of unsuspected distant metastases by pet in apparent stage III non-small-cell lung cancer: implications for radical radiation therapy. *Int J Radiat Oncol Biol Phys*. 2001;50(2):287–293.
2. Travis WD, Garg K, Franklin WA, et al. Evolving concepts in the pathology and computed tomography imaging of lung adenocarcinoma and bronchioloalveolar carcinoma. *J Clin Oncol*. 2005;23(14):3279–3287.
3. Fischer BM, Mortensen J. The future in diagnosis and staging of lung cancer: positron emission tomography. *Respiration*. 2006;73(3):267–276.
4. Chang JM, Lee HJ, Goo JM, et al. False positive and false negative FDG-PET scans in various thoracic diseases. *Korean J Radiol*. 2006;7(1):57–69.
5. Devaraj A, Cook GJ, Hansell DM. PET/CT in non-small cell lung cancer staging-promises and problems. *Clin Radiol*. 2007;62(2):97–108.
6. Lee BE, von Haag D, Lown T, et al. Advances in positron emission tomography technology have increased the need for surgical staging in non-small cell lung cancer. *J Thorac Cardiovasc Surg*. 2007;133(3):746–752.
7. Faria SL, Menard S, Devic S, et al. Impact of FDG-PET/CT on radiotherapy volume delineation in non-small-cell lung cancer and correlation of imaging stage with pathologic findings. *Int J Radiat Oncol Biol Phys*. 2008;70(4):1035–1038.
8. Goudarzi B, Jacene HA, Wahl RL. Diagnosis and differentiation of bronchioloalveolar carcinoma from adenocarcinoma with bronchioloalveolar components with metabolic and anatomic characteristics using PET/CT. *J Nucl Med*. 2008;49(10):1585–1592.
9. Macpherson RE, Higgins GS, Murchison JT, et al. Non-small-cell lung cancer dimensions: CT-pathological correlation and interobserver variation. *Br J Radiol*. 2009;82(977):421–425.
10. Hsu PK, Cheng HF, Yeh YC, et al. Pulmonary sclerosing haemangioma mimicking lung cancer on PET scan. *Respirology*. 2009;14(6):903–906.
11. Beatty JS, Williams HT, Aldridge BA, et al. Incidental PET/CT findings in the cancer patient: how should they be managed? *Surgery*. 2009;146(2):274–281.
12. Chowdhury FU, Sheerin F, Bradley KM, et al. Sarcoid-like reaction to malignancy on whole-body integrated (18)F-FDG PET/CT: prevalence and disease pattern. *Clin Radiol*. 2009;64(7):675–681.
13. Ha JM, Jeong SY, Seo YS, et al. Incidental focal F-18 FDG accumulation in lung parenchyma without abnormal CT findings. *Ann Nucl Med*. 2009;23(6):599–603.
14. Reichert M, Bensadoun ES. PET imaging in patients with coal workers pneumoconiosis and suspected malignancy. *J Thorac Oncol*. 2009;4(5):649–651.
15. Carnochan FM, Walker WS. Positron emission tomography may underestimate the extent of thoracic disease in lung cancer patients. *Eur J Cardiothorac Surg*. 2009;35(5):781–784.

16. Rintoul RC, Tournoy KG, El Daly H, et al. EBUS-TBNA for the clarification of PET positive intra-thoracic lymph nodes-an international multi-centre experience. *J Thorac Oncol*. 2009;4(1):44–48.

17. Vazquez M, Carter D, Brambilla E, et al. International Early Lung Cancer Action Program Investigators. Solitary and multiple resected adenocarcinomas after CT screening for lung cancer: histopathologic features and their prognostic implications. *Lung Cancer*. 2009;64(2):148–154.

18. Yeh DW, Lee KS, Han J, et al. Mediastinal nodes in patients with non-small cell lung cancer: MRI findings with PET/CT and pathologic correlation. *Am J Roentgenol*. 2009;193(3):813–821.

19. Ponnuswamy A, Mediratta N, Lyburn ID, et al. False positive diagnosis of malignancy in a case of cryptogenic organising pneumonia presenting as a pulmonary mass with mediastinal nodes detected on fluorodeoxyglucose-positron emission tomography: a case report. *J Med Case Reports*. 2009;3:124.

20. Barnett PG, Ananth L, Gould MK; Veterans Affairs Positron Emission Tomography Imaging in the Management of Patients with Solitary Pulmonary Nodules (VA SNAP) Cooperative Study Group. Cost and outcomes of patients with solitary pulmonary nodules managed with PET scans. *Chest*. 2010;137(1):53–59.

21. Chirieac LR, Flieder DB. High-resolution computed tomography screening for lung cancer: unexpected findings and new controversies regarding adenocarcinogenesis. *Arch Pathol Lab Med*. 2010;134(1):41–48.

Multimodality Theranostics and Molecular Imaging in the Diagnosis and Treatment of Lung Cancer

► Kirtee Raparia

► Kelvin Wong

► Stephen Wong

► King C. Li

► Philip T. Cagle

Development of image-guided, multimodality diagnostic and therapeutic systems is underway and promises to merge pathology and radiology for improved survival of lung cancer. This novel system could be potentially used for early diagnosis and treatment of peripheral lung cancer, which constitutes more than half of lung cancer cases.[1] Molecular imaging and electromagnetic (EM) tracking can be used to guide a steerable needle that allows image-guided diagnosis along with diagnostic and therapeutic devices including radiofrequency ablation (RFA) needle, fiberoptic fluorescence imaging probe for fluorescence molecular imaging,[2] and laser-induced photothermal therapy; in conjunction with molecular contrast agents including 18F-fluoro-deoxy-glucose, fluorescence molecular imaging contrast agents, and metallic nanoshells (Figs. 20-1 and 20-2). The lung cancer diagnostic and therapeutic system can potentially be used to provide a cost-effective diagnosis and treatment of cancer, in addition to the more established minimally invasive tool such as RFA.

OPTICAL IMAGING FOR IN VIVO MOLECULAR IMAGING

Despite advances in imaging, current techniques such as computerized tomography (CT) cannot visualize tumor morphology and architecture at the cellular level. Currently, in clinical situations a surgical tissue biopsy or needle aspiration is required for histopathologic diagnosis. Because many tumors are heterogeneous, it can be difficult to determine the optimal site to biopsy and sampling error may lead to incorrect diagnoses. Therefore, a minimally invasive technique to provide in vivo data on cellular morphology and molecular expression in real time would radically improve clinical diagnosis and monitoring tumor response. Optical molecular imaging technologies can meet this important clinical need by delivering real-time, in vivo images with subcellular resolution, which can be further enhanced by using targeted optical contrast agents. Nuclear and cellular morphology is observed in thin optical sections, which is similar to conventional

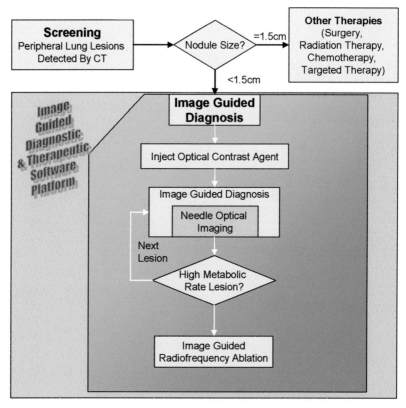

FIGURE 20-1 Image-guided diagnostic and therapeutic workflow for peripheral lung lesions.

histology but without removing tissue, sectioning, and staining. The optical contrast agents can enhance the visualization of the molecular changes, such as expression of oncogenes or tissue-specific receptors. This information can significantly benefit patient care, by providing earlier and more specific detection of disease. The use of molecular imaging also has the potential to develop targeted therapeutics agents.[3]

Optical coherence tomography (OCT) is a novel noninvasive technique, which can detect tissue structure at a resolution of up to 10 to 20 μm. OCT imaging system has been shown to clinically distinguish normal and abnormal cervical tissues, including dysplasia and cancer.[4-7] Confocal scanning laser microscopy has been shown to identify benign and malignant pigmented skin lesions in vivo.[8-10] There is also preliminary data on its role in diagnosing mycosis fungoides.[11] It may also be a promising tool in the diagnosis of nonneoplastic skin lesions such as psoriasis, molluscum contagiosum, discoid lupus erythematosis, folliculitis, and allergic contact dermatitis.[12-17] Real-time confocal reflectance microscopy can also be potentially used to evaluate the margins

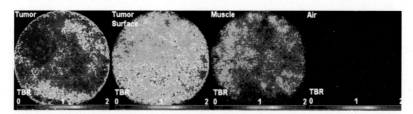

FIGURE 20-2 In vivo fiberoptic microendoscopy of $\alpha_v\beta_3$ expression in A547 lung cancer subcutaneous mouse model. (From Wong KK, Tung CH, Wong ST. In vivo molecular microendoscopy in human lung cancer mouse model. *Proc World Mol Imaging Cong.* 2009.)

in vivo in Mohs surgery for nonmelanoma skin cancers.[18,19] This could avoid the use of frozen sections in these situations, which takes longer time. Confocal microscopy has also been reported to be of significance in detection of oral cavity neoplasia.[20] It also allowed imaging of the urothelium, the superficial and deep portions of the lamina propria, the muscularis propria, and the serosa of the bladder wall of the rats in vivo.[21]

Although there is limited study of these advanced imaging techniques in lung cancer, these may be a promising tool for in vivo imaging of lung lesions. Confocal microscopy has been shown to visualize normal alveolar ducts, alveolar macrophages,[22,23] and human lung cancer cell lines.[24] A recent study of total of 281 OCT images and the corresponding bronchial biopsies suggested that autofluorescence bronchoscopy–guided OCT imaging of bronchial lesions is technically feasible.[25] Quantitative measurement of the epithelial thickness showed that invasive carcinoma was significantly different than carcinoma in situ ($p = 0.004$) and dysplasia was significantly different than metaplasia or hyperplasia ($p = 0.002$) in the bronchial lesions.[25] In another study OCT identified in situ morphologic changes associated with inflammation, squamous metaplasia, and tumor in 15 patients undergoing lung resections for cancer.[26] OCT imaging enabled the characterization of the multilayered histology of the airways, with a maximum penetration depth of up to 2 to 3 mm and 10-μm spatial resolution.[26,27]

Therefore, there is significant clinical potential for confocal microscopy and OCT to be a sensitive and specific method for precancerous and cancerous lesions in the lung. It could be used for clinical diagnosis of the lesions, evaluation of the margins, and to monitor response to therapeutic treatment.

CONTRAST AGENTS FOR MICROENDOSCOPY

With the exception of reflectance confocal microscopy and OCT, most microendoscopes rely on the use of exogenous contrast agents to generate high-contrast images of biological tissues with good signal-to-noise ratio. Several FDA-approved contrast agents such as indocyanine green and fluorescein are in routine clinical use, which provide both absorption- and fluorescence-based contrast. In addition, many targeted contrast agents (tumor specific) are in development for optical molecular imaging.[28–31] The use of these peptide-dye conjugate in optical imaging combines the specificity of ligand/receptor interaction with near-infrared (NIR) fluorescence detection and can be used in diagnosis of cancers. Activatable fluorescence imaging probes to sense enzyme activity have a potential to be used to image protease activity, as well as to study the therapeutic use of protease inhibitors in various diseases in patients.[32–34] Molecular specific imaging using fluorescein isothiocyanate–labeled antibodies[35] for detection of melanomas in mice and indocyanine green N-hydroxysulfosuccinimide ester (ICG-sulfo-OSu)–labeled antibodies[36] in gastric carcinomas have been studied.

Metallic nanoparticles, such as gold, have been extensively used as molecular specific stains in electron microscopy of cells and tissues. Gold particles display electron dense properties and are capable of strong emission of secondary electrons, making them a useful and specific marker in microscopy both at the low and high resolution levels (light and fluorescent microscopy and scanning and transmission electron microscopy).[37–40] The use of the surface plasmon resonance of metallic nanoparticle has been explored for in vivo biological applications.[41] The scattering cross section of gold nanoparticles is extremely high compared to polymeric spheres of the same size, especially in the red. Another interesting optical property of gold nanoparticles for vital optical imaging is the increase in scattering cross section per particle when the particles agglutinate. These changes produce a large optical contrast between isolated gold particles and assemblies of gold particles. This increase in contrast improves the ability to image markers that are not uniquely expressed in diseased tissue but are expressed at higher levels relative to normal tissue (such as EGFR) and to develop highly sensitive labeling procedures that do not require intermediate washing steps to remove single unbound particles.

MULTIMODALITY IMAGE-GUIDED THERAPY SYSTEM

Image-guided therapy is a multidisciplinary approach using a variety of biomedical imaging modalities to see small-sized lesions in a minimum invasive manner and then to direct drugs and devices to these specific target sites in the body. It has the potential to improve patient care across a wide range of diseases. The interventional radiologists have been using this system with success, which includes 16-slice CT scanner, a four-dimensional ultrasound system, a rotational flat detector angiography system, a robotic arm (Kawasaki, Inc.), a portable high-intensity focused ultrasound unit with a transducer that can be mounted to the robotic arm, a portable SPECT camera that can be attached to a robotic arm, and an EM tracking system that can be used to track the needles, microendoscopes, RFA, and other devices.[42] The integration of treatment planning with CT robot systems or EM needle-tip tracking allows for simultaneous visualization and patient-specific tumor ablation. This modality has been applied in liver tumors in animal models,[43,44] kidney cancers,[45] atrial fibrillation,[46] cardiac dyssynchrony,[47] and prostate cancer.[48,49] Studies on the real-time image-guided radiotherapy of lung cancers are limited.[50]

This modality has the potential to locate the lesion with high precision and can diagnose and treat small (<1.5 cm) lung lesion at the same time and eliminate unnecessary surgeries.[1] The implementation of this modality will require a development of software capable of real-time tracking, integration, visualization, analysis, and monitoring of multimodality, image-guided diagnostic and therapeutic application for peripheral lung cancer. Another important component would be an EM tracking device that would enable navigation using CT and ultrasound guidance for biopsy and RFA. Ultimately, the fiberoptic fluorescence imaging coupled with targeted optical contrast agents can be used for the detection and diagnosis of neoplasia in humans. The fluorescent molecular images can give increased cellular-level detail across systems of increasing biological complexity when compared to commercially available confocal reflectance microscope. The information obtained from the real-time monitoring will be used to modify the procedural plan such as making histologic and immunohistologic diagnosis based on real-time microscopic imaging, determining enzyme activities using enzyme-activatable optical imaging probes, obtaining tissue samples from the most appropriate location, and adjusting the location for local ablative therapy to make sure that all the local tumor has been eliminated. After these techniques are successfully performed and tested in in vitro cell cultures, ex vivo and in vivo animal tissue, human biopsy specimens, and normal in vivo human tissue, they could be used in patient diagnosis and management.

IMAGE GUIDED RADIOFREQUENCY ABLATION OF LUNG MALIGNANCIES

RFA is a minimally invasive procedure in which thin needle electrodes are inserted into a lesion under image guidance (ultrasound or CT). Radiofrequency waves are generated from the electrodes to produce heat around the vicinity of the electrodes to induce irreversible thermal damage to the lesion. RFA device was first approved for liver ablation and bone ablation procedures in 2000 and 2002, respectively. Recently, several studies are being conducted to determine the safety and treatment efficacy of RFA devices in lung cancer treatment.[51,52]

RFA can be considered as safe and technically feasible procedure in treating lung cancers with low incidence of complications. A recent study reported most common adverse effect as pneumothorax, occurring in 32% of treatment sessions. Other significant complications included pleuritic chest pain (18%), hemoptysis (7%), pleural effusions (12%), and chest drain insertion (20%).[51] Based on current literature, a phase III multicenter randomized trial (ROSEL) has been initiated to establish the role of stereotactic radiotherapy versus surgery in patients with operable stage IA lung cancer.[53]

GOLD NANOSHELL PHOTOTHERMAL THERAPY OF LUNG CANCER

Metal nanoshells are a class of nanoparticles with tunable optical resonances. The optical properties of gold nanoshells, along with their biocompatibility and their ease of bioconjugation, make them a potentially ideal targeted therapeutic agent. Nanoshells possess absorption cross sections that are six orders of magnitude larger than indocyanine green, making this material a much stronger NIR absorber and therefore a more effective photothermal coupling agent.[54] By tuning the nanoshells to strongly absorb light in the NIR, where optical transmission through tissue is optimal, a distribution of nanoshells in tissue (in vivo or cell lines) can be used to deliver a therapeutic dose of heat by using moderately low exposures of extracorporeally applied NIR light. A nanoshell suspension is injected intravenously, which accumulate in the tumor region due to the enhanced permeability and retention effect. Subsequent NIR illumination causes localized heating and tissue damage within the tumor. This can lead to complete tumor regression. The histologic sections prepared after the treatment show coagulation, cell shrinkage, and loss of nuclear staining indicating irreversible thermal damage.[55] It has been shown recently that the death rates of A549 lung tumor cell lines after gold nanoparticle exposure increased significantly, making them a promising enhancing agent for photothermal therapy of cancer.[56]

In summary, this new paradigm of molecular image-guided therapy is a multimodality image guidance platform which will use all the available information from several imaging modalities. Real-time imaging can be provided by CT and augmented by EM tracking of needles, microendoscope, and other devices such as RFA probes. The EM tracking data can be superimposed on the real-time and preprocedural imaging data, the display of which is modulated by the real-time tracking data. The information obtained from the real-time monitoring can be used to modify the procedural plan such as obtaining tissue sections for histologic and immunohistologic diagnosis based on real-time microscopic imaging, determining enzyme activities using enzyme-activatable optical imaging probes, and adjusting the location for local ablative therapy to make sure that all the local tumor has been eliminated. The in vivo imaging and other data obtained during the procedure can be integrated with tissue analysis data such as histology, immunohistochemistry, functional genomics, and functional proteomics. This type of multiscale data sets can be combined and analyzed using bioinformatics techniques to further our understanding of various neoplastic diseases at cellular level including lung cancer.

References

1. Xue Z, Wong K, Wong ST. Joint registration and segmentation of serial lung CT images for image-guided lung cancer diagnosis and therapy. *Comput Med Imaging Graph*. 2010;34(1):55–60.
2. Wong KK, Tung CH, Wong ST. In vivo molecular microendoscopy in human lung cancer mouse model. *Proc World Mol Imaging Cong*. 2009 (in Press).
3. Shankar LK, Hoffman JM, Bacharach S, et al. Consensus recommendations for the use of 18F-FDG PET as an indicator of therapeutic response in patients in National Cancer Institute Trials. *J Nucl Med*. 2006;47:1059–1066.
4. Zuluaga AF, Follen M, Boiko I, et al. Optical coherence tomography: a pilot study of a new imaging technique for noninvasive examination of cervical tissue. *Am J Obstet Gynecol*. 2005;193:83–88.
5. Sung KB, Richards-Kortum R, Follen M, et al. Fiber optic confocal reflectance microscopy: a new real-time technique to view nuclear morphology in cervical squamous epithelium in vivo. *Opt Express*. 2003;11:3171–3181.
6. Collier T, Lacy A, Richards-Kortum R, et al. Near real-time confocal microscopy of amelanotic tissue: detection of dysplasia in ex vivo cervical tissue. *Acad Radiol*. 2002;9:504–512.

7. Carlson K, Pavlova I, Collier T, et al. Confocal microscopy: imaging cervical precancerous lesions. *Gynecol Oncol.* 2005;99:S84–S88.

8. Langley RG, Rajadhyaksha M, Dwyer PJ, et al. Confocal scanning laser microscopy of benign and malignant melanocytic skin lesions in vivo. *J Am Acad Dermatol.* 2001;45:365–376.

9. Agero AL, Busam KJ, Benvenuto-Andrade C, et al. Reflectance confocal microscopy of pigmented basal cell carcinoma. *J Am Acad Dermatol.* 2006;54:638–643.

10. Curiel-Lewandrowski C, Williams CM, Swindells KJ, et al. Use of in vivo confocal microscopy in malignant melanoma: an aid in diagnosis and assessment of surgical and nonsurgical therapeutic approaches. *Arch Dermatol.* 2004;140:1127–1132.

11. Agero AL, Gill M, Ardigo M, et al. In vivo reflectance confocal microscopy of mycosis fungoides: A preliminary study. *J Am Acad Dermatol.* 2007;57:435–441.

12. Ardigo M, Cota C, Berardesca E, et al. Concordance between in vivo reflectance confocal microscopy and histology in the evaluation of plaque psoriasis. *J Eur Acad Dermatol Venereol.* 2009;23:660–667.

13. Scope A, Benvenuto-Andrade C, Gill M, et al. Reflectance confocal microscopy of molluscum contagiosum. *Arch Dermatol.* 2008;144:134.

14. Ardigo M, Maliszewski I, Cota C, et al. Preliminary evaluation of in vivo reflectance confocal microscopy features of Discoid lupus erythematosus. *Br J Dermatol.* 2007;156:1196–1203.

15. Astner S, Gonzalez E, Cheung A, et al. Pilot study on the sensitivity and specificity of in vivo reflectance confocal microscopy in the diagnosis of allergic contact dermatitis. *J Am Acad Dermatol.* 2005;53: 986–992.

16. Gonzalez S, Rajadhyaksha M, Rubinstein G, et al. Characterization of psoriasis in vivo by reflectance confocal microscopy. *J Med.* 1999;30:337–356.

17. Gonzalez S, Rajadhyaksha M, Gonzalez-Serva A, et al. Confocal reflectance imaging of folliculitis in vivo: correlation with routine histology. *J Cutan Pathol.* 1999;26:201–205.

18. Rajadhyaksha M, Menaker G, Flotte T, et al. Confocal examination of nonmelanoma cancers in thick skin excisions to potentially guide mohs micrographic surgery without frozen histopathology. *J Invest Dermatol.* 2001;117:1137–1143.

19. Gareau DS, Li Y, Huang B, et al. Confocal mosaicing microscopy in Mohs skin excisions: feasibility of rapid surgical pathology. *J Biomed Opt.* 2008;13:054001.

20. Clark AL, Gillenwater AM, Collier TG, et al. Confocal microscopy for real-time detection of oral cavity neoplasia. *Clin Cancer Res.* 2003;9:4714–4721.

21. Koenig F, Gonzalez S, White WM, et al. Near-infrared confocal laser scanning microscopy of bladder tissue in vivo. *Urology.* 1999;53:853–857.

22. Cookson MJ, Davies CJ, Entwistle A, et al. The microanatomy of the alveolar duct of the human lung imaged by confocal microscopy and visualised with computer-based 3D reconstruction. *Comput Med Imaging Graph.* 1993;17:201–210.

23. Pauly JL, Allison EM, Hurley EL, et al. Fluorescent human lung macrophages analyzed by spectral confocal laser scanning microscopy and multispectral cytometry. *Microsc Res Tech.* 2005;67:79–89.

24. Manelli-Oliveira R, Machado-Santelli GM. Cytoskeletal and nuclear alterations in human lung tumor cells: a confocal microscope study. *Histochem Cell Biol.* 2001;115:403–411.

25. Lam S, Standish B, Baldwin C, et al. In vivo optical coherence tomography imaging of preinvasive bronchial lesions. *Clin Cancer Res.* 2008;14:2006–2011.

26. Whiteman SC, Yang Y, Gey van Pittius D, et al. Optical coherence tomography: real-time imaging of bronchial airways microstructure and detection of inflammatory/neoplastic morphologic changes. *Clin Cancer Res.* 2006;12:813–818.

27. Tsuboi M, Hayashi A, Ikeda N, et al. Optical coherence tomography in the diagnosis of bronchial lesions. *Lung Cancer.* 2005;49:387–394.

28. Bugaj JE, Achilefu S, Dorshow RB, et al. Novel fluorescent contrast agents for optical imaging of in vivo tumors based on a receptor-targeted dye-peptide conjugate platform. *J Biomed Opt.* 2001;6:122–133.

29. Ye Y, Bloch S, Xu B, Achilefu S. Novel near-infrared fluorescent integrin-targeted DFO analogue. *Bioconjug Chem.* 2008;19:225–234.

30. Ye Y, Bloch S, Xu B, Achilefu S. Design, synthesis, and evaluation of near infrared fluorescent multimeric RGD peptides for targeting tumors. *J Med Chem.* 2006;49:2268–2275.

31. Achilefu S, Dorshow RB, Bugaj JE, et al. Novel receptor-targeted fluorescent contrast agents for in vivo tumor imaging. *Invest Radiol.* 2000;35:479–485.

32. Faust A, Waschkau B, Waldeck J, et al. Synthesis and evaluation of a novel hydroxamate based fluorescent photoprobe for imaging of matrix metalloproteinases. *Bioconjug Chem.* 2009;20(5):904–912.

33. Bremer C, Tung CH, Weissleder R. In vivo molecular target assessment of matrix metalloproteinase inhibition. *Nat Med.* 2001;7:743–748.

34. Tung CH, Mahmood U, Bredow S, et al. In vivo imaging of proteolytic enzyme activity using a novel molecular reporter. *Cancer Res.* 2000;60:4953–4958.

35. Anikijenko P, Vo LT, Murr ER, et al. In vivo detection of small subsurface melanomas in athymic mice using noninvasive fiber optic confocal imaging. *J Invest Dermatol.* 2001;117:1442–1448.

36. Ito S, Muguruma N, Kusaka Y, et al. Detection of human gastric cancer in resected specimens using a novel infrared fluorescent anti-human carcinoembryonic antigen antibody with an infrared fluorescence endoscope in vitro. *Endoscopy.* 2001;33:849–853.

37. Horisberger M. Colloidal gold: a cytochemical marker for light and fluorescent microscopy and for transmission and scanning electron microscopy. *Scan Electron Microsc.* 1981:9–31.

38. Kneipp J, Kneipp H, McLaughlin M, et al. In vivo molecular probing of cellular compartments with gold nanoparticles and nanoaggregates. *Nano Lett.* 2006;6:2225–2231.

39. Nie S, Emory SR. Probing single molecules and single nanoparticles by surface-enhanced raman scattering. *Science.* 1997;275:1102–1106.

40. Elghanian R, Storhoff JJ, Mucic RC, et al. Selective colorimetric detection of polynucleotides based on the distance-dependent optical properties of gold nanoparticles. *Science.* 1997;277:1078–1081.

41. Lee KS, El-Sayed MA. Gold and silver nanoparticles in sensing and imaging: sensitivity of plasmon response to size, shape, and metal composition. *J Phys Chem B.* 2006;110:19220–19225.

42. Wood BJ, Locklin JK, Viswanathan A, et al. Technologies for guidance of radiofrequency ablation in the multimodality interventional suite of the future. *J Vasc Interv Radiol.* 2007;18:9–24.

43. Levy EB, Zhang H, Lindisch D, et al. Electromagnetic tracking-guided percutaneous intrahepatic portosystemic shunt creation in a swine model. *J Vasc Interv Radiol.* 2007;18:303–307.

44. Banovac F, Tang J, Xu S, et al. Precision targeting of liver lesions using a novel electromagnetic navigation device in physiologic phantom and swine. *Med Phys.* 2005;32:2698–2705.

45. Coleman J, Singh A, Pinto P, et al. Radiofrequency-assisted laparoscopic partial nephrectomy: clinical and histologic results. *J Endourol.* 2007;21:600–605.

46. Thiagalingam A, Manzke R, D'Avila A, et al. Intraprocedural volume imaging of the left atrium and pulmonary veins with rotational X-ray angiography: implications for catheter ablation of atrial fibrillation. *J Cardiovasc Electrophysiol.* 2008;19:293–300.

47. Tournoux FB, Manzke R, Chan RC, et al. Integrating functional and anatomical information to facilitate cardiac resynchronization therapy. *Pacing Clin Electrophysiol.* 2007;30:1021–1022.

48. Xu S, Kruecker J, Turkbey B, et al. Real-time MRI-TRUS fusion for guidance of targeted prostate biopsies. *Comput Aided Surg.* 2008;13:255–264.

49. Singh AK, Kruecker J, Xu S, et al. Initial clinical experience with real-time transrectal ultrasonography-magnetic resonance imaging fusion-guided prostate biopsy. *BJU Int.* 2008;101:841–845.

50. Lin T, Cervino LI, Tang X, et al. Fluoroscopic tumor tracking for image-guided lung cancer radiotherapy. *Phys Med Biol.* 2009;54:981–992.

51. Zhu JC, Yan TD, Glenn D, et al. Radiofrequency ablation of lung tumors: feasibility and safety. *Ann Thorac Surg.* 2009;87:1023–1028.

52. Chang JY, Dong L, Liu H, et al. Image-guided radiation therapy for non-small cell lung cancer. *J Thorac Oncol.* 2008;3:177–186.

53. Hurkmans CW, Cuijpers JP, Lagerwaard FJ, et al. Recommendations for implementing stereotactic radiotherapy in peripheral stage IA non-small cell lung cancer: report from the Quality Assurance Working Party of the randomised phase III ROSEL study. *Radiat Oncol.* 2009;4:1.

54. O'Neal DP, Hirsch LR, Halas NJ, et al. Photo-thermal tumor ablation in mice using near infrared-absorbing nanoparticles. *Cancer Lett.* 2004;209:171–176.

55. Hirsch LR, Stafford RJ, Bankson JA, et al. Nanoshell-mediated near-infrared thermal therapy of tumors under magnetic resonance guidance. *Proc Natl Acad Sci USA.* 2003;100:13549–13554.

56. Liu X, Lloyd MC, Fedorenko IV, et al. Enhanced imaging and accelerated photothermalysis of A549 human lung cancer cells by gold nanospheres. *Nanomedicine.* 2008;3:617–626.

Molecular Pathology

Molecular Diagnostics of Lung Cancer

21

▶ Sanja Dacic

The diagnosis of lung carcinoma is largely based on morphology. Ancillary tools such as histochemical stains and immunohistochemistry are used in occasional cases. Our understanding of lung carcinoma carcinogenesis at the genetic level has significantly expanded over the last few decades, but only several observations have been implemented into molecular diagnostics of lung cancer. Development of invasive lung carcinoma is a result of sequential accumulation of genetic and epigenetic changes which are also reflected at the morphological level. However, every tumor does not harbor the same mutations in the same genes, and the different tumors acquire mutations in a different sequence. This represents a fundamental limitation in diagnostic sensitivity and specificity of genetic analysis regardless of the testing approach. This chapter will focus on applications of molecular assays that are currently used to address some diagnostically problematic areas including differentiation between primary and metastatic tumors, origin of tumors occurring in lung allografts, diagnosis of salivary gland tumors, and potential classification of poorly differentiated carcinomas.

PRIMARY VERSUS METASTATIC TUMORS

The distinction between a primary lung carcinoma and lung metastasis in patients with prior history of extrathoracic malignancy can be established on clinical grounds or by immunohistochemistry in some cases. The presence of multiple pulmonary nodules is usually considered as evidence of metastatic disease. However, in patients who present with a solitary lung nodule, particularly if they have history of squamous cell carcinoma, this distinction may be extremely difficult. Histologic criteria that are used by surgical pathologists include the comparison of histologic grade and identification of premalignant changes in the respiratory epithelium. The accuracy of this approach is uncertain. The correct diagnosis has practical importance for choice of therapy. The surgical approach and adjuvant therapy are usually different in these situations. Furthermore, patients with early-stage non–small cell lung carcinoma usually have better prognosis than patients with metastatic carcinoma. Several molecular assays can be used including PCR-based DNA clonality assays, mutational analysis, SNPs, and gene expression assays to distinguish between these two possibilities.

DNA-Clonality Assays

The clonal origin of a tissue may be assessed by analysis of somatic genetic alterations (e.g., loss of heterozygosity [LOH]) or chromosome X inactivation pattern (X-linked clonality analysis).[1] These PCR clonality assays are based on microsatellite analysis. Microsatellites represent a highly polymorphic and repetitive noncoding DNA sequences widely distributed in the human genome. Several microsatellites have been used for DNA fingerprinting and are very useful in genetic linkage analysis. If the selected polymorphic region is related to known tumor suppressor gene, a possibility of mutation or function dysregulation of the corresponding gene can be determined based on observed alterations of microsatellite markers. Therefore, the assumption is that the LOH of a given genetic marker is linked to loss of tumor suppressor genes. Comparison of patterns of LOH between two tumors can help to determine whether the tumors are clonally similar (metastases) or different (independent primaries) (Fig. 21-1).[2–4] There are several issues that should be

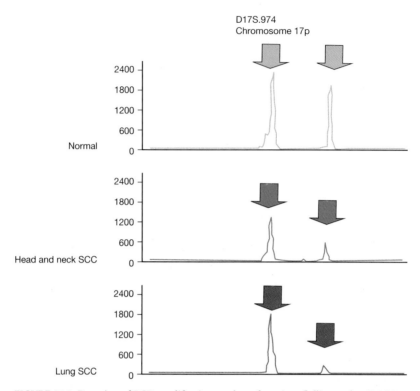

FIGURE 21-1 Detection of PCR amplification products for microsatellite marker D17S.974 located on chromosome 17p by capillary electrophoresis. The allelic peak height ratios were calculated in the normal and tumor samples. Squamous cell carcinoma of the lung and head and neck exhibited a concordant profile of allelic loss.

addressed.[5] First, LOH assay requires matched normal DNA in order to determine whether an individual is heterozygous (informative) or homozygous (noninformative) for a particular chromosomal locus. Normal DNA may be obtained from morphologically normal-appearing tissue or from the patient's leukocytes, which may not be readily available. The second issue is reliability of the results. Some authors report that LOH assay can definitely establish whether tumor represents a metastasis or a new primary lung cancer in 91% of cases.[3] In our experience, a number of selected microsatellite markers and selection of chromosomal loci may influence the results and interpretation. Other considerations include tumor cell heterogeneity, sample size, tissue control, artifactual allelic dropout, cost, and turnaround time.

X-linked clonality analysis can be used only for clonality analysis in informative females, does not assess tumor heterogeneity, and does not provide any data on the precise genetic alteration responsible for clonal proliferation. In females, each X chromosome may be inactivated through a random methylation process early in embryogenesis. Once established in a particular cell, the methylation pattern is invariably transmitted to all the progenies. Hence, a unique nonrandom pattern of methylation is expected in malignant tumors, since all cells are supposed to derive from the same precursor. DNA probes can detect polymorphisms at particular X-linked loci to allow distinctions between the maternal X chromosome and paternal X chromosomes in a female subject. The active X chromosome may be distinguished from the inactive X chromosome by its state of methylation or by gene expression. Ideally, half the cells in a polyclonal reactive tissue will have inactivated the paternally derived X chromosome and half will have inactivated the maternally derived X chromosome. A monoclonal or clonal population of cells by contrast will have exclusively inactivated one X chromosome. There are several polymorphic foci that have been used to assess clonality by this assay. The X-linked human androgen receptor gene (HUMARA gene) is particularly well suited for analysis because it has a high rate of heterozygosity ("informativeness" >90%)

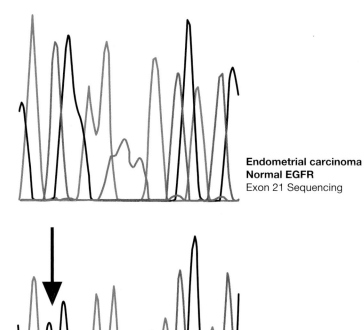

FIGURE 21-2 An example of EGFR mutational analysis in a patient with a history of endometrial adenocarcinoma presenting with a solitary lung nodule. The distinction cannot be made based on morphology and immunohistochemistry.

Endometrial carcinoma
Normal EGFR
Exon 21 Sequencing

Lung nodule
Mutant EGFR
Exon 21 Sequencing
(T→G transversion)

and consistent patterns of methylation. While nonrandom patterns of X chromosome inactivation may occur in up to 25% of female subjects (skewed lyonization), assessment of the HUMARA assay can be helpful in assessing selective highly concentrated cellular elements. This assay is technically challenging and is less suitable for the clinical practice than LOH assay.

Mutational Analysis

Several reports in literature indicate significance of DNA mutational analysis of p53 and other genes by DNA direct sequencing or other mutation detection techniques.[6,7] Our recent experience indicates that detection of *EGFR* mutations may not only predict patients' response to TKI therapies but also can be of diagnostic importance. Somatic mutations of *EGFR* unique to lung adenocarcinoma have been independently reported by several groups. Although several reports indicated the presence of these mutations in colorectal carcinomas and head and neck carcinomas, recent reports question those results. The differentiation of lung adenocarcinoma from endometrial carcinoma, breast, or pancreatic adenocarcinomas may be difficult based on morphology and immunohistochemistry. *EGFR* mutations in exons 18 to 21 may be extremely useful in making this distinction (Fig. 21-2). Unfortunately, these mutations occur in only 10% of Western population. On the other hand, up to 50% of Asian patients may harbor these mutations, and therefore, this assay may be more suitable for diagnostic use in this subset of patients.

ORIGIN OF TUMORS IN LUNG ALLOGRAFTS

The origins of malignancies that develop after transplantation of lung allografts are not always clear. In our experience, the most common malignancies in lung allografts are primary lung carcinomas. However, more challenging cases are metastatic carcinomas to the lung, which may represent either incidentally transmitted occult tumors from clinically healthy donors to the recipients or metastasis of a recipient's primary tumor outside of the lung. To resolve the question of donor

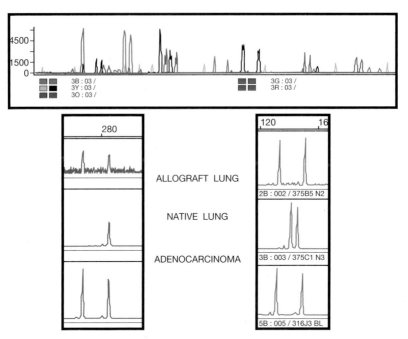

FIGURE 21-3 Molecular analysis of adenocarcinoma arising in lung allograft. Paraffin-embedded tissue of adenocarcinoma and the recipient's native lung was microdissected and amplified by multiplex PCR using AmpFLSTR kit, which amplifies 16 STR loci. The PCR products were detected by capillary electrophoresis. The allele sizes of the STR loci overlap in size but are detectable by the use of different fluorescent labels (**top panel**). The results indicate that the tumor is of donor's origin.

versus recipient tumor origin, DNA typing can be performed.[8,9] There are several commercially available diagnostic kits containing short tandem repeats (STRs). Population statistics for these genetic loci have been determined and are used in the calculation of genetic profile frequencies. DNA typing is performed as a multiplex PCR, which involves adding more than one set of PCR primers to the reaction in order to target multiple locations throughout the genome. This is an ideal technique for DNA typing because the probability of identical alleles in two individuals decreases with an increase in the number of polymorphic loci examined. Many commercial DNA typing kits also have the amelogenin gene, which is located on the X and Y chromosomes and is useful in determining the sex of an individual. The assay includes analysis and comparison of genomic DNA from the tumor in question and the recipient DNA (either from tissue or peripheral blood). If tumor and recipient DNA match, then the tumor is of recipient origin; if they are different, the tumor came from the donor (Fig. 21-3).

MOLECULAR DIAGNOSIS OF BRONCHIAL MUCOEPIDERMOID CARCINOMA

The t(11;19)(q21;p13) is the major chromosomal abnormality observed in salivary gland mucoepidermoid carcinomas.[10–13] This translocation involves two genes: _mucoepidermoid carcinoma translocated 1_ (*MECT1*) gene located on chromosomes 19p13 and a _mammalian mastermind-like 2_ (*MAML2*) located on 11q21.[10,12,13] *MECT1-MAML2* fuses exon 1 of *MECT1* with exons 2 to 5 of *MAML2* (Fig. 21-4). *MECT1* is a coactivator of cyclic AMP responsive element binding protein. *MAML2* is an essential coactivator of NOTCH receptor transcriptional activation and signaling. The translocation disrupts NOTCH signaling, activating transcription of NOTCH target genes, and stimulates aberrant activation of downstream cyclic AMP/cyclic AMP responsive element binding protein-signaling genes. Similar to head and neck mucoepidermoid

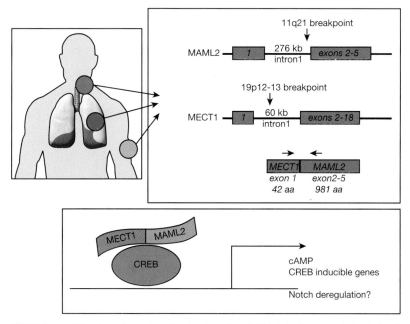

FIGURE 21-4 The t(11;19) translocation involves the MECT1 (also known as TORC 1) and the MAML2 gene. The translocation disrupts NOTCH, signaling activating transcription for NOTCH targeted genes, and stimulates aberrant activation of downstream cyclic MAP/cAMP responsive element binding protein signaling genes.

carcinomas, this translocation is exclusively seen in bronchopulmonary mucoepidermoid carcinomas when compared to primary lung squamous, adenosquamous, and adenocarcinomas.[14]

Several assays could be used to detect this genetic abnormality including conventional cytogenetics, dual-color break-apart FISH probe, and RT-PCR. Recently, Behboudi et al.[10] demonstrated that the translocation results in the expression of a 110-kD fusion protein that could be detected by immunohistochemistry. The authors generated a polyclonal antibody to the fusion protein and showed in a small subset of salivary gland mucoepidermoid carcinomas that positive staining correlated with the molecular identification of the translocation. FISH assay detects only *MAML2* gene rearrangement and does not indicate the fusion partner or completely exclude inversions. FISH seems to be a more sensitive but less specific approach for the diagnosis of *MAML2* rearrangement than RT-PCR analysis, most likely due to formalin fixation interfering with RNA integrity.

MOLECULAR DIAGNOSIS OF UNDIFFERENTIATED CARCINOMAS

Two commercial diagnostic tests, qRT-PCR-based and gene expression assays, are presently available for analysis of origin of undifferentiated carcinomas (Fig. 21-5).[15,16] Gene expression diagnostic test uses a high-density oligonucleotide array with 1668 gene probe sets of markers which can identify 15 different tissue types, including the lung (Pathwork Tissue of Origin Test, Pathwork Diagnostics, Sunnyvale, California).[15,17] This test could be performed on a fresh or formalin-fixed paraffin embedded tissue. FDA has approved its use on a fresh tissue. The test is determining the similarity of gene expression patterns between tumors of unknown origin and cancers from 1 of 15 known origins. For each specimen, the algorithm reduces the highly complex expression data into 15 separate similarity scores. These continuous scores (scale 0–100) are reported to the pathologist, who then establishes whether or not a particular tissue type is present in the specimen. A reported specificity for this test is 89% and sensitivity 99%. The test is associated with the

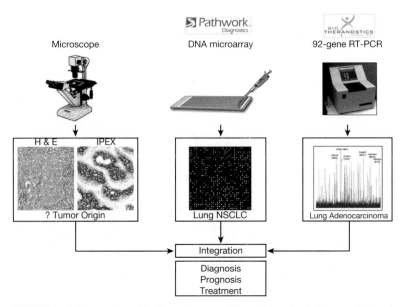

FIGURE 21-5 Two commercial diagnostic tests, qRT-PCR-based (BioTheranostics) and gene expression assays (Pathwork Diagnostics), are presently available for analysis of origin of undifferentiated carcinomas, including lung carcinomas.

high cost. Although non–small cell lung tumors are present on this platform, a histologic subtype is not specified. That would be extremely important since different histologic types of lung carcinomas have different gene expression profiles.

The second assay that is commercially available but not FDA approved is a 92-gene panel RT-PCR for classifying 32 tumor classes (Theros Cancer TYPE ID, BioTheranostics).[16] The authors essentially converted a large microarray database to the RT-PCR platform, which should be suitable for clinical laboratory. The overall success rate is 87% and varies for different tumor types. This assay includes lung small cell and non–small cell carcinomas including adenocarcinomas/large cell carcinomas and squamous cell carcinomas.

MOLECULAR TESTING FOR TARGETED THERAPIES

DNA Mutational Analysis

Multiple approaches for assessment of *EGFR* status in lung carcinoma have been introduced into clinical practice including DNA mutational analysis, FISH/chromogenic in situ hybridization (CISH), and immunohistochemistry. Since *EGFR* gene mutations are the best predictor of a patient's response to EGFR TKI, various DNA mutational assays have been described (Table 21-1). Sangen DNA direct sequencing is the most common mutational technique used by many laboratories. This assay may not detect mutations if tumor cells represent <25% of the sample, which may be an issue with a small biopsy and cytology specimens.

Many other more sensitive mutation detection techniques have been reported. Similar to DNA direct sequencing, these assays perform better on fresh tissue samples. Some of these more sensitive assays (e.g., SSCP, DHPLC) can screen large number of samples in a short period of time but require direct sequencing for result confirmation. A significance of low-abundance mutations detected in heterogeneous samples with these more sensitive assays is uncertain. In addition to *EGFR* mutations, screening for *KRAS* mutations is also implemented in the clinical practice. *EGFR* and *KRAS* mutations are mutually exclusive, and *KRAS* mutations that lead to substitutions of amino acids for glycines at positions 12 and 13 can be identified in up to 30% of

Table 21-1	Methods for detection of EGFR mutations in lung cancer specimens		
Technique	Sensitivity (% Mutant DNA)	Mutations Identified	Comprehensive Detection of Deletions and Insertion
Direct sequencing	25	Known and new	Yes
PCR-SSCP	10	Known and new	Yes
TaqMan PCR	10	Known only	No
Loop-hybrid mobility shift assay	7.5	Known only	Yes
Cycleave PCR	5	Known only	Yes
PCR-RFLP and length analysis	5	Known only	Yes
MALDI-TOF MS-based genotyping	5	Known only	No
PNA-LNA PCR clamp	1	Known only	No
Scorpions ARMS	1	Known only	No
dHPLC	1	Known and new	Yes
Single-molecule sequencing	0.2	Known and new	Yes
Mutant-enriched PCR	0.2	Known only	No
SMAP	0.1	Known only	No

ARMS, amplified refractory mutation system; dHPLC, denaturing high-performance liquid chromatography; MALDI-TOF MS, matrix-assisted laser desorption/ionization time-of-flight mass spectrometry; PNA-LNA, peptide nucleic acid-locked nucleic acid; SSCP, single-strand conformation polymorphism.
Source: Modified from *Clin Cancer Res.* 2007;13:4954–4955.

adenocarcinomas.[18,19] At the present, there are no guidelines in terms of specimen selection, methods, and interpretation criteria that would represent a standard of patient care.[19]

FISH/CISH

Even though most laboratories accepted DNA mutational methods as most reliable assays that predict responders to *EGFR* tyrosine kinase inhibitors, it is still uncertain if *EGFR* FISH or CISH may provide additional clinically useful information.[20–24] The complicating factor is that *EGFR* mutations are frequently associated with increased *EGFR* gene copy numbers. Interpretation criteria for *EGFR* FISH have neither been standardized nor validated yet. The group from University of Colorado proposed a scoring system for FISH-positive samples taking into consideration classical amplification and polysomy (Table 21-2).[24,25] The importance of distinguishing increased copy number of chromosome 7 without *EGFR* gene amplification (high polysomy) and with *EGFR* gene amplification is still uncertain, and additional studies are needed to validate the significance of those criteria. Many reported studies indicated that *EGFR* FISH results correlate with *EGFR* gene mutations, but the correlation is not absolute. It is important to mention that EGFR-FISH positivity was not limited to *EGFR*-mutated group only, but it was also present in tumors harboring *KRAS* mutations and in *EGFR* and *KRAS* wild-type tumors.[26] This observation suggests that EGFR FISH cannot be solely used as a method to predict a patient's response to EGFR-TKI.

Table 21-2	UCCC criteria for stratification of NSCLC patients according to the EGFR FISH assay

EGFR FISH Positive

- Specimens with EGFR gene amplification, defined as
  - (a) EGFR gene to CEP 7 ratio > 2
  - (b) Small gene cluster (4–10 copies) or innumerable tight gene cluster in >10% of the tumor cells independent of the EGFR to CEP 7 ratio
  - (c) Larger and brighter EGFR signals than CEP 7 signals in >10% of the tumor cells while EGFR signals are smaller than the CEP 7 signals in the adjacent stromal and reactive cells independent of the EGFR to CEP 7 ratio
  - (d) >15 copies of the EGFR signals in >10% of tumor cells independent of the EGFR to CEP 7 ratio
- Specimens with ≥40% of cells displaying ≥4 copies of the EGFR signal

EGFR FISH Negative

- Specimens without gene amplification as defined above and with <40% of cells displaying >4 copies of the EGFR signal

Source: Varella-Garcia M. Stratification of non–small cell lung cancer patients for therapy with epidermal growth factor receptor inhibitors: the EGFR fluorescence in situ hybridization assay. *Diagn Pathol.* 2006;1:19.

EGFR Immunohistochemistry

EGFR immunohistochemistry results highly depend on the antibody type procedure protocols, and interpretation criteria.[27–29] Recently, mutation-specific rabbit monoclonal antibodies detecting two most common EGFR mutations (exon 19 deletions and exon 21 L858 mutation) have been reported.[30] This simple assay should be further validated, because it may provide a rapid and cost-effective clinical test to identify lung cancer patients responsive to EGFR-based therapies.

References

1. Diaz-Cano SJ, Blanes A, Wolfe HJ. PCR techniques for clonality assays. *Diagn Mol Pathol.* 2001;10:24–33.
2. Beer DG, Kardia SLR, Huang C-C, et al. Gene-expression profiles predict survival of patients with lung adenocarcinoma. *Nat Med.* 2002;8:816–824.
3. Leong PP, Rezai B, Koch WM, et al. Distinguishing second primary tumors from lung metastases in patients with head and neck squamous cell carcinoma. *J Natl Cancer Inst.* 1998;90:972–977.
4. Schwartz LH, Ozsahin M, Zhang GN, et al. Synchronous and metachronous head and neck carcinomas. *Cancer.* 1994;74:1933–1938.
5. Tomlinson IPM, Lambros MBK, Roylance RR. Loss of heterozygosity analysis: practically and conceptually flawed? *Genes, Chromosomes Cancer.* 2002;34:349–353.
6. Lau DH, Yang B, Hu R, et al. Clonal origin of multiple lung cancers: K-ras and p53 mutations determined by nonradioisotopic single-strand conformation polymorphism analysis. *Diagn Mol Pathol.* 1997;6:179–184.
7. Yang HK, Linnoila RI, Conrad NK, et al. TP53 and RAS mutations in metachronous tumors from patients with cancer of the upper aerodigestive tract. *Int J Cancer.* 1995;64:229–233.
8. Budowle B, Sprecher CJ. Concordance study on population database samples using the PowerPlex 16 kit and AmpFlSTR Profiler Plus kit and AmpFlSTR COfiler kit. *J Forensic Sci.* 2001;46:637–641.

9. Collins PJ, Hennessy LK, Leibelt CS, et al. Developmental validation of a single-tube amplification of the 13 CODIS STR loci, D2S1338, D19S433, and amelogenin: the AmpFlSTR Identifiler PCR Amplification Kit. *J Forensic Sci.* 2004;49:1265–1277.

10. Behboudi A, Enlund F, Winnes M, et al. Molecular classification of mucoepidermoid carcinomas-prognostic significance of the MECT1-MAML2 fusion oncogene. *Genes, Chromosomes Cancer.* 2006;45: 470–481.

11. Nordkvist A, Gustafsson H, Juberg-Ode M, et al. Recurrent rearrangements of 11q14–22 in mucoepidermoid carcinoma. *Cancer Genet Cytogenet.* 1994;74:77–83.

12. Okabe M, Miyabe S, Nagatsuka H, et al. MECT1-MAML2 fusion transcript defines a favorable subset of mucoepidermoid carcinoma. *Clin Cancer Res.* 2006;12:3902–3907.

13. Tonon G, Gehlhaus KS, Yonescu R, et al. Multiple reciprocal translocations in salivary gland mucoepidermoid carcinomas. *Cancer Genet Cytogenet.* 2004;152:15–22.

14. Achcar RDOD, Nikiforova MN, Dacic S, et al. Mammalian mastermind like 2 11q21 gene rearrangement in bronchopulmonary mucoepidermoid carcinoma. *Hum Pathol.* 2009;40:854–860.

15. Dumur CI, Lyons-Weiler M, Sciulli C, et al. Interlaboratory performance of a microarray-based gene expression test to determine tissue of origin in poorly differentiated and undifferentiated cancers. *J Mol Diag.* 2008;10:67–77.

16. Ma X-J, Patel R, Wang X, et al. Molecular classification of human cancers using a 92-gene real-time quantitative polymerase chain reaction assay. *Arch Pathol Lab Med.* 2006;130:465–473.

17. Monzon FA, Lyons-Weiler M, Buturovic LJ, et al. Multicenter validation of a 1,550-gene expression profile for identification of tumor tissue of origin. *J Clin Oncol.* 2009;27:2503–2508.

18. Ahrendt SA, Decker PA, Alawi EA, et al. Cigarette smoking is strongly associated with mutation of the K-ras gene in patients with primary adenocarcinoma of the lung. *Cancer.* 2001;92:1525–1530.

19. Eberhard DA, Johnson BE, Amler LC, et al. Mutations in the epidermal growth factor receptor and in KRAS are predictive and prognostic indicators in patients with non-small-cell lung cancer treated with chemotherapy alone and in combination with erlotinib. *J Clin Oncol.* 2005;23:5900–5909.

20. Cappuzzo F, Hirsch FR, Rossi E, et al. Epidermal growth factor receptor gene and protein and gefitinib sensitivity in non-small-cell lung cancer. *J Natl Cancer Inst.* 2005;97:643–655.

21. Chang JW-C, Liu H-P, Hsieh M-H, et al. Increased epidermal growth factor receptor (EGFR) gene copy number is strongly associated with EGFR mutations and adenocarcinoma in non-small cell lung cancers: a chromogenic in situ hybridization study of 182 patients. *Lung Cancer.* 2008;61:328–339.

22. Gallegos Ruiz MI, Floor K, Vos W, et al. Epidermal growth factor receptor (EGFR) gene copy number detection in non-small-cell lung cancer; a comparison of fluorescence in situ hybridization and chromogenic in situ hybridization. *Histopathology.* 2007;51:631–637.

23. Hirsch FR, Varella-Garcia M, McCoy J, et al. Increased epidermal growth factor receptor gene copy number detected by fluorescence in situ hybridization associates with increased sensitivity to gefitinib in patients with bronchioloalveolar carcinoma subtypes: a Southwest Oncology Group Study. *J Clin Oncol.* 2005;23:6838–6845.

24. Sholl LM, John Iafrate A, Chou Y-P, et al. Validation of chromogenic in situ hybridization for detection of EGFR copy number amplification in nonsmall cell lung carcinoma. *Modern Pathol.* 2007;20: 1028–1035.

25. Varella-Garcia M. Stratification of non-small cell lung cancer patients for therapy with epidermal growth factor receptor inhibitors: the EGFR fluorescence in situ hybridization assay. *Diagn Pathol.* 2006;1:19.

26. Dacic S, Yongli S, Yousem SA, et al. Clinico-pathologic predictors of EGFR/KRAS mutational status in primary lung carcinomas. *Modern Pathol.* 2010;23:159–168.

27. Clark GM, Zborowski DM, Culbertson JL, et al. Clinical utility of epidermal growth factor receptor expression for selecting patients with advanced non-small cell lung cancer for treatment with erlotinib. *J Thoracic Oncol.* 2006;1:837–846.

28. Hirsch FR, Dziadziuszko R, Thatcher N, et al. Epidermal growth factor receptor immunohistochemistry: comparison of antibodies and cutoff points to predict benefit from gefitinib in a phase 3 placebo-controlled study in advanced nonsmall-cell lung cancer. *Cancer.* 2008;112:1114–1121.

29. Han S-W, Kim T-Y, Jeon YK, et al. Optimization of patient selection for gefitinib in non-small cell lung cancer by combined analysis of epidermal growth factor receptor mutation, K-ras mutation, and Akt phosphorylation. *Clin Cancer Res.* 2006;12:2538–2544.

30. Yu J, Kane S, Wu J, et al. Mutation-specific antibodies for the detection of EGFR mutations in non-small-cell lung cancer. *Clin Cancer Res.* 2009;15:3023–3028.

22

Molecular Targeted Therapy of Lung Cancer

▶ Sanja Dacic

T he most frequently targeted pathways in non–small cell lung carcinomas (NSCLC) have involved the epidermal growth factor receptor (EGFR), vascular endothelial growth factor (VEGF), and the VEGF receptor (VEGFR). Recently reported clinical trials using agents targeting these molecules showed their potential to affect the treatment of patients with NSCLC (Table 22-1).

EGFR

The EGFR signaling network plays a central role in the development of many cancers including NSCLC. EGFR (HER-1/ErbB1) is a member of the ErbB family of tyrosine kinase receptors (TKs), which includes HER-1/ErbB1, HER-2/neu/ErbB2, HER-3/ErbB3, and HER-4/ErbB4. It is composed of extracellular (ligand binding), transmembrane, and intracellular (tyrosine-kinase) domain. Upon ligand binding and receptor homodimerization or heterodimerization and activation, activated EGFR signals downstream to the PI3K/AKT and RAS/RAF/MAPK pathways (Fig. 22-1). These intracellular signaling pathways regulate key processes such as apoptosis and proliferation. EGFR is expressed in a large proportion of epithelial tumors and its role in lung cancer has been known for decades.

Therapies Targeting EGFR

Two treatment strategies to target EGFR have been developed: monoclonal antibodies directed against the extracellular ligand-binding domain of the EGFR (e.g., cetuximab)[1–3] and small molecule TK inhibitors (TKIs) (e.g., gefitinib and erlotinib).[4–7] Initial clinical trials reported objective responses to EGFR TKIs in 10% to 27% of unselected NSCLC patients after failure of chemotherapy. Several clinical features were found to be associated with increased response rate to EGFR TKIs including female gender, never smokers, Asian ethnicity, and adenocarcinoma histology. Several groups of investigators independently identified somatic mutations in the exons 18 to 21 of the TK domain of EGFR in responders to TKI therapies.[8–10] These mutations occur in approximately 10% of Western and up to 50% of Asian patients. The most common are in-frame deletions in exon 19 (45%), followed by a point mutation (CTG to CGG) in exon 21 at nucleotide 2573 which results in substitution of leucine by arginine at codon 858 (L858R) (41%). Other less common mutations which are associated with sensitivity to EGFR TKIs include G719 mutations in exon 18 and the L861 mutations in exon 21. In recent prospective clinical trials of gefitinib or erlotinib, response rates of EGFR-mutated cases ranged from 65% to 90%. In most studies, patients with EGFR mutations and a response to erlotinib showed a longer progression-free survival and a trend towards improved overall survival.

EGFR Mutations and Morphology

The correlation between morphology and *EGFR* mutations is still controversial but indicates that the histologic subtype of NSCLC should be explicitly reported in pathology reports. Initial studies indicated that *EGFR* mutations are most frequently observed in bronchioloalveolar

Table 22-1	Investigational agents in non–small cell lung cancer		
Agent	**Target(s)**	**Class**	**Latest Phase of Development**
Erlotinib	EGFR	TKI	FDA approved for NSCLC in second- and third-line treatment
Gefitinib	EGFR	TKI	Phase 3[a]
Cetuximab	EGFR	Monoclonal antibody	Phase 3
Sorafenib	VEGFR-1,-2,-3; B-Raf; PDGFR-B; c-Kit	TKI	Phase 3
Sunitinib	VEGFR-1,-2; PDGFR; c-Kit	TKI	Phase 3
Cediranib	VEGFR-1,-2,-3	TKI	Phase 2
Bevacizumab	VEGF	Monoclonal antibody	FDA approved for NSCLC first line in combination with carboplatin and paclitaxel
Vandetanib	VEGFR-2, EGFR, RET	TKI	Phase 3
CP-751871	IGF-1R	Monoclonal antibody	Phase 3
NOV-002	Glutathione mimetic	Oxidized glutathione conjugated to cisplatin	Phase 3

[a]Initially FDA approved was rescinded after a phase 3 trial failed to confirm an overall survival benefit.
EGFR, epidermal growth factor receptor; FDA, U.S. Food and Drug Administration; IGF-1R, insulin-like growth factor receptor; NSCLC, non-small cell lung cancer; PDGFR, platelet-derived growth factor receptor; TKI, tyrosine kinase inhibitor; VEGF, vascular endothelial growth factor; VEGFR, VEGF receptor.
Source: Bean J, Brennan C, Shih J-Y, et al. MET amplification occurs with or without T790M mutations in EGFR mutant lung tumors with acquired resistance to gefitinib or erlotinib. *Proc Natl Acad Sci USA.* 2007;104:20932–20937.

carcinomas (BAC).[11–14] However, studies that applied strict 2004 WHO definition of BAC failed to demonstrate this association. Subsequently, several reports showed that mixed subtype of invasive adenocarcinoma with a BAC component were commonly associated with *EGFR* mutations, although other studies did not confirm this correlation. More recent studies found a link between papillary differentiation and *EGFR* mutations.[15,16] In our experience, there is a large overlap in histologic growth patterns between different adenocarcinomas with a different mutational profile. *EGFR* mutations are extremely rare in large cell carcinomas, small cell carcinomas, and large cell neuroendocrine carcinomas.

Primary Resistance to EGFR Inhibitors

Genetic mutations in the gene encoding proteins involved in the *EGFR* signaling cascade (*KRAS, HER2, BRAF, PI3K, LKB1, SHP2*) seem to exist as mutually exclusive somatic mutations, with the possible exception of those in PI3K.[17] *KRAS* mutations are predictor of failure of EGFR TKI therapy. They occur most often in adenocarcinomas of smokers and are adverse prognostic factor.[18–20] Mucinous differentiation in mixed subtypes of adenocarcinomas and mucinous type of BAC strongly correlates with *KRAS* mutations.[21,22] *HER2* mutations are very similar to *EGFR* mutations, affecting adenocarcinomas with BAC morphology in women, never smokers and may predict sensitivity to other targeted therapies.[23] It has been reported that mutation of the *BRAF* gene occurs in about 1% to 3% of lung adenocarcinomas.[23] Because of the low incidence, it is not clear how patients with *BRAF* mutation respond to EGFR-TKIs. Animal models and early clinical

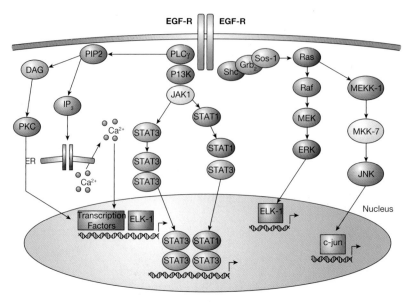

FIGURE 22-1 EGFR signaling pathway.

trials demonstrated that tumors harboring *BRAF* mutation (V600E) showed regression induced by a specific MEK inhibitor, CI-104045. [24,25]

Therefore, clinical testing in lung adenocarcinomas goes beyond *EGFR* mutation status, and some clinical laboratories are putting into practice a comprehensive mutational profiles for lung adenocarcinoma (Fig. 22-2). [26]

Secondary Resistance to EGFR Inhibitors

The T790M *EGFR* mutation was initially considered to confer secondary resistance toTKIs. [27–29] Using more sensitive mutation-detection techniques, it was shown that this mutation may coexist with L858R mutations, which indicated that T790M might confer pretreatment (primary) resistance to EGFR TKIs. Importantly, the presence of T790M at such a low frequency did not preclude significant responses to therapy with TKIs among patients with sensitivity-conferring *EGFR* mutations, but it was associated with a significant difference in median progression-free

FIGURE 22-2 Summary of existing and proposed molecular tests in lung adeno-carcinomas in clinical practice.

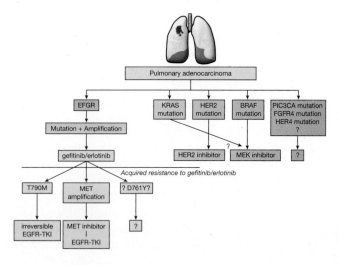

survival. This mutation resembles a series of mutations that occur in the *BCR–ABL* gene that are linked to resistance to the TKI, imatinib. A novel T854A mutation responsible for acquired resistance in a patient with EGFR-mutant adenocarcinomas has been reported.[30]

Amplification of *MET* has recently been identified as a second mechanism of EGFR TKI resistance.[31] The incidence of *MET* amplification in TKI-resistant tumor specimens was 21%, but only 3% in specimens from a cohort who had never received TKI treatment.[32] Somatic *EGFR* mutations and *MET* amplification are not mutually exclusive events, and therefore, additional studies will be needed to clarify the role of MET in *de novo* and/or acquired resistance.

VEGF

Antivascular treatment represents a novel type of molecular-based antitumor therapies. The most important molecule in physiologic and pathologic angiogenesis is VEGF.[33] VEGF is recognized by two receptors found on the surface of endothelial cells, VEGFR-1 (FLT-1) and VEGFR-2 (KDR). VEGFR-2 plays the primary role in the activation of endothelial cells. VEGF activates signaling pathways important in vascular permeability, endothelial cell proliferation, endothelial cell migration, and cell survival (Fig. 22-3).[34] Overexpression of VEGF by tumor cells and elevated levels in blood have been associated with tumor progression and poor prognosis in NSCLC. As with the EGFR, monoclonal antibodies targeting VEGF (bevacizumab) and small molecule tryosine kinase inhibitors of VEGFR (sorafenib, sunitinib, cediranib) have been developed.[33,35,36] As a result of the ECOG E4599 trial with bevacizumab, the US FDA approved its use in combination with carboplatin and paclitaxel for the initial systemic treatment of patients with unresectable, locally advanced, recurrent or metastatic, nonsquamous NSCLC.[37]

From laboratory standpoint, there is no currently available assay that could be used to predict tumor response to anti-VEGF therapies. Because of fatal hemorrhages in patients with squamous cell carcinomas, these therapies are used only in nonsquamous NSCLC. Therefore, surgical pathologists have to make every effort to precisely histologically subclassify NSCLC in the pathology reports.

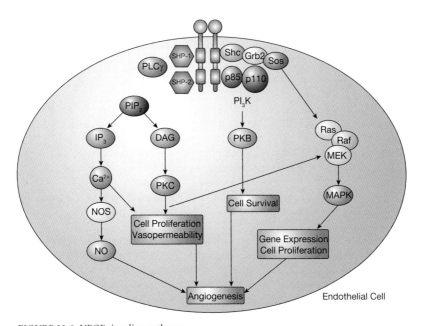

FIGURE 22-3 VEGF signaling pathway.

COMBINED EGFR AND VEGF INHIBITION

It is believed that because of nonoverlapping toxicity of anti-EGFR and anti-VEGFR agents, strategies targeting both pathways may be beneficial in advanced NSCLC.[38,39] Two strategies were employed including combination of single agents (e.g., erlotinib or cetuximab and bevacizumab) or the use of a single multitargeted agent (e.g., vandetanib). First clinical trials showed mixed results in advanced NSCLC. Although vandetanib seems to have some effects, it remains unclear whether this is simply a result of its anti-EGFR effects. Although initial results are unclear, it is certain that agents targeting EGFR and VEGF have become valuable tools in the treatment of NSCLC and that clinical trials investigating the activity of these agents will continue.

ALK

Anaplastic large cell lymphoma kinase gene (*ALK*) was originally identified in anaplastic large cell lymphomas (ALCLs) with t(2;5)(p23;35) translocation.[40,41] *ALK* encodes a TK that is normally expressed only in select neuronal cell types. In *ALK*-rearranged ALCLs, the intracytoplasmic portion of *ALK* is fused to the N-terminal portion of nucleophosmin resulting in a chimeric protein with constitutive kinase activity. Several other balanced translocations involving *ALK* have been discovered in ALCLs; however, the various resulting chimeric proteins all retain the ALK kinase domain.

    Recently, *ALK*-rearrangements were identified in rare NSCLC cell lines and in primary NSCLC isolated among the Japanese and Chinese populations.[42,43] The majority of the *ALK*-rearrangements within NSCLCs result from an interstitial deletion and inversion in chromosome 2p and result in the *EML4-ALK* fusion gene and gene product. More recently, so-called variant 3 of EML4-ALK rearrangement was identified in some patients with NSCLC and in the human NSCLC cell line H2228. The presence of EML4-ALK seems to be mutually exclusive to that of EGFR and KRAS mutations in NSCLC.[44] Murine tumors and human cell lines expressing EML-*ALK* are sensitive to inhibitors that target *ALK* enzymatic activity. Together these data indicate that, like *EGFR*, *ALK* is an important novel molecular target in lung carcinoma.[45] Various methods have been used for detection of EML4-ALK rearrangements including FISH, RT-PCR, and immunohistochemistry.[44] Recently, it has been reported that the presence of EML4-ALK rearrangements is associated with signet ring differentiation in lung adenocarcinomas.[46]

References

1. Pirker R, Pereira JR, Szczesna A, et al. Cetuximab plus chemotherapy in patients with advanced non-small-cell lung cancer (FLEX): an open-label randomised phase III trial. *Lancet*. 2009;373: 1525–1531.
2. Robert F, Blumenschein G, Herbst RS, et al. Phase I/IIa study of cetuximab with gemcitabine plus carboplatin in patients with chemotherapy-naive advanced non-small-cell lung cancer. *J Clin Oncol*. 2005;23:9089–9096.
3. Thienelt CD, Bunn PA, Jr., Hanna N, et al. Multicenter phase I/II study of cetuximab with paclitaxel and carboplatin in untreated patients with stage IV non-small-cell lung cancer. *J Clin Oncol*. 2005;23: 8786–8793.
4. Fukuoka M, Yano S, Giaccone G, et al. Multi-institutional randomized phase II trial of gefitinib for previously treated patients with advanced non-small-cell lung cancer (The IDEAL 1 Trial) [corrected] [erratum appears in *J Clin Oncol*. 2004 Dec 1;22(23):4811]. *J Clin Oncol*. 2003;21:2237–2246.
5. Giaccone G, Herbst RS, Manegold C, et al. Gefitinib in combination with gemcitabine and cisplatin in advanced non-small-cell lung cancer: a phase III trial–INTACT 1. *J Clin Oncol*. 2004;22:777–784.
6. Herbst RS, Giaccone G, Schiller JH, et al. Gefitinib in combination with paclitaxel and carboplatin in advanced non-small-cell lung cancer: a phase III trial–INTACT 2. *J Clin Oncol*. 2004;22:785–794.

7. Herbst RS, Prager D, Hermann R, et al. TRIBUTE: a phase III trial of erlotinib hydrochloride (OSI-774) combined with carboplatin and paclitaxel chemotherapy in advanced non-small-cell lung cancer. *J Clin Oncol*. 2005;23:5892–5899.

8. Lynch TJ, Bell DW, Sordella R, et al. Activating mutations in the epidermal growth factor receptor underlying responsiveness of non-small-cell lung cancer to gefitinib. *New Engl J Med*. 2004;350: 2129–2139.

9. Paez JG, Janne PA, Lee JC, et al. EGFR mutations in lung cancer: correlation with clinical response to gefitinib therapy. *Science*. 2004;304:1497–1500.

10. Pao W, Miller V, Zakowski M, et al. EGF receptor gene mutations are common in lung cancers from "never smokers" and are associated with sensitivity of tumors to gefitinib and erlotinib. *Proc Natl Acad Sci US A*. 2004;101:13306–13311.

11. Blons H, Cote J-F, Le Corre D, et al. Epidermal growth factor receptor mutation in lung cancer are linked to bronchioloalveolar differentiation. *Amer J Surg Pathol*. 2006;30:1309–1315.

12. Hirsch FR, Varella-Garcia M, McCoy J, et al. Increased epidermal growth factor receptor gene copy number detected by fluorescence in situ hybridization associates with increased sensitivity to gefitinib in patients with bronchioloalveolar carcinoma subtypes: a Southwest Oncology Group Study. *J Clin Oncol*. 2005;23:6838–6845.

13. Yatabe Y, Kosaka T, Takahashi T, et al. EGFR mutation is specific for terminal respiratory unit type adenocarcinoma. *Amer J Surg Pathol*. 2005;29:633–639.

14. Zakowski MF, Hussain S, Pao W, et al. Morphologic features of adenocarcinoma of the lung predictive of response to the epidermal growth factor receptor kinase inhibitors erlotinib and gefitinib. *Arch Pathol Lab Med*. 2009;133:470–477.

15. Motoi N, Szoke J, Riely GJ, et al. Lung adenocarcinoma: modification of the 2004 WHO mixed subtype to include the major histologic subtype suggests correlations between papillary and micropapillary adenocarcinoma subtypes, EGFR mutations and gene expression analysis. *Amer J Surg Pathol*. 2008;32: 810–827.

16. Ninomiya H, Hiramatsu M, Inamura K, et al. Correlation between morphology and EGFR mutations in lung adenocarcinomas Significance of the micropapillary pattern and the hobnail cell type. *Lung Cancer*. 2009;63:235–240.

17. Linardou H, Dahabreh IJ, Bafaloukos D, et al. Somatic EGFR mutations and efficacy of tyrosine kinase inhibitors in NSCLC. *Nat Rev Clin Oncol*. 2009;6:352–366.

18. Ahrendt SA, Decker PA, Alawi EA, et al. Cigarette smoking is strongly associated with mutation of the K-ras gene in patients with primary adenocarcinoma of the lung. *Cancer*. 2001;92:1525–1530.

19. Eberhard DA, Johnson BE, Amler LC, et al. Mutations in the epidermal growth factor receptor and in KRAS are predictive and prognostic indicators in patients with non-small-cell lung cancer treated with chemotherapy alone and in combination with erlotinib. *J Clin Oncol*. 2005;23:5900–5909.

20. Riely GJ, Kris MG, Rosenbaum D, et al. Frequency and distinctive spectrum of KRAS mutations in never smokers with lung adenocarcinoma. *Clin Cancer Res*. 2008;14:5731–5734.

21. Finberg KE, Sequist LV, Joshi VA, et al. Mucinous differentiation correlates with absence of EGFR mutation and presence of KRAS mutation in lung adenocarcinomas with bronchioloalveolar features. *J Mol Diagn*. 2007;9:320–326.

22. Marchetti A, Buttitta F, Pellegrini S, et al. Bronchioloalveolar lung carcinomas: K-ras mutations are constant events in the mucinous subtype. *J Pathol*. 1996;179:254–259.

23. Shigematsu H, Takahashi T, Nomura M, et al. Somatic mutations of the HER2 kinase domain in lung adenocarcinomas. *Cancer Res*. 2005;65:1642–1646.

24. Friday BB, Yu C, Dy GK, et al. BRAF V600E disrupts AZD6244-induced abrogation of negative feedback pathways between extracellular signal-regulated kinase and Raf proteins. *Cancer Res*. 2008;68: 6145–6153.

25. Marks JL, Gong Y, Chitale D, et al. Novel MEK1 mutation identified by mutational analysis of epidermal growth factor receptor signaling pathway genes in lung adenocarcinoma. *Cancer Res*. 2008;68: 5524–5528.

26. Dacic S. EGFR assays in lung cancer. *Adv Anatomic Pathol*. 2008;15:241–247.

27. Balak MN, Gong Y, Riely GJ, et al. Novel D761Y and common secondary T790M mutations in epidermal growth factor receptor-mutant lung adenocarcinomas with acquired resistance to kinase inhibitors. *Clin Cancer Res*. 2006;12:6494–6501.

28. Janne PA. Challenges of detecting EGFR T790M in gefitinib/erlotinib-resistant tumours. *Lung Cancer*. 2008;60(suppl 2):S3–S9.

29. Ji H, Wang Z, Perera SA, et al. Mutations in BRAF and KRAS converge on activation of the mitogen-activated protein kinase pathway in lung cancer mouse models. *Cancer Res.* 2007;67: 4933–4939.

30. Bean J, Riely GJ, Balak M, et al. Acquired resistance to epidermal growth factor receptor kinase inhibitors associated with a novel T854A mutation in a patient with EGFR-mutant lung adenocarcinoma. *Clin Cancer Res.* 2008;14:7519–7525.

31. Engelman JA, Zejnullahu K, Mitsudomi T, et al. MET amplification leads to gefitinib resistance in lung cancer by activating ERBB3 signaling. *Science.* 2007;316:1039–1043.

32. Bean J, Brennan C, Shih J-Y, et al. MET amplification occurs with or without T790M mutations in EGFR mutant lung tumors with acquired resistance to gefitinib or erlotinib. *Proc Natl Acad Sci USA.* 2007;104:20932–20937.

33. Pennell NA, Mekhail T. Investigational agents in the management of non-small cell lung cancer. *Curr Oncol Rep.* 2009;11:275–284.

34. Bergers G, Benjamin LE. Tumorigenesis and the angiogenic switch. *Nat Rev Cancer.* 2003;3:401–410.

35. Bremnes RM, Camps C, Sirera R. Angiogenesis in non-small cell lung cancer: the prognostic impact of neoangiogenesis and the cytokines VEGF and bFGF in tumours and blood. *Lung Cancer.* 2006;51: 143–158.

36. Johnson DH, Fehrenbacher L, Novotny WF, et al. Randomized phase II trial comparing bevacizumab plus carboplatin and paclitaxel with carboplatin and paclitaxel alone in previously untreated locally advanced or metastatic non-small-cell lung cancer. *J Clin Oncol.* 2004;22:2184–2191.

37. Ramalingam SS, Dahlberg SE, Langer CJ, et al. Outcomes for elderly, advanced-stage non small-cell lung cancer patients treated with bevacizumab in combination with carboplatin and paclitaxel: analysis of Eastern Cooperative Oncology Group Trial 4599. *J Clin Oncol.* 2008;26:60–65.

38. Gettinger S. Targeted therapy in advanced non-small-cell lung cancer. *Semin Respir Crit Care Med.* 2008;29:291–301.

39. Herbst RS, Sandler A. Bevacizumab and erlotinib: a promising new approach to the treatment of advanced NSCLC. *Oncologist.* 2008;13:1166–1176.

40. Lamant L, Meggetto F, al Saati T, et al. High incidence of the t(2;5)(p23;q35) translocation in anaplastic large cell lymphoma and its lack of detection in Hodgkin's disease. Comparison of cytogenetic analysis, reverse transcriptase-polymerase chain reaction, and P-80 immunostaining. *Blood.* 1996;87: 284–291.

41. Morris SW, Kirstein MN, Valentine MB, et al. Fusion of a kinase gene, ALK, to a nucleolar protein gene, NPM, in non-Hodgkin's lymphoma.[erratum for *Science.* 1994 Mar 4;263(5151):1281–1284; PMID: 8122112]. *Science.* 1995;267:316–317.

42. Rikova K, Guo A, Zeng Q, et al. Global survey of phosphotyrosine signaling identifies oncogenic kinases in lung cancer. *Cell.* 2007;131:1190–1203.

43. Soda M, Choi YL, Enomoto M, et al. Identification of the transforming EML4-ALK fusion gene in non-small-cell lung cancer. *Nature.* 2007;448:561–566.

44. Mano H. Non-solid oncogenes in solid tumors: EML4-ALK fusion genes in lung cancer. *Cancer Sci.* 2008;99:2349–2355.

45. Shaw AT, Yeap BY, Mino-Kenudson M, et al. Clinical features and outcome of patients with non-small-cell lung cancer who harbor EML4-ALK. *J Clin Oncol.* 2009; 27:4247–4253.

46. Rodig SJ, Mino-Kenudson M, Dacic S, et al. Unique clinicopathologic features characterize ALK-rearranged lung adenocarcinoma in the western population. *Clin Cancer Res.* 2009;15:5216–5223.

Molecular Prognostic Markers of Lung Cancer

23

▶ Sanja Dacic

M any studies have examined potentially prognostic genetic changes in lung carcinoma using different methodologies from immunohistochemistry to gene expression profiling. However, no clinically useful prognostic gene markers were found. This chapter will review some of the most commonly investigated prognostic markers.

CELL CYCLE REGULATORS

p53

A tumor suppressor gene, *p53*, is the most studied gene in all types of cancer, including lung cancer. A prognostic significance of this gene in lung cancer is contradictory. This is probably caused by different detection methods used to identify *p53* alterations. Immunohistochemistry can detect missense mutant *p53* proteins but may not detect the protein products of nonsense, deletion, or truncation mutants.[1-4] The frequency of *p53* mutations or positive IHC staining is higher in squamous cell carcinoma (60%–70%) than in adenocarcinoma (50%–70%).[5] *p53* mutations are unique in NSCLC of smokers with an excess of G:C to T:A transversions. Lack of prognostic significance of altered immunoexpression of *p53* in NSCLC was more frequently reported. Several studies using *p53* mutation analysis found a poorer prognosis for NSCLC with *p53* mutations. Studies using both approaches, IHC and mutational analysis, failed to demonstrate a prognostic significance. Overall, conflicting results preclude the use of *p53* gene alterations as prognostic markers for NSCLC in clinical practice.

Ras-Raf-Mek

The Ras proteins are members of a large superfamily of GTP-binding proteins involved in signal transduction regulating cell growth. The *Ras-Raf-Mek* pathway is involved in signaling downstream from *EGFR*. Activating *KRAS* mutations are present in up to 30% of lung adenocarcinomas.[5] Most *KRAS* mutations in lung adenocarcinomas are smoking-related G:T transversions and affect exon 12 (in 90% of patients) or exon 13.[5] *KRAS* point mutations may occur in never smokers (about 15%) and they are unrelated to tobacco carcinogens, typically G12D.[6] A recent meta-analysis demonstrated that NSCLC patients with *KRAS* mutations have a worse overall survival.[7] *KRAS* has the potential to be used as a predictive marker for the efficacy of EGFR-TKI therapies and as a prognostic marker in NSCLC.

ERCC1

ERCC1 is 1 of 16 genes that encode the proteins of the nucleotide excision repair complex. The nucleotide excision repair pathway recognizes and repairs cisplatin-induced DNA adducts. Small, retrospective clinical studies have repeatedly reported an association between low levels of ERCC1 mRNA in several cancers and improved clinical outcome among patients treated with platinum-containing regimens, particularly in advanced NSCLC.[8,9] Recently, the International

Adjuvant Lung Trial (IALT) demonstrated that patients who had NSCLC with no detectable ERCC1 by immunohistochemistry had longer disease-free survival after cisplatinum-based chemotherapy than patients with ERCC1-positive tumors.[10] Median overall survival was 14 months longer in ERCC1-negative tumors treated with chemotherapy than in those not receiving chemotherapy. There were no differences in survival between ERCC1-positive tumors in respect to chemotherapy treatment. Another recent study also showed that ERCC1 expression as measured by automated quantitative analysis of immunofluorescence is a determinant of survival in stage I NSCLC. These findings suggest that ERCC1 expression could be potentially used as a prognostic marker.

GENE EXPRESSION PROFILES

A number of prognostic gene expression signatures have been reported to predict survival in NSCLC.[11] Chen et al.[12] reported a 5-gene signature that correlated with clinical outcome in 125 randomly selected patients who underwent surgical resection for NSCLC and did not receive adjuvant chemotherapy. The five selected genes were *DUSP6* (dual specificity phosphatase 6), *MMD* (monocyte-to-macrophage differentiation-associated protein), *STAT1* (signal transducer and activator of transcription 1), *ERBB3* (v-erb b2 avian erythroblastic leukemia viral oncogene homolog 3), and *LCK* (lymphocyte-specific protein tyrosine kinase). In another study by Potti et al.,[13] authors used the lung metagene model to predict the risk of recurrence in a cohort of 89 patients with early-stage NSCLC. The lung metagene model represents the dominant average pattern of expression of the gene cluster across the tumor sample. Reported results included a metagene represented with a single molecular process such as angiogenesis. Other key metagenes represented a combination of the BRAF, phosphatidylinositol 3′ quinase, TP53, and MYC signaling pathways.

Beer et al.[14] reported a 50-gene signature that separated patients into low and high risk and predicted survival of stage I lung adenocarcinoma patients. The signature was also able to identify patients with poor prognosis independent of stage.

In a more recent study, the same authors validated prognostic significance of 35-gene signature for stratification of stage 1A lung adenocarcinoma patients into distinct prognostic subgroups.[15] This lung cancer prognostic signature was independent of traditional clinicopathologic factors, including patient age, clinical stage, tumor differentiation, and tumor grade. The signature had better prognostic performance than other lung cancer signatures, including the 5-gene signature reported by Chen et al. and the 133-gene signature reported by Potti et al. Most importantly, the gene expression and protein expression of the identified biomarkers were validated by real-time reverse transcription-PCR and Western blots analysis of clinical specimens, with TAL2 and ILF3 as potential prognostic markers.

These studies demonstrate that the microarray technologies promise the discovery of prognostic novel markers. There are several disadvantages that have limited their application in routine clinical laboratory, such as cost and reproducibility. RT-PCR can overcome the problems with microarray analysis and is emerging as the optimal method of choice for clinical laboratory.

miRNA

MicroRNAs are a family of endogenous, small (approximately 22 nucleotides in length), noncoding, functional RNAs. miRNAs are expressed in a tissue-specific manner, and changes in miRNA expression within a tissue type can be correlated with disease status. Yanaihara et al.[16] demonstrated in lung adenocarcinomas that high hsa-mir-155 and low hsa-let-7a-2 expression correlated with poor survival by univariate analysis as well as multivariate analysis for hsa-mir-155. Yu et al.[17] identified a signature of 5 miRNAs (let-7a, miR-221, miR-137, miR-372, miR-182) that predicted treatment outcome in NSCLC patients. Patients with a high-risk score for these 5 miRNAs had an increased relapse rate and shortened survival times. Our understanding of biologic role and possible prognostic significance of miRNAs in cancers should be further investigated.

References

1. Custodio AB, Gonzalez-Larriba JL, Bobokova J, et al. Prognostic and predictive markers of benefit from adjuvant chemotherapy in early-stage non-small cell lung cancer. *J Thorac Oncol.* 2009;4:891–910.
2. Mitsudomi T, Hamajima N, Ogawa M, et al. Prognostic significance of p53 alterations in patients with non-small cell lung cancer: a meta-analysis. *Clin Cancer Res.* 2000;6:4055–4063.
3. Steels E, Paesmans M, Berghmans T, et al. Role of p53 as a prognostic factor for survival in lung cancer: a systematic review of the literature with a meta-analysis. *Eur Respir J.* 2001;18:705–719.
4. Zhu CQ, Shih W, Ling CH, et al. Immunohistochemical markers of prognosis in non-small cell lung cancer: a review and proposal for a multiphase approach to marker evaluation. *J Clin Pathol.* 2006;59: 790–800.
5. Herbst RS, Heymach JV, Lippman SM. Lung cancer. *N Engl J Med.* 2008;359:1367–1380.
6. Riely GJ, Kris MG, Rosenbaum D, et al. Frequency and distinctive spectrum of KRAS mutations in never smokers with lung adenocarcinoma. *Clin Cancer Res.* 2008;14:5731–5734.
7. Mascaux C, Iannino N, Martin B, et al. The role of RAS oncogene in survival of patients with lung cancer: a systematic review of the literature with meta-analysis. *Brit J Cancer.* 2005;92:131–139.
8. Altaha R, Liang X, Yu JJ, et al. Excision repair cross complementing-group 1: gene expression and platinum resistance. *Int J Mol Med.* 2004;14:959–970.
9. Lord RVN, Brabender J, Gandara D, et al. Low ERCC1 expression correlates with prolonged survival after cisplatin plus gemcitabine chemotherapy in non-small cell lung cancer. *Clin Cancer Res.* 2002;8:2286–2291.
10. Olaussen KA, Dunant A, Fouret P, et al. DNA repair by ERCC1 in non-small-cell lung cancer and cisplatin-based adjuvant chemotherapy. *New Engl J Med.* 2006;355:983–991.
11. Singhal S, Miller D, Ramalingam S, et al. Gene expression profiling of non-small cell lung cancer. *Lung Cancer.* 2008;60:313–324.
12. Chen H-Y, Yu S-L, Chen C-H, et al. A five-gene signature and clinical outcome in non-small-cell lung cancer. *New Engl J Med.* 2007;356:11–20.
13. Potti A, Mukherjee S, Petersen R, et al. A genomic strategy to refine prognosis in early-stage non-small-cell lung cancer [erratum appears in *N Engl J Med.* 2007 Jan 11;356(2):201–202]. *New Engl J Med.* 2006;355:570–580.
14. Beer DG, Kardia SLR, Huang C-C, et al. Gene-expression profiles predict survival of patients with lung adenocarcinoma. *Nat Med.* 2002;8:816–824.
15. Guo NL, Wan Y-W, Tosun K, et al. Confirmation of gene expression-based prediction of survival in non-small cell lung cancer. *Clin Cancer Res.* 2008;14:8213–8220.
16. Yanaihara N, Caplen N, Bowman E, et al. Unique microRNA molecular profiles in lung cancer diagnosis and prognosis. *Cancer Cell.* 2006;9:189–198.
17. Yu S-L, Chen H-Y, Chang G-C, et al. MicroRNA signature predicts survival and relapse in lung cancer. *Cancer Cell.* 2008;13:48–57.

Staging

Problems in the Staging of Lung Cancer

24

▶ Philip T. Cagle

THE TNM STAGING SYSTEM

The stage, or anatomic extent, of a cancer at the time of diagnosis is one of the most important factors in predicting prognosis, selecting therapy, and stratifying patients for clinical trials and other research protocols.[1–21] To be useful, a staging system must be as objective and reproducible as possible. There are multiple staging systems of which the tumor-node-metastasis (TNM) system is most commonly used, based on a combination of primary tumor size and local invasiveness (T), extent of nodal metastases (N), and presence or absence of distant metastases (M). The specific stage of a patient is derived from the combined TNM and patients in the same stage group are expected to have similar prognosis and be candidates for similar approaches to treatment. Generally, the higher the stage (or the T, N, or M individually), the worse the prognosis.[1–19] This staging system is developed and maintained by the American Joint Committee on Cancer (AJCC) and the Union Internationale Contre le Cancer (UICC) and is periodically updated (the 7th edition went into effect in January 2010[17]; see Chapter 25). Traditionally, TNM stage has been thus far the single most important factor in determining survival of lung cancer patients.[19–21]

TNM staging may be either clinical or pathologic. Clinical staging, designated with the prefix "c," is based on clinical and imaging findings prior to any treatment, including history and physical examination, computed tomography (CT) scan, positron emission tomography (PET) scan, integrated CT-PET, magnetic resonance imaging, as well as surgical staging procedures such as mediastinoscopy (see Chapters 18 and 19). Pathologic staging, designated with the prefix "p," is based in most cases on gross and histologic examination of cancer resection specimens by the surgical pathologist. Obviously, the latter means that a treatment procedure, surgical resection, has occurred before staging is performed leading some critics to state that pathologic staging is at a disadvantage because clinical staging can be done prior to any treatment decision and used for those decisions. However, even after resection, vital information about prognosis and follow-up therapy can be gleaned from pathologic staging. On the other hand, the criteria for pathologic staging can be met without complete resection of a cancer if the highest T and N categories or the M1 category of the cancer can be histologically confirmed on biopsy or other specimens that do not involve complete resection of the primary cancer.[17,18]

The first TNM staging system for lung cancer was adopted in 1973 by the AJCC and in 1974 by the UICC. This first TNM staging system was proposed by Dr. Clifton Mountain and was based on a database of 2,155 patients from MD Anderson Cancer Center in Houston. The last revision of the lung cancer TNM staging system, prior to 2010, was in 1997 and was based on a database of 5,319 patients from MD Anderson Cancer Center. By 1997, standardization of the regional lymph node stations was established. Although these versions of the TNM staging system were generally valid, they were considered limited because the database is restricted to a single institution and the sample size is comparatively small, especially when broken down into subgroups. There was also some bias toward surgically treated patients.[10,12,13]

Although the TNM system has been widely used for non–small cell lung carcinomas, an alternative staging system has been widely used for small cell lung carcinoma, the Veterans Administration Lung Study Group System. In this system, patients are categorized into one of two stage groups: limited-stage disease or extensive-stage disease.[10,12,13,19–21]

In addition to the criticisms just mentioned above, the 1997 TNM staging system had a number of other criticisms, some general and some specific to practical details. The International Association for the Study of Lung Cancer (IASLC) initiated a large multinational study in 1999 to define and validate a new TNM staging system with extensive analysis of a larger, more representative database. The IASLC proposals were published in the *Journal of Thoracic Oncology* in 2007 and were subsequently approved and adopted by the AJCC and UICC. Based on a much larger group of patients (81,015 after exclusions) from 45 sources in 20 countries on four continents, the IASLC study validated the TNM descriptors on the basis of patient survival.[4–18] The new TNM staging for lung cancer was published in the 7th edition of the *AJCC Staging Manual* in October 2009 and implemented in January 2010.[17] This new TNM staging system is described in more detail in the subsequent chapter (see Chapter 25).

PROBLEMS IN LUNG CANCER STAGING

Compared to previous TNM staging systems for lung cancer, the new TNM staging system provides a validated, evidence-based system derived from a much larger database that is more representative of the world as a whole rather than a single institution. Details about the current TNM staging system including a number of practical issues are enumerated in Chapter 25. Even though the new TNM staging system addresses many criticisms of the previous TNM staging system, there are certain general shortcomings with any TNM staging system and certain practical challenges in pathologic staging of lung cancer that still arise that are not directly caused by the staging system itself.[17–19,22,23] The remainder of this chapter attempts to define these general shortcomings and practical challenges of lung cancer staging.

GENERAL SHORTCOMINGS OF PATHOLOGIC TNM STAGING OF LUNG CANCER

Exclusion of Nonanatomic Information

One broad criticism is that TNM staging is based purely on anatomic extent of disease and does not take into account other nonanatomic information which may significantly impact prognosis and treatment choices and perhaps potentially even be of greater importance than anatomic stage.[17–19,22,23] In particular for pathologic staging, the plethora of molecular studies of lung cancer, including molecular prognostic markers (Chapter 23) and the introduction of molecular targeted therapies (Chapter 22), has resulted in criticisms that molecular features of a cancer may be far more important than anatomic extent of disease in determining biologic behavior and, thus, prognosis and treatment. While this may prove true in the future, currently much more study on much larger numbers of patients are needed before specific molecular profiles can be validated as a new nonanatomic staging system or integrated into the current anatomic-based system.

Pathologic Versus Clinical Staging

Although the criteria for each stage are the same in both the clinical and pathologic staging, the information available to the individual doing the staging may vary. For example, the pathologist examining a cancer resection specimen may not have information about a distant metastasis that has been identified on imaging studies. On the other hand, the pathologist may discover a metastasis upon histologic examination of a lymph node that was not suspected on a clinical/radiologic basis. Pathologic staging is more accurate than clinical staging, but, with a few exceptions in which sufficient information is compiled from biopsies to permit pathologic staging, it requires that a treatment, namely surgical resection, be performed. Since most lung cancer patients present with advanced disease and, therefore, do not have surgical resections, pathologic staging is often not performed.

Dependence on Sampling by the Surgeon

An obvious limitation of pathologic staging is that it is dependent on adequate sampling by the surgeon. For example, N is dependent on the lymph node station involved and if the surgeon does not sample mediastinal or subcarinal lymph node stations, the pathologist cannot assess them. Generally, this problem is solved if surgeons follow guidelines in providing the appropriate samples for pathologic staging.

PRACTICAL CHALLENGES IN PATHOLOGIC STAGING OF LUNG CANCER

Determining Tumor Size

Many lung cancers have a nonneoplastic peritumoral reaction around the periphery of the tumor that may include interstitial fibrosis and inflammatory infiltrates (interstitial pneumonia), intra-alveolar collections of macrophages (desquamative interstitial pneumonia-like reaction or pseudo-desquamative interstitial pneumonia), and acute, organizing, or endogenous lipid pneumonia.[18,19,22–25] These nonneoplastic reactions may be grossly firm and discolored, giving a gross impression that they are part of the cancer and that the actual cancer is larger than what it truly is. Therefore, gross measurements of lung cancers should be verified with the histology to determine the actual tumor size.

Extent of Associated Atelectasis or Obstructive Pneumonitis

The presence and extent of tumor-associated atelectasis or obstructive pneumonitis influences T and, thus, stage group, depending on whether it extends to the hilar region but does not involve the entire lung (pT2a) or involves the entire lung (T3). It may be possible to assess the extent of tumor-associated atelectasis or obstructive pneumonitis in a pneumonectomy specimen, but accurate pathologic assessment may not be possible in less extensive resections. In these cases, correlation with imaging studies is recommended.

Distance from Carina

When a lung cancer involves the main bronchus, it is designated pT2a if it involves main bronchus, 2 cm or more distal to the carina; designated pT3 if it involves the main bronchus, <2 cm distal to the carina but without involvement of the carina; and designated pT4 if it involves the carina. Involvement of a main bronchus may be observed by the pathologist in specimens with central cancers, but the specimen typically does not permit assessment of the distance to the carina since it is not sampled. Therefore, evaluation of the distance of a central cancer from the carina often requires input from the radiologist, surgeon, or bronchoscopist.

Superficial Spreading Tumors

Superficial spreading tumors extending proximally to the main bronchus and with invasion limited to the bronchial wall are rare. However, regardless of their size, these cancers are pT1.

Assessment of Surgical Margins

The type of surgical margins depends on the type of surgical resection specimen and should generally be inked to avoid ambiguity on histologic examination. Surgical margins are often examined at frozen section. Lobectomies and pneumonectomies have bronchial and vascular margins and may occasionally have parenchymal margins with staple lines. Wedge resections have a parenchymal margin with staple lines. The visceral pleura is not a surgical margin. However, some specimens may have additional margins associated with extrapulmonary tissues such as parietal pleura or chest wall resected en bloc with the lung including when visceral pleura is adherent to parietal pleura.

Bronchial margins are often examined by frozen section at the time of lobectomy or pneumonectomy. Bronchial margins may be positive for cancer in any of four patterns: direct extension of the cancer, lymphatic spread of cancer, invasion of peribronchial tissues, and carcinoma in situ. Since residual carcinoma in situ at the bronchial margin is reported not to change patient survival, it is up to the surgeon to determine whether or not to take additional bronchial margin in this circumstance.

Histologic Prognostic Factors that Do Not Alter TNM

It has been reported that lymphovascular invasion is an unfavorable prognostic finding in lung cancer specimens. Lymphovascular invasion may be histologically obvious in some cases and equivocal in other cases. Immunostains such as D2-40 for lymphatic endothelial cells and CD31 or CD34 for vascular endothelial cells may be helpful. However, although presumed to be an unfavorable prognostic sign, lymphovascular invasion does not alter pT, pN, or TNM stage group.

A lung cancer metastasis to a lymph node may extend outside the lymph node capsule (extranodal extension). It has been reported that extranodal extension of a mediastinal lymph node is an unfavorable prognostic finding in lung cancer specimens, but it does not alter pN or TNM group.

Multiple Tumor Nodules

It is not unusual for lung cancers to present as multiple tumor nodules, in the same lobe, same lung but different lobe, or opposite lung. The presence of multiple tumor nodules in a resection specimen can be ambiguous as to whether one is dealing with multiple separate primary cancers or metastases from one primary cancer. Although molecular profiling may offer better solutions in the future, current criteria for diagnosing separate synchronous primary cancers as opposed to metastases rely on histologic features. They are (a) physically distinct and separate tumors with different histologic cell type or (b) physically distinct and separate tumors with similar histology which show an origin from carcinoma in situ, have no carcinoma in lymphatics common to both tumors, and have no extrapulmonary metastases at the time of diagnosis. When there are multiple separate synchronous primaries, the largest cancer (largest T) is reported and the suffix "m" (for multiple) or number of tumors is reported in parentheses (e.g., pT3[m]).

When physically distinct and separate tumor nodules are of similar histology but do not show an origin from carcinoma in situ, have carcinoma in lymphatics common to both tumors, and have extrapulmonary metastases, it is presumed that one tumor is a metastasis from the other. If such tumors are found in the same lobe, they are classified as T3, and they are classified as T4 if in ipsilateral separate lobes, consistent with survival data.

There are several problems in assessing whether a cancer is a synchronous primary or a metastasis using the above criteria. Lung cancers are typically heterogeneous and, therefore, different histology may predominate in a metastasis. Identifying lymphovascular invasion is dependent on sampling and may still be difficult to recognize when present.

Effects of Neoadjuvant Therapy

Surgical resection and pathologic staging may occur subsequent to adjuvant chemotherapy, radiation therapy, or both. The extent to which a cancer regresses as a result of neoadjuvant therapy impacts prognosis. If a cancer is resected and pathologically staged after the patient has received neoadjuvant therapy, the "y" prefix should be used to indicate that this is tumor stage after neoadjuvant therapy (ypTNM group).

Recurrent Tumor

If a lung cancer has recurred after a documented disease-free interval and pathologic staging is performed on a new resection specimen, the "r" prefix should be used (rTNM).

Visceral Pleura Invasion

The new TNM staging system addresses several previous ambiguities regarding staging of pleural involvement, but the histologic difficulties in interpretation may still make this a difficult assessment. [18,22-25] The visceral pleura has an external elastic layer (also referred to as the external elastic lamina) that is often, but not always, visible on H&E-stained sections and often, but not always, highlighted with elastic stains such as VVG (Figs. 24-1 and 24-2). If the cancer does not penetrate the visceral pleura external elastic layer, then visceral pleural invasion is absent (Figs. 24-3 and 24-4). There does not appear to be a difference in prognosis between tumors that invade into the visceral pleura (penetrate the external elastic layer but do not extend to the surface) and those that invade through visceral pleura to the surface. If a tumor penetrates the external elastic layer of the visceral pleura, with or without extension to the visceral pleural surface, visceral pleural invasion is present and a tumor that is otherwise pT1 tumor is increased to pT2 (Figs. 24-5 and 24-6).

Although this criterion is simple enough to define, in actual histologic sections, it is often difficult to differentiate a well-formed visceral pleura elastic layer when there is pleural fibrosis present. The pleura has elastic fibers that merge with the underlying lung, and in pathologic conditions, as with an invasive cancer, there may be fibroelastotic changes of the visceral pleura and underlying lung with elastic fiber distortion, destruction, and duplication. Although elastic stains

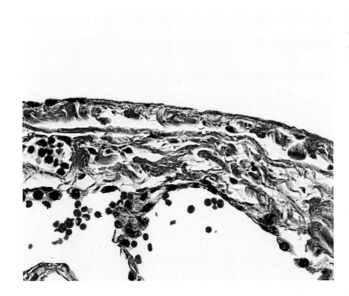

FIGURE 24-1 The external elastic layer or lamina appears as a relatively thick, eosinophilic, refractile line within the connective tissue of the visceral pleura.

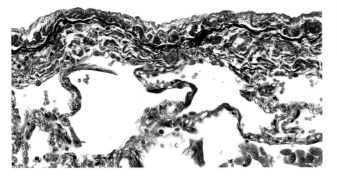

FIGURE 24-2 Elastic stain (VVG) highlights the external elastic layer as a relatively thick black line within the connective tissue of the visceral pleura.

FIGURE 24-3 This adenocarcinoma is observed to be entirely beneath the distinctly visible external elastic layer and, thus, no pleural invasion is present.

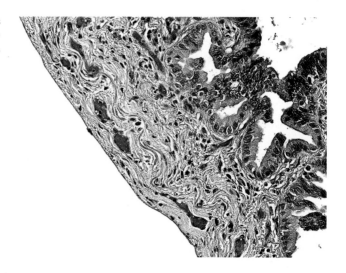

FIGURE 24-4 Elastic stain (VVG) confirms that the adenocarcinoma in Figure 24.3 does not penetrate the black-staining external elastic layer.

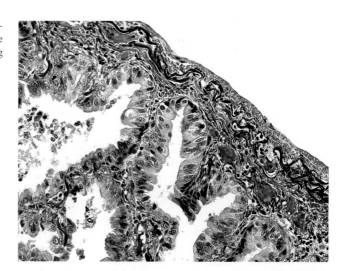

FIGURE 24-5 Malignant glands are observed on both sides of a partially disrupted external elastic layer consistent with invasion of the visceral pleura.

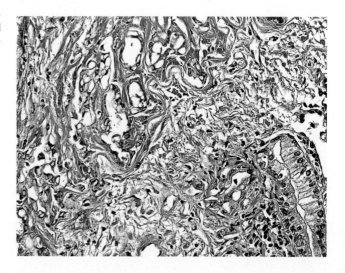

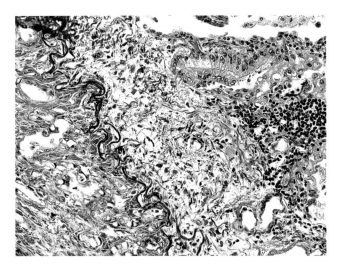

FIGURE 24-6 Elastic stain (VVG) highlights the external elastic layer demonstrating adenocarcinoma on both sides of the elastic layer confirming invasion of the visceral pleura.

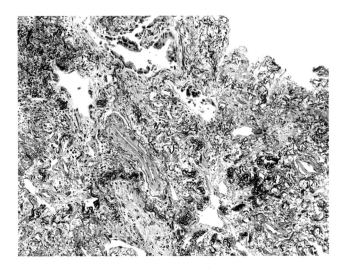

FIGURE 24-7 Elastic stain (VVG) displays a jumble of fragmented elastic fibers due to fibroelastotic changes of the visceral pleura in response to the cancer. The external elastic layer is difficult to discern because of the fragmentation, distortion, and duplication of elastic fibers. Visceral pleural invasion is presumed present but is difficult to confirm.

have been advocated to help assess invasion of the visceral pleura elastic layer, determination of invasion may still be difficult (Fig. 24-7).

References

1. American Joint Committee for Cancer Staging and End Results Reporting: Classification and Staging of Lung Cancer of Site. Chicago: American Joint Committee for Cancer Staging and End Results Reporting, 1976.
2. International Union Against Cancer (UICC): Lung tumors ICDO-0162. In: Hermanek P, Sobin LH, eds. *TNM Classification of Malignant Tumors.* 4th ed. Berlin: Springer-Verlag; 1987:70–73.
3. Mountain CF, Libshitz HI, Hermes KE. *Lung Cancer Handbook For Staging And Imaging.* 2nd ed. Houston: Clifton F. Mountain Foundation; 1997.
4. Goldstraw P, Crowley J, Chansky K, et al. The IASLC Lung Cancer Staging Project: proposals for the revision of the TNM stage groupings in the forthcoming (seventh) edition of the TNM Classification

of malignant tumours. *J Thorac Oncol.* 2007 Aug;2(8):706–714 [erratum in *J Thorac Oncol.* 2007 Oct;2(10):985].

5. Groome PA, Bolejack V, Crowley JJ, et al. IASLC Lung Cancer Staging Project: validation of the proposals for revision of the T, N, and M descriptors and consequent stage groupings in the forthcoming (seventh) edition of the TNM classification of malignant tumours. *J Thorac Oncol.* 2007;2(8): 694–705.

6. Postmus PE, Brambilla E, Chansky K, et al. The IASLC Lung Cancer Staging Project: proposals for revision of the M descriptors in the forthcoming (seventh) edition of the TNM classification of lung cancer. *J Thorac Oncol.* 2007;2(8):686–693.

7. Rusch VW, Crowley J, Giroux DJ, et al. The IASLC Lung Cancer Staging Project: proposals for the revision of the N descriptors in the forthcoming seventh edition of the TNM classification for lung cancer. *J Thorac Oncol.* 2007;2(7):603–612.

8. Rami-Porta R, Ball D, Crowley J, et al. The IASLC Lung Cancer Staging Project: proposals for the revision of the T descriptors in the forthcoming (seventh) edition of the TNM classification for lung cancer. *J Thorac Oncol.* 2007;2(7):593–602.

9. Travis WD, Giroux DJ, Chansky K, et al. The IASLC Lung Cancer Staging Project: proposals for the inclusion of broncho-pulmonary carcinoid tumors in the forthcoming (seventh) edition of the TNM Classification for Lung Cancer. *J Thorac Oncol.* 2008;3(11):1213–1223.

10. Rami-Porta R, Chansky K, Goldstraw P. Updated lung cancer staging system. *Future Oncol.* 2009; 5(10):1545–1553.

11. Vallières E, Shepherd FA, Crowley J, et al. The IASLC Lung Cancer Staging Project: proposals regarding the relevance of TNM in the pathologic staging of small cell lung cancer in the forthcoming (seventh) edition of the TNM classification for lung cancer. *J Thorac Oncol.* 2009;4(9):1049–1059.

12. Detterbeck FC, Boffa DJ, Tanoue LT. The new lung cancer staging system. *Chest.* 2009;136(1): 260–271.

13. Tanoue LT, Detterbeck FC. New TNM classification for non-small-cell lung cancer. *J Thorac Oncol.* 2009;4(4):437–443.

14. Ruffini E, Filosso PL, Bruna MC, et al. Recommended changes for T and N descriptors proposed by the International Association for the Study of Lung Cancer—Lung Cancer Staging Project: a validation study from a single-centre experience. *Eur J Cardiothorac Surg.* 2009;36(6):1037–1044.

15. Giroux DJ, Rami-Porta R, Chansky K, et al. The IASLC Lung Cancer Staging Project: data elements for the prospective project. *J Thorac Oncol.* 2009;4(6):679–683.

16. Rusch VW, Asamura H, Watanabe H, et al. The IASLC lung cancer staging project: a proposal for a new international lymph node map in the forthcoming seventh edition of the TNM classification for lung cancer. *J Thorac Oncol.* 2009;4(5):568–577.

17. Edge SB, Byrd DR, Compton CC, et al., eds. *AJCC Cancer Staging Manual.* 7th ed. New York, NY: Springer; 2009.

18. Butnor KJ, Beasley MB, Cagle PT, et al. Protocol for the examination of specimens from patients with primary non-small cell carcinoma, small cell carcinoma, or carcinoid tumor of the lung. *Arch Pathol Lab Med.* 2009;133(10):1552–1559.

19. Cagle PT. Carcinoma of the lung. In: Churg AM, Myers JL, Tazelaar HD, et al., eds. *Pathology of the Lung.* 3rd ed. New York, NY: Thieme Medical Publishers; 2005:413–479.

20. Flieder DB, Hammar SP. Common non-small cell carcinomas and their variants. In: Tomashefski J, Cagle PT, Farver C, et al., eds. *Dail and Hammar's Pulmonary Pathology.* 3rd ed. Vol 2. New York: Springer; 2008:216–307.

21. Jones KD. Malignant epithelial neoplasms. In: Cagle PT, Allen TC, Beasley MB, eds. *Diagnostic Pulmonary Pathology.* 2nd ed. New York, NY: Informa; 2008:611–626.

22. Marchevsky AM. Problems in pathologic staging of lung cancer. *Arch Pathol Lab Med.* 2006;130(3): 292–302.

23. Flieder DB. Commonly encountered difficulties in pathologic staging of lung cancer. *Arch Pathol Lab Med.* 2007;131(7):1016–1026.

24. Butnor KJ, Cooper K. Visceral pleural invasion in lung cancer: recognizing histologic parameters that impact staging and prognosis. *Adv Anat Pathol.* 2005;12(1):1–6.

25. Butnor KJ, Vollmer RT, Blaszyk H, et al. Interobserver agreement on what constitutes visceral pleural invasion by non-small cell lung carcinoma: an internet-based assessment of international current practices. *Am J Clin Pathol.* 2007;128(4):638–647.

New Staging System for Lung Cancer

▶ Philip T. Cagle

THE NEW TNM STAGING SYSTEM FOR LUNG CANCER

As noted in the previous chapter, the TNM staging system for lung cancer, last revised in 1997, was criticized because it was based on a limited number of patients (5,319) from one institution (MD Anderson Cancer Center). This meant that many subgroups of patients were small and that evidence-based criteria and validation of stage groupings were not ideal. Likewise, there were questions of whether the findings at one institution could be applied to multiple institutions throughout the world. In 1999, the International Association for the Study of Lung Cancer (IASLC) began an ambitious project to study a larger, more representative database to propose criteria for a revised TNM staging system. Their proposals were published in the *Journal of Thoracic Oncology* in 2007 and later adopted by American Joint Committee on Cancer (AJCC) and the Union Internationale Contre le Cancer.[1-13] In October 2009, the new TNM staging for lung cancer was published in the 7th edition of the *AJCC Staging Manual*, and it was put into practice in January 2010.[14,15]

After exclusions for various reasons, 81,015 patients from 45 sources in 20 countries on four continents were included. These included 67,725 patients with non–small cell lung carcinoma (NSCLC) and 13,290 cases of small cell carcinoma. Of the NSCLC cases, 53,640 were clinically staged, 33,933 were pathologically staged, and 20,006 cases were both clinically and pathologically staged. The geographic sources of the NSCLC cases were 40,059 from Europe, 12,178 from North America, 10,216 from Asia, and 5,272 from Australia.[1-15]

The new TNM staging system classified T, N, and M categories into stage groups according to similar survivals which resulted in some changes from the 1997 TNM staging system. However, many aspects of the 1997 staging system were found to be reliable and, for example, the N categories were found to clearly identify prognostically distinct groups of patients.[1-15] In contrast to previous editions, TNM staging of small cell carcinoma and carcinoid tumors is included using the same TNM staging as for the NSCLC.[6,8] In addition, the IASLC has proposed new international lymph node map to reconcile differences between older maps.[13-15]

There are criticisms of the new staging system. Not all previous ambiguities have been addressed and it remains a staging system based on anatomic extent of disease without other nonanatomic prognostic criteria such as molecular pathology. Subsequent division of the 81,015 patients into subgroups based on differing TNM categories means that each of these subgroups had smaller numbers of patients, of course, than the impressive total. Also, although an obvious improvement over representation from just one institution, there are still issues of biases introduced by differences between countries and regions of the world in terms of diagnosis, therapy, outcomes, and level of participation. Overall, however, the new TNM staging system is considered a vast improvement in terms of database size, wider representation, objective, evidence-based evaluation, and validation of TNM categories and stage groupings.[1-15]

Table 25-1 is a summary of the observations and revisions for the TNM descriptors for lung cancer proposed by the IASLC study. Table 25-2 provides the new pathology TNM descriptors for lung cancer, and Table 25-3 summarizes the stage groupings for the 7th edition of the *AJCC Cancer Staging Manual*.

Table 25-1	Observations and revisions for TNM descriptors for lung cancer proposed by IASLC

Changes to T Descriptors[5]

Several changes to the T descriptors were proposed by the IASLC as follows:
Subclassify T1 as T1a and T1b by size
Subclassify T2 as T2a and T2b by size
Reclassify T2 tumors larger than 7 cm as T3
Reclassify T4 tumors by additional nodules in the primary lobe as T3
Reclassify M1 by additional nodules in the ipsilateral lung (different lobe) as T4

Changes to N Categories[4]

Found to be valid in IASLC database
N0, N1, N2, and N3 clearly identify prognostically distinct groups of patients
Patients fall into three prognostically distinct categories, depending on the extent of nodal metastases:
Single-zone N1
Multiple-zone N1
Single-zone N2
Multiple-zone N2
Suggests that the overall disease burden, rather than just the anatomical location of lymph node involvement, may have the most important influence on outcome
Warrants future study

Changes to M Descriptors[3]

Reclassify pleural dissemination (malignant pleural effusions, pleural nodules) from T4 to M1a
M1a: Cases with malignant pleural effusions and cases with nodules in the contralateral lung
M1b: Cases with distant metastases
Cases with nodule(s) in the ipsilateral lung (nonprimary lobe), currently staged M1, should be reclassified as T4M0

Table 25-2	pTNM descriptors for lung cancer (per the 7th edition AJCC cancer staging manual[14,15])

Primary Tumor (pT)	
pTX	Cannot be assessed, or tumor proven by presence of malignant cells in sputum or bronchial washings but not visualized by imaging or bronchoscopy
pT0	No evidence of primary tumor
pTis	Carcinoma in situ
pT1a	Tumor 2 cm or less in greatest dimension, surrounded by lung or visceral pleura, without bronchoscopic evidence of invasion more proximal than the lobar bronchus (i.e., not in the main bronchus); or superficial spreading tumor of any size with its invasive component limited to the bronchial wall, which may extend proximally to the main bronchus

(Continued)

Table 25-2	pTNM descriptors for lung cancer (per the 7th edition AJCC cancer staging manual[14,15]) (Continued)
pT1b	Tumor > 2 cm, but 3 cm or less in greatest dimension, surrounded by lung or visceral pleura, without bronchoscopic evidence of invasion more proximal than the lobar bronchus (i.e., not in the main bronchus)
pT2a	Tumor > 3 cm, but 5 cm or less in greatest dimension surrounded by lung or visceral pleura, without bronchoscopic evidence of invasion more proximal than the lobar bronchus (i.e., not in the main bronchus); or tumor 5 cm or less in greatest dimension with any of the following features of extent: involves main bronchus; 2 cm or more distal to the carina; invades the visceral pleura; associated with atelectasis or obstructive pneumonitis that extends to the hilar region but does not involve the entire lung
pT2b	Tumor > 5 cm, but 7 cm or less in greatest dimension
pT3	Tumor > 7 cm in greatest dimension
	Tumor of any size that directly invades any of the following: chest wall (including superior sulcus tumors), diaphragm, phrenic nerve, mediastinal pleura, parietal pericardium; or tumor of any size in the main bronchus <2 cm distal to the carina but without involvement of the carina; or tumor of any size associated with atelectasis or obstructive pneumonitis of the entire lung; or tumor of any size with separate tumor nodule(s) in the same lobe
pT4	Tumor of any size that invades any of the following: mediastinum, heart, great vessels, trachea, recurrent laryngeal nerve, esophagus, vertebral body, carina or tumor of any size with separate tumor nodule(s) in a different lobe of ipsilateral lung
Regional Lymph Nodes (pN)	
pNX	Cannot be assessed
pN0	No regional lymph node metastasis
pN1	Metastasis in ipsilateral peribronchial and/or ipsilateral hilar lymph nodes, and intrapulmonary nodes, including involvement by direct extension
pN2	Metastasis in ipsilateral mediastinal and/or subcarinal lymph node(s)
pN3	Metastasis in contralateral mediastinal, contralateral hilar, ipsilateral or contralateral scalene, or supraclavicular lymph node(s)
Distant metastasis (pM)	
Not applicable	
pM1a	Separate tumor nodule(s) in contralateral lung; tumor with pleural nodules or malignant pleural (or pericardial) effusion
pM1b	Distant metastases outside the lung/pleura

Source: Butnor KJ, Beasley MB, Cagle PT, et al. Members of the Cancer Committee, College of American Pathologists. Protocol for the examination of specimens from patients with primary non–small cell carcinoma, small cell carcinoma, or carcinoid tumor of the lung. *Arch Pathol Lab Med.* 2009 Oct;133(10):1552–1559.

Table 25-3	TNM stage groupings for lung cancer (per the 7th edition AJCC cancer staging manual[14,15])		
Stage IA	T1a	N0	M0
	T1b	N0	M0
Stage IB	T2a	N0	M0
Stage IIA	T1a	N1	M0
	T1b	N1	M0
	T2a	N1	M0
	T2b	N0	M0
Stage IIB	T2b	N1	M0
	T3	N0	M0
Stage IIIA	T1a	N2	M0
	T1b	N2	M0
	T2a	N2	M0
	T2b	N2	M0
	T3	N1-2	M0
	T4	N0-1	M0
Stage IIIB	T1a	N3	M0
	T1b	N3	M0
	T2a	N3	M0
	T2b	N3	M0
	T3	N3	M0
	T4	N2-3	M0
Stage IV	Any T	Any N	M1a or M1b

Source: Butnor KJ, Beasley MB, Cagle PT, et al. Members of the Cancer Committee, College of American Pathologists. Protocol for the examination of specimens from patients with primary non–small cell carcinoma, small cell carcinoma, or carcinoid tumor of the lung. *Arch Pathol Lab Med.* 2009 Oct;133(10):1552–1559.

References

1. Goldstraw P, Crowley J, Chansky K, et al. The IASLC Lung Cancer Staging Project: proposals for the revision of the TNM stage groupings in the forthcoming (seventh) edition of the TNM Classification of malignant tumours. *J Thorac Oncol.* 2007 Aug;2(8):706–714 [erratum in: *J Thorac Oncol.* 2007 Oct;2(10):985].

2. Groome PA, Bolejack V, Crowley JJ, et al. IASLC Lung Cancer Staging Project: validation of the proposals for revision of the T, N, and M descriptors and consequent stage groupings in the forthcoming (seventh) edition of the TNM classification of malignant tumours. *J Thorac Oncol.* 2007;2(8): 694–705.

3. Postmus PE, Brambilla E, Chansky K, et al. The IASLC Lung Cancer Staging Project: proposals for revision of the M descriptors in the forthcoming (seventh) edition of the TNM classification of lung cancer. *J Thorac Oncol.* 2007;2(8):686–693.

4. Rusch VW, Crowley J, Giroux DJ, et al. The IASLC Lung Cancer Staging Project: proposals for the revision of the N descriptors in the forthcoming seventh edition of the TNM classification for lung cancer. *J Thorac Oncol.* 2007;2(7):603–612.

5. Rami-Porta R, Ball D, Crowley J, et al. The IASLC Lung Cancer Staging Project: proposals for the revision of the T descriptors in the forthcoming (seventh) edition of the TNM classification for lung cancer. *J Thorac Oncol.* 2007;2(7):593–602.

6. Travis WD, Giroux DJ, Chansky K, et al. The IASLC Lung Cancer Staging Project: proposals for the inclusion of broncho-pulmonary carcinoid tumors in the forthcoming (seventh) edition of the TNM Classification for Lung Cancer. *J Thorac Oncol.* 2008;3(11):1213–1223.

7. Rami-Porta R, Chansky K, Goldstraw P. Updated lung cancer staging system. *Future Oncol.* 2009;5(10):1545–1553.

8. Vallières E, Shepherd FA, Crowley J, et al. The IASLC Lung Cancer Staging Project: proposals regarding the relevance of TNM in the pathologic staging of small cell lung cancer in the forthcoming (seventh) edition of the TNM classification for lung cancer. *J Thorac Oncol.* 2009;4(9):1049–1059.

9. Detterbeck FC, Boffa DJ, Tanoue LT. The new lung cancer staging system. *Chest.* 2009;136(1): 260–271.

10. Tanoue LT, Detterbeck FC. New TNM classification for non-small-cell lung cancer. *J Thorac Oncol.* 2009;4(4):437–443.

11. Ruffini E, Filosso PL, Bruna MC, et al. Recommended changes for T and N descriptors proposed by the International Association for the Study of Lung Cancer—Lung Cancer Staging Project: a validation study from a single-centre experience. *Eur J Cardiothorac Surg.* 2009;36(6):1037–1044.

12. Giroux DJ, Rami-Porta R, Chansky K, et al. The IASLC Lung Cancer Staging Project: data elements for the prospective project. *J Thorac Oncol.* 2009;4(6):679–683.

13. Rusch VW, Asamura H, Watanabe H, et al. The IASLC lung cancer staging project: a proposal for a new international lymph node map in the forthcoming seventh edition of the TNM classification for lung cancer. *J Thorac Oncol.* 2009;4(5):568–577.

14. Edge SB, Byrd DR, Compton CC, et al., eds. *AJCC Cancer Staging Manual.* 7th ed. New York, NY: Springer; 2009.

15. Butnor KJ, Beasley MB, Cagle PT, et al. Protocol for the examination of specimens from patients with primary non-small cell carcinoma, small cell carcinoma, or carcinoid tumor of the lung. *Arch Pathol Lab Med.* 2009;133(10):1552–1559.

Preneoplastic and Preinvasive Lesions

Bronchial Squamous Dysplasia and Carcinoma In Situ

26

▶ Keith M. Kerr

T his chapter will review squamous dysplasia and carcinoma in situ (SD/CIS), recognized in the WHO classification of lung tumors as precursor lesions for the development of bronchogenic squamous cell carcinoma.[1] The evolution, morphology, differential diagnosis, and molecular biology of these lesions will be considered, as well as some comment on the clinical relevance of the lesions, particularly with respect to lung cancer screening. SD/CIS are regarded as preinvasive lesions since they have some, but not all, of the morphological features of malignancy; by definition, they lack hallmark invasion yet have the potential for its development. Occasionally, these lesions are referred to as preneoplastic and their importance is that the relative risk of these lesions becoming invasive is high. Almost certainly, SD/CIS does not arise de novo from bronchial respiratory epithelium. It is hypothesized that SD transforms into CIS, but SD itself also has likely precursor lesions.

Animal models have been extensively used to study the process of malignant transformation in bronchial epithelium. While many of these models do not absolutely reflect the situation in the human bronchial tree, primarily since, setting aside the obvious species differences, experiments have tended to involve the use of much higher doses of irritants or carcinogens and concern models of disease with a time course orders of magnitude shorter that that seen in the human, they have, nonetheless, given useful insight into what probably happens in the human airway.[2] A consistent finding in many of these models is the initial induction of inflammation and respiratory cell injury, followed by a proliferative/reparative reaction. Metaplasia occurs soon after; usually, this is squamous metaplasia. Ultimately dysplasia supervenes.

BRONCHIAL CARCINOGENESIS

It is very likely that a similar sequence of events occurs in the human. As will be discussed later, the most important etiological factor in the development of SD/CIS is tobacco smoke. As well as containing 50 to 60 recognized carcinogens, there are around 4,000 other chemical substances in tobacco smoke, some of which are responsible for chronic irritation of the tracheobronchial epithelium.[3,4] This irritation leads to a number of morphological changes, which are described below. These changes include mucous cell hyperplasia, basal cell hyperplasia, and squamous metaplasia; all may be regarded as reactive or adaptive changes in the respiratory mucosa, leading to an epithelium better able to cope with the prevailing "toxic" environment. While a role for mucous cell hyperplasia in the evolution of SD/CIS is not clear, basal cell hyperplasia and squamous metaplasia are both implicated as "precursors" for the development of SD. It is likely that these reactive lesions represent epithelia, which have in some ways "begun" the molecular and morphological evolution toward malignancy.

The emergence of a phenotypically malignant cell population is the result of the accumulation, in that cell population, and most critically in the stem cells, of a number of key genetic changes or abnormalities. Lesions such as SD and CIS are a morphological representation of the accumulation of many of these genetic changes; it is presumed that a few more are required for the fully invasive malignant phenotype to evolve. It has been estimated that between 3 and

12 critical genetic changes must occur, in a specific order, for malignancy to develop.[5] In fact, as discussed below, many more changes than this actually accumulate as dysplasia and CIS evolve and it is crucial that none of the accumulated changes are fatal to the cells affected. The chances of the required genetic changes occurring in the correct cells (cells with stem-like properties), in the correct sequence, are actually very small. Cancer is a "statistical" disease. Doll correctly described the evolution of cancer as "…largely a matter of luck: bad luck…."[6]

Following the concept of field carcinogenesis, which applies well in the case of the bronchus, and indeed the peripheral lung epithelium (see Chapter 27), multiple foci of preinvasive change are usually present in the affected tracheobronchial tree.[7] Each lesion probably represents a patch of altered epithelium which has accumulated some but not all of the crucial genetic changes required for the full malignant phenotype. Each patch may well represent independent clonal expansion of an altered stem cell population; such cells are believed to reside in the bronchial gland ducts and at intracartilagenous boundaries in the large airways mucosa. More patches will exist with fewer genomic changes and therefore less morphological abnormality; fewer areas will have evolved genetically further and show more severe atypia or even CIS. In some patients, one of these lesions "makes it" to invasive carcinoma; occasionally, patients develop two or even more foci of independently evolving malignancy (synchronous primary tumors). Some of these genetic changes, which are consistently found in SD/CIS but less often in basal cell hyperplasia and squamous metaplasia, may also be found in morphologically normal respiratory epithelium of tobacco smokers, as discussed below. This is presumably evidence that the earliest genetic changes precede the evolution of morphological change.

Bronchial carcinogenesis has been associated with exposure to ionizing radiation or certain chemicals, and the role of air pollution is still debated, but more is known about tobacco-related carcinogenesis. Of the numerous carcinogens found in tobacco smoke, the two most important groups are the polycyclic aromatic hydrocarbons and the N-nitrosamines.[3,4] While the former have been particularly associated with bronchial carcinogenesis and N-nitrosamines, especially a substance known as NNK, with peripheral lung adenocarcinogenesis, the effects of these compounds are not anatomically exclusive. Many of the compounds in tobacco smoke actually require chemical modification to become active carcinogens. It is something of a paradox that xenobiotic metabolizing enzymes (XMEs) that have a physiological role in detoxification of foreign chemical compounds may actually activate procarcinogens in tobacco smoke. Other enzymes are involved in further chemical modification of these activated carcinogenic compounds, inactivating them and facilitating their elimination. The ultimate "carcinogenic effect" of particular tobacco carcinogens will, therefore, depend on the relative efficiency of the so-called type 1 XMEs, such as many of the cytochrome P450s which activate procarcinogens and the type 2 XMEs, including glutathione-S-transferases which detoxify active carcinogens. If activation is efficient and detoxification is poor, carcinogenesis is more likely; vice versa would see a situation mitigating against tumor development. This is a simplification of a complex process involving many different carcinogens and numerous different enzymes. Many of these enzymes exist in different isoforms. Some isoforms are more or less efficient than others in their catalytic actions. It follows that an individual's ability to detoxify or chance of suffering cytogenetic damage from tobacco carcinogens will depend on the particular enzyme gene polymorphisms he or she has inherited. There is growing evidence of particular combinations of polymorphisms (genotypes), which are associated with greater risk of developing lung cancer.[8] Polymorphisms of the nicotinic acetylcholine receptor gene cluster are also associated with an apparent variable risk in developing lung cancer. These polymorphisms appear to determine variability in nicotine addiction and may stimulate greater tobacco consumption in some individuals.

PREINVASIVE LESIONS OF BRONCHIAL MUCOSA

Goblet Cell Hyperplasia

Some have suggested, largely on the basis of animal studies, that hyperplastic mucinous cells in the bronchial epithelium may transform into squamous metaplasia and dysplasia; at best, this is speculation. Certainly, this lesion is one of the adaptive changes seen in tobacco smokers and one

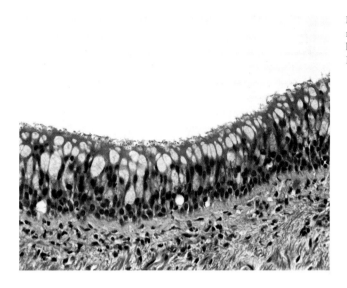

FIGURE 26-1 Goblet cell hyperplasia. The mucosa in this lobar bronchial mucosa has an excess of goblet cells (compare with Fig. 26-2).

of the key changes leading to the mucous hypersecretory state which defines chronic bronchitis (Fig. 26-1). Goblet cell hyperplasia is manifest in the central cartilaginous airways as small foci where, instead of occasional goblet cells admixed with other differentiated columnar cells in normal epithelium, there are patches of numerous goblet cells crowded together, sometimes giving a slightly raised or tufted appearance to the affected epithelium. There is no cytological atypia.

Basal Cell Hyperplasia

Basal cell hyperplasia is defined by the presence of three or more layers of basal cells in the respiratory epithelium (Fig. 26-2). Sometimes, there may be many more layers of cells almost completely replacing the epithelium but leaving a columnar cell layer on the surface. These cells are regular with small, round to oval nuclei and there is no atypia. Despite the hyperplastic terminology mitoses are very uncommon. Tangential cutting of the bronchial epithelium can give a false impression of basal cell hyperplasia, but in such a case, the basement membrane is also apparently thickened and the surface columnar cells do not appear vertically sectioned. It may be very difficult to discriminate between basal cell hyperplasia and some patterns of mild dysplasia. The basal cell layer may be demonstrated using immunohistochemistry and antibodies to p63 protein or cytokeratin 5/6.

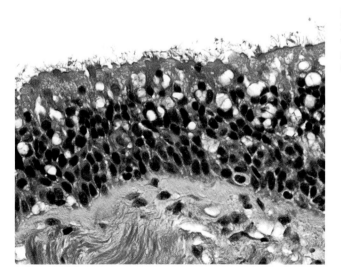

FIGURE 26-2 Basal cell hyperplasia. Increased layers of basal cells (compare with Fig. 26-1). Basal cell nuclei are slightly enlarged but there is no significant atypia.

SQUAMOUS METAPLASIA

This is recognized when the bronchial epithelium is replaced by a differentiated squamous epithelium comprising basal cells, a zone of larger prickle cells and superficial flattening of cells with keratinization (Fig. 26-3). As with basal cell hyperplasia, there should be no cytological atypia. In the proposed evolution of SD and CIS, squamous metaplasia is seen as the stage immediately preceding SD. Squamous metaplasia is an adaptation by the airway epithelium to chronic irritation and as well as tobacco smoke; it has been associated with air pollution, irradiation, smoking marijuana, and many chronic inflammatory or infective situations involving airways or lung cavities.[2,9] Long-standing airway intubation may lead to squamous metaplasia at points of trauma, it is associated with vitamin A deficiency, and it is quite common for a thin layer of squamous metaplastic epithelium to cover relatively long-standing endobronchial tumors such as carcinoid tumors, lipomas, or endobronchial hamartomas (Fig. 26-4). Squamous metaplasia may also be seen in alveolated lung in the context of organizing diffuse alveolar damage or usual interstitial pneumonia.

Squamous metaplasia as described above is not an obligate precursor for SD. Fully mature squamous metaplasia is not so common. More often, evidence of squamous differentiation

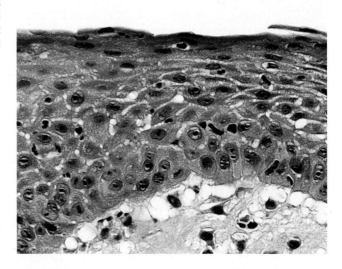

FIGURE 26-3 Complete, full-thickness squamous metaplasia of the bronchial mucosa. A relatively unusual lesion, it shows a marked prickle cell layer and superficial maturation with keratinization.

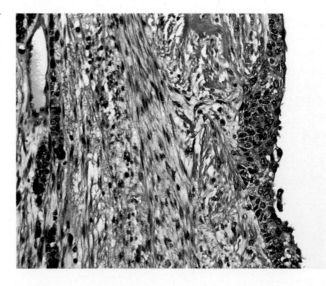

FIGURE 26-4 Squamous metaplasia of the epithelium overlying a typical bronchial carcinoid tumor. In this context the squamous epithelium may become extremely thin.

(prickle cells) is seen in expanded zones of basal cell hyperplasia, surmounted by differentiated columnar cells. This could be considered immature squamous metaplasia and dysplasia may occur in this setting without full-thickness squamous change.

SQUAMOUS DYSPLASIA AND CARCINOMA IN SITU

Much of the early work on these lesions and their association with bronchogenic carcinoma and tobacco smoking came from the autopsy studies of Auerbach et al.[10] Interest in SD/CIS has increased recently as a result of the expanding use of autofluorescence bronchoscopy (AFB) to detect and localize bronchial mucosal abnormality, as discussed below.

The strongest known etiological factor for SD/CIS is tobacco smoking.[11] Other studies have been carried out on patient cohorts exposed to airborne irradiation (radon—uranium miners) or chemicals such as chromates but much of these data were confounded by patients also smoking.[12] There is some evidence of a dose-response relationship between amount smoked and the number and grade of dysplastic lesions that may be found. It is somewhat controversial but smoking cessation may be associated with lesion regression. Associations with air pollution are difficult to prove. SD/CIS is commoner in males than females; this may be related to gender differences in smoking habits. The macroscopic features of SD/CIS are rarely appreciated, either by pathologists or bronchoscopists. Most lesions are invisible in pathological material, partly due to the subtle changes they induce but also because of the quality of material and the intercurrent pathology that is often present. SD/CIS lesions are most often found on the spurs of airway carinae. Lesions may cause loss of the rugal folds of the mucosa, opacification and roughening of the surface and occasionally result in slightly elevated plaques. Extensive disease can, at least theoretically, lead to retention pneumonia if there is replacement of enough normal ciliated respiratory epithelium to interrupt the mucociliary flow. Lesions are generally quite small. CIS lesions have been described at between 2 and 17 mm in diameter with a mean diameter of around 8 to 9 mm. SD lesions tend to be smaller, mostly measuring around 1.5 to 5 mm in greatest dimension (Fig. 26-5).[13,14]

Histologically, there are four grades of disease defined within the WHO classification of SD/CIS; mild, moderate and severe dysplasia, and carcinoma in situ.[1] This is, thus, a relatively complex classification, and though following those originally proposed for other organ sites such as the cervix, there have been suggestions that a two-tier system of low- and high-grade dysplasia would be better. The classification is based upon the identification of architectural and cytological changes distributed within a full-thickness squamous epithelium. All the possible features may not necessarily be present and may vary from microscopic field to field within a lesion.

FIGURE 26-5 A small, localized lesion of mild squamous dysplasia, flanked on either side by respiratory mucosa.

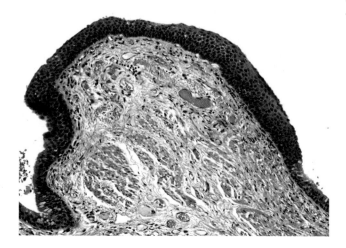

The dysplastic epithelium is notionally divided into lower (basal), middle, and upper thirds for the purposes of assessing the distribution of changes.

Mild dysplasia concerns changes confined to the basal third of the squamous epithelium. The epithelium itself may be mildly thickened, but maturation is complete with superficial flattening of cells above a clear prickle cell zone (Fig. 26-6). The basal cell layer may be expanded but only within the lower third of the epithelium. In this zone, there may be minimal alteration of cell size and shape, nuclei are orientated vertically, and nuclear chromatin is finely granular. Both nucleoli and mitoses are inconspicuous.

Moderate dysplasia is diagnosed when there is less subtle cytological change, which extends into the middle third of the epithelium. This thicker epithelium still shows maturation but superficial flattening of cells and prickle cells are confined to the upper third. The basal cell zone extends to involve the middle third of the epithelium where vertically orientated nuclei show still finely granular chromatin, but nuclear angulation and grooving may be appreciated. Nucleoli remain inconspicuous but mitosis may be found, confined to the lower third of the epithelium (Fig. 26-7). Cells are larger and there is some pleomorphism.

FIGURE 26-6 High-power image of mild squamous dysplasia. There is minimal nuclear irregularity of the basal cells.

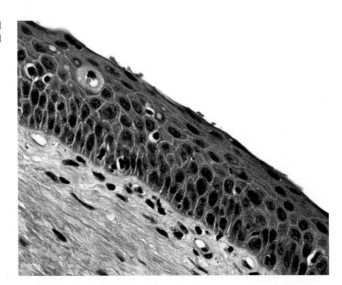

FIGURE 26-7 This area of moderate dysplasia shows basal third mitoses, more pleomorphism than in Figure 26-6, but clear evidence of superficial third maturation.

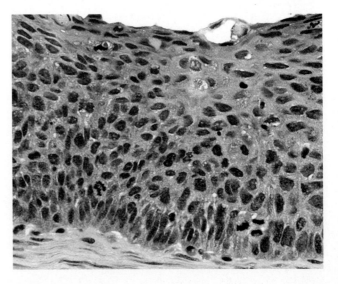

Severe dysplasia shows atypia extending throughout the epithelial layers (Fig. 26-8). The epithelium may be notably thickened. Maturation is minimal but the most superficial cell layers may be flattened and prickle cells are rarely identified. The basal cell zone of cells with vertically orientated nuclei extends well into the upper third of the epithelium. There is now marked increase in cell size and pleomorphism. Nuclei have coarse, uneven chromatin; nuclear angulation and grooving are regularly seen. Nucleoli are prominent and mitoses may be encountered in the lower and middle thirds of the epithelium.

Carcinoma in situ is identified when there is marked cytological atypia and complete loss of maturation, such that if this chaotic epithelium were inverted, it would look much the same (Fig. 26-9). CIS lesions may be markedly thickened but, paradoxically, may also comprise a rather thin epithelium, making assessment difficult. Papillary architecture has been described in CIS, but caution should be taken before making a diagnosis of CIS in this situation. The WHO classification regards all papillary lesions as invasive. In CIS, mitotic figures may be found throughout the epithelium.

As the degree of atypia increases so may the thickness of the basement membrane. In severe SD and CIS, the basement membrane may become irregular, or even appear absent, but this is not

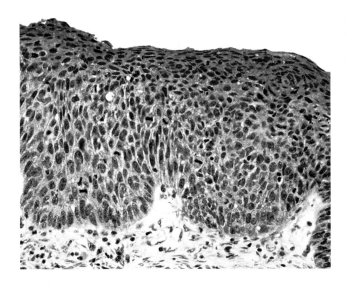

FIGURE 26-8 High-power image of severe dysplasia shows mitoses extending into the middle third of the epithelium, atypia extending to the upper third but still very superficial evidence of maturation.

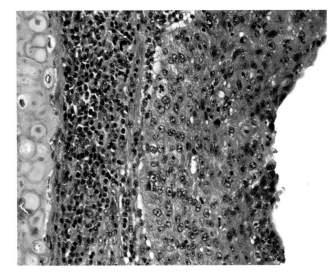

FIGURE 26-9 Squamous cell carcinoma in situ shows no maturation and marked pleomorphism. Mitotic figures may occur anywhere in the epithelium.

a reliable indicator of invasion. The vascularity of the stroma deep to SD/CIS may also increase. This has been regarded by some as a sign of impending invasion. A notable pattern of vascularity is seen in so-called angiogenic squamous dysplasia (ASD). In this lesion, tufts of capillary vessels protrude into the overlying squamous epithelium, which may be variably atypical (Fig. 26-10). The capillaries are usually surrounded by prominent hyaline basement membrane–like material and the epithelium over the apex of the vascular tuft may be very thin.[15] The lesions may result in localized protruberance of the epithelium, giving it a papillomatous appearance; this lesion has also been referred to as micropapillomatosis (Fig. 26-11).[16] ASD shows variable atypia that can be very difficult to grade according to the WHO scheme, and similar changes may be observed in nonatypical pseudostratified respiratory epithelium. ASD appears to be associated with smoking and does show molecular features consistent with neoplasia and angiogenesis.

Atypical squamous cells may be detected in sputum samples and in bronchial washings or brushings. Some complex classification systems have been proposed for squamous atypia in exfoliative bronchial cytology samples and these have been related to the WHO histological classification. As would be expected, this is based upon detailed cell and nuclear characteristics and the

FIGURE 26-10 This is angiogenic squamous dysplasia (ASD). The capillary vessels that sprout into the squamous epithelium show prominent endothelial cells and are surrounded by hyaline eosinophilic material.

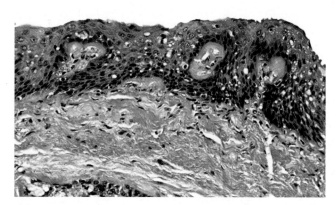

FIGURE 26-11 In this extreme and relatively unusual example of ASD, the application of the term micropapillomatosis would be appropriate. This particular case is from a bronchial biopsy sample.

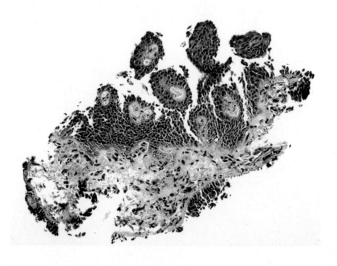

tinctorial cytoplasmic features of basophilia and orangeophilia. Without considerable experience these classifications are difficult to apply. Sputum cytology has poor sensitivity, even for detecting invasive bronchial carcinoma, as well as SD/CIS, and while atypia *somewhere* in the bronchial tree can be detected in some cases, there is no way of localizing the lesion. Various artifacts and reactive changes may also lead to false-positive diagnosis of dysplasia.

DIAGNOSIS OF SD/CIS: PROBLEM AREAS

Unfamiliarity with the lesions described above can make this diagnosis a challenge. Unless the pathologist works in a centre with high volumes of lung cancer patients or one where AFB is practiced, experience of these lesions may be limited. Given that most SD/CIS lesions are invisible to the bronchoscopist and that many bronchoscopists will only biopsy visible abnormality, most SD/CIS lesions encountered are chance findings. They may also be seen if airways around a squamous cell carcinoma are sampled during the gross examination of a surgically resected case. There is very little data in the literature on the reproducibility of the WHO classification. One study has suggested it is reproducible; others have challenged this view.[17,18] More work is required in this area.

The WHO criteria are based on the assessment of a full-thickness squamous epithelium, allowing its division into upper, middle, and lower thirds. This can be very difficult in a sample showing a very thin epithelium or where there is poor orientation of the epithelium in a small bronchial biopsy sample. It is relatively common for atypical epithelium to have a persistent layer of differentiated columnar cells on the surface, making application of the "thirds" rule difficult. Even severe cytological atypia may be seen beneath attenuated but clearly visible ciliated or mucous cells (Fig. 26-12). Residual columnar cells may, if necessary, be highlighted by either a mucin stain or immunohistochemistry, using antibodies to cytokeratin 7, which will stain the residual columnar cells, or cytokeratin 5/6, which will stain SD/CIS. This overlying differentiated epithelium probably represents one of two processes; most often, this is the result of dysplasia developing in immature squamous metaplasia/basal cell hyperplasia, without the presence of full-thickness squamous metaplasia. It is also possible, especially with severe dysplasia or carcinoma in situ, that there may be some lateral, intraepithelial spread of the lesion, undermining adjacent respiratory epithelium.

Sometimes the surface of dysplastic epithelium is rather ragged and it is clear that superficial cell layers have been lost, perhaps the result of trauma during endoscopy or bronchial brushing/washing to obtain cytology samples. This also makes assessment of dysplasia difficult. In some

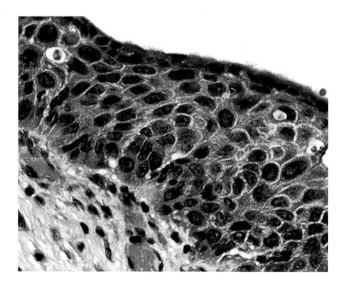

FIGURE 26-12 Here there is moderate to severe cytological atypia of squamous cells with well-developed intercellular bridges, yet there is a clear layer of persisting but attenuated ciliated columnar cells on the epithelial surface. The latter respiratory epithelial cells often have an eosinophilic tincture that should not be mistaken for superficial cell keratinization.

instances, it appears as if the residual respiratory epithelium mentioned above is particularly prone to being shed, as if the interface between the dysplastic and differentiated zones is discohesive. In cases where, for whatever reason, a proper assessment of the WHO criteria cannot be made, it is acceptable to attempt a simpler classification in a two-tier system, low-grade dysplasia (hyperplasia, metaplasia and mild dysplasia) and high-grade dysplasia (moderate dysplasia or worse) being classified on the available evidence, be that architecture or cytology.

DIFFERENTIAL DIAGNOSIS OF SD/CIS

Depending on the particular case, it may be necessary to discriminate SD/CIS either from invasive squamous cell carcinoma or from a variety of reactive or metaplastic lesions.[19] Invasion is obviously the key discriminating feature between CIS and squamous cell carcinoma. The individual cytological features are no different between CIS and invasive squamous cell carcinoma, and in the context of a small bronchial biopsy sample, the diagnosis of invasion relies upon the recognition of infiltration of any subepithelial stroma that is present in the sections. If this stroma is absent and only naked strips or fragments of malignant-looking squamous epithelium are seen, a confident diagnosis of invasive carcinoma is impossible. The interface between CIS and the underlying connective tissue is generally smooth. Mention has already been made of the variable state of the basement membrane and how it is not particularly helpful in this diagnostic situation. Strips of CIS epithelium lacking stroma retain their smooth outlines. Fragments of invasive carcinoma are more often irregularly shaped; nodules, clumps, or islands of epithelium may be seen. Apart from the particular case of ASD, CIS epithelium is not vascularized. Invasive carcinoma may well have a capillary blood supply, though this can be hard to identify as the capillaries are accompanied by little or no connective tissue. CIS epithelium does not undergo necrosis; focal necrosis may be seen in invasive disease. There is more tendency for the epithelium in invasive carcinoma to show a range of different architectures; basaloid areas, foci of keratinization or even squamous pearl formation. CIS epithelium is, by definition, cytologically heterogeneous, but such variation in architecture is not usually a feature.

Clinical information is, as always, useful. It may be very helpful to know what the bronchcoscopist saw, before the biopsy was performed. Of course, a history of an endobronchial mass lesion does not confirm a diagnosis of carcinoma in the absence of histological evidence of invasion. In situ disease may extend into bronchial gland ducts and replace bronchial gland acini (Fig. 26-13). This can give a false impression of invasion. If attention is paid to the location of these foci of atypical cells, adjacent to cartilage, their shape, taking the outline of the replaced ducts or gland

FIGURE 26-13 Squamous cell carcinoma in situ extending to involve the submucosal bronchial glands and their ducts. Lumenal mucin persists in some acini. These epithelial foci exhibit severe cytological features but the architecture of the gland acini and occasional glandular cells are preserved, helping to distinguish this change from invasive disease. This particular example was found in a bronchial mucosal biopsy sample.

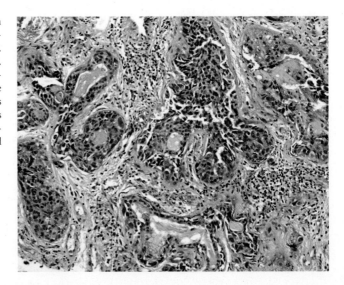

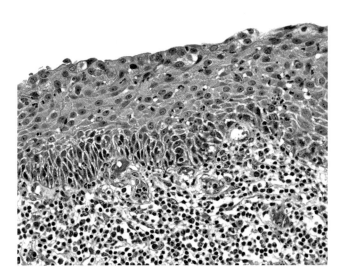

FIGURE 26-14 This example of squamous metaplasia was found lining a chronically infected bronchiectatic cavity. There is marked subepithelial and intra-epithelial inflammation. The mild nuclear irregularity should be considered a reactive phenomenon and not dysplasia.

lobules, and the presence of any residual serous or mucous cells, then a misdiagnosis of carcinoma may be avoided. Inevitably, there will be cases where a confident diagnosis of invasion cannot be made. Given the implications of a malignant diagnosis in prognostic and therapeutic terms, it is better to err on the side of caution. A phrase such as "at least carcinoma in situ" may be useful to help convey suspicion of invasion but reticence to commit to this diagnosis in the absence of adequate evidence. Discussion with the physician is often helpful and repeat biopsy may be necessary to secure a diagnosis.

At the opposite end of the spectrum of SD/CIS, distinction between mild dysplasia and either squamous metaplasia or basal cell hyperplasia may be extremely difficult, even if the samples are well prepared and properly orientated on the stained sections. The cytological changes that define mild dysplasia are very subtle and require thin sections of high quality for their identification. Atypical cells may be seen in reactive, hyperplastic respiratory epithelium, and if the expansion of the basal cell layer is marked, distinction between this and mild dysplasia is extremely difficult; indeed, the distinction in theoretical terms is moot. Hyperplastic or squamous metaplastic epithelium lining lung cysts, chronic inflammatory cavities, or ectatic bronchi may develop cytological atypia when there is marked inflammation; the presence of the inflammatory infiltrate supports attribution of any cytological atypia to a reactive change, as opposed to "true" dysplasia (Fig. 26-14). Similar reactive changes may be found in the airways serving an area of infected lung. Respiratory epithelium or that lining bronchial glands or their ducts may become atypical after chemotherapy or radiotherapy. The cytopathic effects of viral infection may give rise to individual cells with bizarre nuclei. Overdiagnosis of mild dysplasia is probably less of a problem for the patient. Mild dysplasia causes no symptoms, does not require treatment, and, as discussed in the next section, has a limited potential for progression. Accurate diagnosis is, of course, always desirable and is of particular importance in the context of research studies or trials where the natural history and or treatment of SD/CIS are being studied.

PREVALENCE AND CLINICAL IMPLICATIONS OF SD/CIS

The earliest descriptions of SD/CIS derive from autopsy studies carried out by Auerbach et al.[10,12] In a number of papers, they described the frequency and distribution of lesions that conform to current descriptions of SD/CIS in smokers, uranium workers, patients with bronchogenic carcinoma, and patients with pneumonia.[10,12,20,21] SD/CIS was more prevalent, more extensive, and of higher grade in those who smoked more; especially so in those with concurrent bronchial carcinoma, usually squamous cell but small cell carcinomas were not infrequent. They found SD/CIS in 40% of smokers who did not have carcinoma, in 92% of those with lung cancer, and in 96% of uranium miners with lung cancer. These studies were conducted in the 1950 to 1970s when smoking habits and the nature of cigarettes were undoubtedly different from those of today.

Disease prevalence has also been studied using sputum cytology to identify cytological atypia in bronchi. Most of these studies have been designed to detect carcinoma as opposed to preinvasive disease and have targeted groups at high risk of developing malignancy. In as much as this cytological method can detect and grade disease, mild, moderate, and severe dysplasia have been reported in high-risk patients in approximately 50%, 25%, and 5% of cases, respectively.[22] When comparison was made, the false-negative rates are high and significant false-positive rates are also recognized.

AFB has renewed considerable interest in SD/CIS as improved methods for screening for lung cancer are sought.[23] AFB is carried out using a blue or violet light source and special image detection systems that allow the identification of areas of abnormal bronchial mucosa due to a loss of the normal green autoflourescence (Figs. 26-15 and 26-16). When compared to normal "white light" bronchoscopy (WLB), AFB allows the detection of many more bronchial lesions;

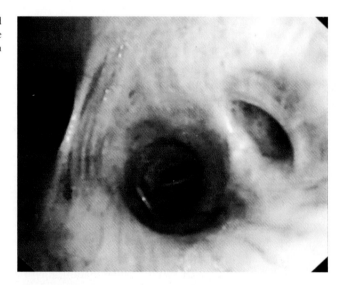

FIGURE 26-15 The view under standard WLB shows no obvious lesion. (Image courtesy of Dr. Robert Rintoul, Papworth Hospital, Cambridge, UK.)

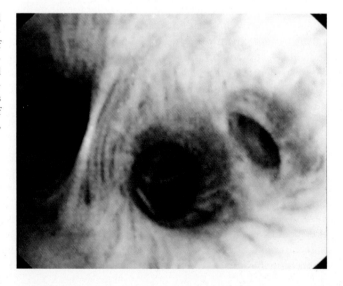

FIGURE 26-16 The same airway viewed using autofluoresence demonstrates preservation of the green autofluorescence of "normal" mucosal but loss of this appearance over the carina between the central and right-sided airway orifice. The reddish patch demonstrated mild squamous dysplasia on biopsy. (Image courtesy of Dr. Robert Rintoul, Papworth Hospital, Cambridge, UK.)

data vary but figures of between 6- and 18-fold improvement are quoted for AFB in detecting SD/CIS. A recent study found WLB had a sensitivity of 65% for detecting SD/CIS while AFB had 90% sensitivity.[24] Specificity is, however, a problem. Many of the areas abnormal at AFB, when biopsied, show inflammation, nonspecific changes or even morphologically normal mucosa. Despite these problems, AFB is a very useful tool in the detection of SD/CIS and its use is recommended in guidelines for the management of preinvasive bronchial disease. In a contemporary study (late 1990s) of at-risk smokers without lung cancer, moderate dysplasia was detected in 14% of subjects, severe dysplasia in 6.5%, and CIS in 1.8%. One or other of these abnormalities was found in 31% of males and 14% of females in the study.[25] Other studies have reported rates of around 5% for "high-grade" preinvasive disease. Studies vary greatly in terms of subjects and their risk profile, biopsy practice, and AFB technology used.

SD/CIS: IMPLICATIONS OF THE DIAGNOSIS

There are considerable difficulties in making longitudinal observations of the same SD/CIS lesions over time in order to gather data on likelihood of disease progression. Sputum cytology only detects cytological atypia but cannot locate the disease. Many follow-up studies have had as their end point the development of invasive carcinoma but any tumor that developed was not necessarily at the site of previously diagnosed SD/CIS. One could argue that if a reliable measure of risk of lung cancer is found, it does not actually matter where the tumor develops. Issues relating to the sensitivity and diagnostic accuracy of sputum cytology in this context, and the inability to localize disease have already been discussed. Various studies have shown that the incidence of subsequent lung cancer in patients with low- and high-grade sputum atypia range from as low as 4% up to 45%, respectively, but as before, study cohorts vary greatly as do follow-up periods.[2,26] The mean age of patients at diagnosis rises with increasing sputum atypia, and the mean time period between diagnosis of atypia and subsequent carcinoma falls. One study reported intervals of 4.8, 2.9, and 2.5 years, respectively, for moderate SD, severe SD, and CIS diagnosed by sputum cytology to be followed by a diagnosis of lung cancer.[27]

If, however, we wish to learn more about the biology of SD/CIS and understand the implications of this diagnosis for the patient, in terms of risk of developing malignancy, then more particular longitudinal studies are required. AFB offers the best opportunity to carry out such work since it is possible to both detect and localize SD/CIS.[23] In theory, it is possible to observe lesions over time through repeat AFB examinations and many such studies are now published. These are not without problems. In some of the studies, CIS lesions were treated in various ways. None of the SD/CIS lesions can be accurately diagnosed without biopsy. The biopsy procedure may remove the lesion completely or induce inflammation in any remaining parts of the lesion, which, in turn, could either cause regression or promote progression of the disease. Repeat biopsy could miss the visible lesion. All of these factors conspire to make interpretation of the numerous published studies rather difficult and probably explain the considerable variation in reported results. Some conclusions may be drawn from these studies: (a) Progression of SD/CIS to invasive carcinoma may occur; (b) higher grade disease probably carries a greater risk of progression than lower grade disease; (c) any grade of disease may regress to a lower grade of disease or disappear completely; and this is more likely with low-grade disease; (d) lesions may wax and wane; (e) lesion stability, even with CIS, may occur over long periods; and (f) correlation between smoking cessation and lesion regression is not strong. There are also emerging data relating various molecular biological factors in SD/CIS to their risk of progression to invasive disease. These will be considered in the next section.

MOLECULAR BIOLOGY OF SD/CIS

Both the increase in material available from AFB studies and advances in molecular techniques have led to a considerable increase in the published literature concerning the molecular biology of SD/CIS.[2,28–30] While there is an enormous amount of data available, it is less clear which are the key molecular changes in this evolution of disease, but some sort of picture is beginning to emerge. Much of the literature in this area has concerned the expression of individual genes, looking for the gene product using immunohistochemistry. Fewer studies have considered other aspects of individual gene "status" such as deletion, amplification, mutation, or epigenetic alteration such as gene promoter methylation.[2,5,11,31–33] Pan-genomic studies have also been carried out.[34] These include the study of chromosomal gains and losses using comparative genomic hybridization or techniques looking for loss of hetrozygosity (LOH) of particular chromosomal loci. The latter is important since gene deletion may be an important mechanism for loss of tumor suppressor gene (TSG) function and LOH studies may identify possible loss of known or putative TSGs. Global mRNA expression studies are also beginning to report interesting data.[35–37] Interpretation of these data must be related to accurate and consistent classification of different grades of SD/CIS. This will allow a better understanding of the molecular basis of SD/CIS evolution and progression and facilitate studies designed to predict the risk of progression of disease based upon molecular characteristics. This may also help identify markers for disease identification through screening and targets for therapeutic intervention.

Increased cell proliferation is a hallmark not only of invasive but also of preinvasive disease. Mitosis is also a mechanism through which some genetic alterations occur, during carcinogenesis. Hyperproliferation is one of the earliest epithelial changes, laying down a basis for further genomic alteration leading to malignancy. As would be expected given the morphological changes seen in basal cell hyperplasia and SD/CIS, there is abundant evidence, based upon the immunohistochemical identification of cell cycle related proteins using antibodies against Ki67 or MCM2, that cell cycle activity is increased in SD/CIS.[38,39] The expression of these proteins reflects the expansion of the proliferative compartment in the epithelium, to occupy the lower, middle, or upper thirds of the epithelium, depending on the grade of disease. There is some evidence that the degree of proliferative activity mirrors smoking activity and diminishes with smoking cessation.

p53 is a key gene, important in the regulation of many cellular functions including cell proliferation and cell death through apoptosis. *p53* acts as a TSG by promoting apoptosis, especially when cells suffer genetic damage, and by inducing G1-S arrest, so limiting cell proliferation. *p53* is one of the commonest genes to be altered in human cancer. Changes in this gene and both its upstream regulators and downstream targets and effectors have been recorded in SD/CIS. *p53* function may be lost through gene deletion or mutation (LOH). Wild-type *p53* protein is rapidly degraded so it is rarely detectable in normal cells but dysregulation of gene function may lead to abnormal protein accumulation. Increased levels of *p53* protein can be demonstrated immunohistochemically, rarely in normal respiratory epithelium in smokers, occasionally in hyperplasia and metaplasia, and regularly in SD/CIS, expression increasing as disease grade increases.[40,41] Not all lesions even of severe SD or CIS express *p53*; increased expression is likely to be seen in SD/CIS if concurrent squamous cell carcinoma also shows stainable *p53*. *p53* mutation is rare and has generally only been found in severe SD or CIS lesions. LOH at 17p13, the site of the *p53* gene, is found in some examples of severe SD or CIS but not in earlier lesions. *p63* is a *p53* regulator and like its target shows evidence of increased protein expression and gene amplification in high-grade disease. Bcl2 and bax mediate the antiapoptotic effects of *p53*. Proapoptotic bax decreases and antiapoptotic bcl2 may increase in some SD/CIS lesions. There appears to be an increase in the bcl2:bax ratio as disease progresses; alterations may be seen in low-grade disease and are independent of *p53* status. Studies of related proteins such as mdm2, p14arf, and NPM in SD/CIS have been inconclusive.[42]

The *p16ink4-cyclinD1-CDK4-RB* pathway is important in maintaining G1-S arrest in cells, a function in part regulated by p53 via p21(waf1/cip1). Dysregulation of this pathway seems to be important in the evolution of SD/CIS and appears to occur early, through upregulation of cyclin D1, loss of p16 function, and loss of p21, but rarely, if ever, through loss of RB function.[43] This latter change seems to be much more important in the development of small cell carcinoma. Upregulation of cyclin D1 has been described in hyperplastic and metaplastic lesions, becoming more frequent with increasing dysplasia. Loss of stainable p16 seems to occur a little later, when lesions are dysplastic. Hypermethylation of the *P16* gene complex promoter is a common mechanism of gene silencing and is smoking related. This change has been recorded in morphologically normal epithelium of smokers, in hyperplasia and metaplasia, as well as SD/CIS, prevalence increasing as disease progresses.[44] p16 gene function can also be lost through LOH at 9p21; this has been recorded very occasionally in hyperplastic lesions but more so in dysplasia and very often in CIS.

The HER family of cell membrane–bound tyrosine kinases are important catalysts of many downstream signaling pathways controlling cell cycle activity, cell proliferation, cell death, and angiogenesis. Ligand-receptor binding leads to a number of events culminating in activation of the internal kinase domain. Epidermal growth factor receptor (EGFR—HER1) is the most frequently studied of this family in SD/CIS. Many studies have demonstrated upregulation of EGFR protein even at the earliest stages with increasing amounts found as dysplasia evolves. EGFR levels appear to mirror cell cycle activity in SD/CIS and diminish on smoking cessation. Phosphorylated AKT and K-RAS are potential downstream targets in different EGFR-mediated signaling pathways. While there is no evidence that alteration of KRAS is involved in SD/CIS, increasing expression of phosphorylated AKT has been found during evolution and progression of SD/CIS.[45]

The morphological description of increased capillary proliferation in association with SD/CIS, including ASD, is reflected in evidence of molecular changes that promote angiogenesis. These changes include upregulation of vascular endothelial growth factor (VEGF) and increased expression of VEGF receptor proteins neuropilin 1, KDR, and flt1. Angiogenenic activity may be limited by competitive binding of other ligands such as some semaphorins. Semaphorin 3F may thus act as a TSG, and this gene may be lost as a result of 3p21.3 LOH observed in some SD/CIS lesions.[30]

Cell senescence is in part mediated by progressive telomere shortening that occurs each time a cell divides. Cessation of this process will prevent p53-mediated physiological cell loss via apoptosis and is characteristic of many human tumors, including lung carcinomas. This is mediated by activation of telomerase ribonucleoprotein complexes. There are a number of different measures of this increased molecular activity in tumor cells, relating to increased expression of several genes involved in this process. Human telomerase reverse transcriptase (hTERT) has been more frequently studied in SD/CIS and a progressive increase in activity of hTERT is seen from hyperplasia to CIS; almost all CIS lesions show increases in hTERT mRNA levels.[46]

The general increase in metabolic activity and gene expression in SD/CIS is reflected in an increase in a number of other transcription factors and other genes/proteins being expressed during this evolution of disease. Factors such as nuclear factor kappa B, upstream stimulatory factors 1 and 2, c-ETS-1, heat shock proteins 10 and 60, heterologous ribonucleoprotein B1, and maspin have all been shown to be overexpressed in SD/CIS and related lesions to a variable extent. Generally speaking, the higher the grade of disease, the more likely these factors are to be upregulated.[2] Other TSGs such as retinoic acid receptor beta (*RARbeta*) and the fragile histidine triad (*FHIT*) have been studied in SD/CIS and losses have been found, mostly in higher grade lesions. Both these genes are located on chromosome 3p and these losses are amongst a number which occur in 3p, which are consistent findings in many lung cancers and appear to be important in the evolution of SD/CIS.[2,11,29,33] Many of these losses have been found, admittedly at low frequency, in morphologically normal respiratory epithelium in smokers. Loci affected include 3p14.2 (*FHIT*), 3p21 (*RASSF1A, FUS-1, SEMA3B*), 3p22–24 (*BAP-1*), and 3p25. As disease progresses and becomes more atypical, so do the extent and frequency of these losses. Loss of 9p21 (*P16*) and 8q21-23 may also appear early while 17p13 (*P53*) loss appears later. Loss at 3p12 (*DUTT1*) may also be a later event, while losses at 13p14 (*RB*) and 5q (*APC*) are late infrequent findings.

Chromosomal aneuploidy can be demonstrated and is more apparent as disease progresses. Among the changes noted have been 3q24 amplification, chromosome 3 polysomy, chromosome 7 aneusomy, amplification at 8p21 and 8q22 in CIS, and gains at 1q25-32, 12q23-24.2, and 17q12-22, also in CIS but not in earlier lesions.

TSG silencing through smoking-induced promoter hypermethylation has been mentioned above with regard to the p16 gene. Other genes that have been found with hypermethylated promoters in SD/CIS include *RARbeta, FHIT, RASSF1A, H-cadherin, ECAD, DAPK, and MGMT*.

Gene expression array analysis of morphologically normal microdissected bronchial epithelium has shown differentially expressed genes between smokers and nonsmokers. Some oncogenes and TSGs are involved, but many of the upregulated genes in smokers were XMEs presumably involved in the metabolism of smoke toxins but also with the potential for carcinogen activation, as discussed above. Smoking cessation seems to see some but not all the genes revert to normal expression levels; however, this may take some considerable time.

Proteomic analyses have also shown differential protein expression profiles between metaplasia, dysplasias, and CIS and changes in microRNAs have been described.[47,48] The significance of these new data remains illunderstood. Many of these molecular changes such as gene mutation or patterns of LOH have been used to show multiple preinvasive lesions from the same patient are not clonally related. This supports the concept of field carcinogenesis in the central airways with multiple independently arising foci of disease developing in a much larger, unstable, at-risk epithelial compartment. Studies looking at the ability of molecular markers to predict the risk of progression of disease have been few and the results variable. This is possibly due to the inconsistent findings concerning the lesion's natural history. p16, p53, cyclin D1, bcl2:bax, and hTERT status have all been related to risk of disease progression and positive results have been reported.[41,43,49,50] It is not clear in some of these studies whether the molecular feature is a predictor of progression risk, independent of lesion grade. None of these markers is ready for clinical use.

CONCLUSION

A number of preinvasive lesions of the bronchial epithelium are recognized and have been described above. SD/CIS is a precursor lesion for invasive squamous cell carcinoma. The precise sequence of lesion evolution prior to the development of SD is a matter of some debate but it seems that complete squamous metaplasia is not an obligatory stage in the pathway. Much is known regarding the molecular changes that accompany the evolution and progression of SD/CIS; less is known about the relative importance of various changes. Loss of function of p16 and p53 are amongst likely key factors in what is essentially a smoking-induced disease.

An understanding of the differential diagnosis of SD/CIS will assist in the accurate and consistent classification of disease. The distinction between CIS and invasive disease is most important because of the prognostic and therapeutic implications for the patient. A diagnosis of hyperplasia, metaplasia, or dysplasia is of uncertain significance for the patient. Often these lesions are found in conjunction with invasive carcinoma when their importance is less. Until we know more about the risks and rate of progression of SD/CIS, the clinical significance of this finding will remain uncertain.

A better understanding of the biology of SD/CIS will be derived from, but also facilitate, the design and conduct of lung cancer screening trials. AFB is not a primary screening tool but is a valuable way to locate SD/CIS in patients identified as being at risk of lung cancer. It remains to be seen whether molecular factors can be used as screening tools to identify more at-risk groups. Early detection and treatment of disease remains the best hope of making improvements in the outcomes for patients with this most common and fatal form of cancer.

References

1. Franklin WA, Wistuba II, Geisinger, et al. Squamous dysplasia and carcinoma in situ. In: Travis WD, Brambilla E, Muller-Hermelink HK, et al., eds. *World Health Organisation Classification of Tumours. Pathology and Genetics of Tumours of the Lung, Pleura, Thymus and Heart.* Lyon: IARC press; 2004:68–72.
2. Kerr KM, Fraire AE. Pre-invasive disease. In: Tomashefski JF, Cagle PT, Farver CF, et al., eds. *Dail and Hammar's Pulmonary Pathology.* New York, NY: Springer; 2008:II:158–215.
3. Hecht SS. Tobacco smoke carcinogens and lung cancer. *J Natl Cancer Inst.* 1999;91:1194–1210.

4. Hecht SS. Cigarette smoking: cancer risks, carcinogens and mechanisms. *Langenbecks Arch Surg.* 2006;391:603–613.

5. Mao L. Molecular abnormalities in lung carcinogenesis and their potential clinical implications. *Lung Cancer.* 2001;34:S27–S34.

6. Doll R. Commentary: the age distribution of cancer and a multistage theory of carcinogenesis. *Int J Epidemiol.* 2004;33:1183–1184.

7. Braakhuis BJ, Tabor MP, Kummer JA, et al. A genetic explanation of Slaughter's concept of field cancerization: evidence and clinical implications. *Cancer Res.* 2003;63:1727–1730.

8. Lee KM, Kang D, Clapper ML, et al. CYP1A1, GSTM1, and GSTT1 polymorphisms, smoking, and lung cancer risk in a pooled analysis among Asian populations. *Cancer Epidemiol Biomarkers Prev.* 2008;17:1120–1126.

9. Valentine EH. Squamous metaplasia of the bronchus; a study of metaplastic changes occurring in the epithelium of the major bronchi in cancerous and noncancerous cases. *Cancer.* 1957;10:272–279.

10. Auerbach O. Pathogenesis of lung cancer. *Cancer.* 1961;7:11–21.

11. Wistuba II, Mao L, Gazdar, AF. Smoking molecular damage in bronchial epithelium. *Oncogene.* 2002;21:7298–7306.

12. Auerbach O, Saccomanno G, Kuschner M, et al. Histologic findings in the tracheobronchial tree of uranium miners and non-miners with lung cancer. *Cancer.* 1978;42:483–489.

13. Nagamoto N, Saito Y, Sato M, et al. Clinicopathological analysis of 19 cases of isolated carcinoma in situ of the bronchus. *Am J Surg Pathol.* 1993;17:1234–1243.

14. Lam S, MacAulay C, LeRiche JC, et al. Detection and localization of early lung cancer by fluorescence bronchoscopy. *Cancer.* 2000;89:2468–2473.

15. Keith RL, Miller YE, Gemmill RM, et al. Angiogenic squamous dysplasia in bronchi of individuals at high risk for lung cancer. *Clin Cancer Res.* 2000;6:1616–1625.

16. Meert A-P, Feoli F, Martin B, et al. Angiogenesis in preinvasive, early invasive bronchial lesions and micropapillomatosis and correlation with EGFR expression. *Histopathology.* 2007;50:311–317.

17. Nicholson AG, Perry LJ, Cury PM, et al. Reproducibility of the WHO/IASLC grading system for pre-invasive squamous lesions of the bronchus: a study of inter-observer and intra-observer variation. *Histopathology.* 2001;38:202–208.

18. Venmans BJ, Van der Linden JC, Elbers JRJ, et al. Observer variability in histopathological reporting of bronchial biopsy specimens: Influence on the results of autofluorescence bronchoscopy in detection of bronchial neoplasia. *J Bronchol.* 2000;7:210–214.

19. Kerr KM, Popper HH. The differential diagnosis of pulmonary pre-invasive lesions. *Eur Respir Mon.* 2007;39:37–62.

20. Auerbach O, Stout AP, Hammond EC, et al. Changes in bronchial epithelium in relation to cigarette smoking and in relation to lung cancer. *N Engl J Med.* 1961;265:255–267.

21. Auerbach O, Stout AP, Hammond EC, et al. Changes in bronchial epithelium in relation to sex, age, residence, smoking and pneumonia. *N Engl J Med.* 1962;267:111–119.

22. Kennedy TC, Franklin WA, Prindiville SA, et al. High prevalence of occult endobronchial malignancy in high risk patients with moderate sputum atypia. *Lung Cancer.* 2005;49:187–191.

23. Banerjee AK. Preinvasive lesions of the bronchus. *J Thorac Oncol.* 2009;4:545–551.

24. Ikeda N, Honda H, Hayashi A, et al. Early detection of bronchial lesions using newly developed video-endoscopy-based autofluorescence bronchoscopy. *Lung Cancer.* 2006;52:21–27.

25. Lam S, Kennedy T, Unger M, et al. Localization of bronchial intraepithelial lesions by fluorescence bronchoscopy. *Chest.* 1998;113:696–702.

26. Frost JK, Ball WC, Levin ML, et al. Sputum cytopathology: use and potential in monitoring the workplace environment by screening for biological effects of exposure. *J Occup Med.* 1986;28:692–703.

27. Saccomanno G, Saunders RP, Archer VE, et al. Cancer of the lung—The cytology of sputum prior to the development of carcinoma. *Acta Cytol.* 1965;9:413–423.

28. Kerr KM. Morphology and genetics of preinvasive pulmonary disease. *Curr Diag Pathol.* 2004;10:259–268.

29. Wistuba II, Gazdar AF. Lung cancer preneoplasia. *Annu Rev Pathol.* 2006;1:331–348.

30. Lantuejoul S, Salameire D, Salon S, et al. Pulmonary preneoplasia—sequential molecular carcinogenic events. *Histopathology.* 2009;54:43–54.

31. Wistuba II, Behrens C, Virmani AK, et al. Allelic losses at chromosome 8p21–23 are early and frequent events in the pathogenesis of lung cancer. *Cancer Res.* 1999;59:1973–1979.

32. Ma J, Gao M, Lu Y, et al. Gain of 1q25–32, 12q23–24.3, and 17q12–22 facilitates tumourigenesis and progression of human squamous cell lung cancer. *J Pathol.* 2006;210:205–213.

33. Wistuba II, Behrens C, Milchgrub S, et al. Sequential molecular abnormalities are involved in the multistage development of squamous cell lung carcinomas. *Oncogene.* 1999;18:643–650.

34. Woenckhaus M, Klein-Hitpass L, Grepmeier U, et al. Smoking and cancer-related gene expression in bronchial epithelium and non-small-cell-lung cancers. *J Pathol.* 2006;210:192–204.

35. Zhang L, Lee JJ, Tang H, et al. Impact of smoking cessation on global gene expression in the bronchial epithelium of chronic smokers. *Cancer Prev Res.* 2008;1:112–118.

36. Chari R, Lonergan KM, Ng RT, et al. Effect of active smoking on the human bronchial epithelium transcriptome. *BMC Genomics.* 2007;8:297.

37. Boelens MC, van den Berg A, Fehrmann RS, et al. Current smoking-specific gene expression signature in normal bronchial epithelium is enhanced in squamous cell lung cancer. *J Pathol.* 2009;218:182–191.

38. Meert AP, Martin B, Verdebout JM, et al. EGFR, c-erbB-2 and ki-67 in NSCLC and preneoplastic bronchial lesions. *Anticancer Res.* 2006;26:135–138.

39. Tan D-F, Huberman JA, Hyland A, et al. MCM2—a promising marker for premalignant lesions of the lung: a cohort study. *BMC Cancer.* 2001;1:6–14.

40. Bennett WP, Colby TV, Travis WD, et al. p53 protein accumulates frequently in early bronchial neoplasia. *Cancer Res.* 1993;53:4817–4822.

41. Brambilla E, Gazzeri S, Lantuejoul S, et al. P53 mutant immunophenotype and deregulation of p53 transcription pathway (bcl2, bax and waf1) in precursor bronchial lesions of lung cancer. *Clin Cancer Res.* 1998;4:1609–1618.

42. Mascaux C, Bex F, Martin B, et al. The role of NPM, p14arf and MDM2 in precursors of bronchial squamous cell carcinoma. *Eur Respir J.* 2008;32:678–686.

43. Brambilla E, Gazzeri S, Moro D, et al. Alterations of Rb pathway (Rb-p16INK4-cyclin D1) in preinvasive bronchial lesions. *Clin Cancer Res.* 1999;5:243–250.

44. Lamy A, Sesboue R, Bourguignon J, et al. Aberrant methylation of the CDKN2A/P16*INK4A* gene promoter region in preinvasive bronchial lesions: A prospective study in high-risk patients without invasive cancer. *Int J Cancer.* 2002;100:189–193.

45. Massion PP, Taflan PM, Shyr Y, et al. Early involvement of the phosphatidylinositol 3-kinase/Akt pathway in lung cancer progression. *Am J Respir Crit Care Med.* 2004;170:1088–1094.

46. Lantuejoul S, Soria JC, Morat L, et al. Telomere shortening and telomerase reverse transcriptase expression in preinvasive bronchial lesions. *Clin Cancer Res.* 2005;11:2074–2082.

47. Rahman SM, Shyr Y, Yildiz PB, et al. Proteomic patterns of preinvasive bronchial lesions. *Am J Respir Crit Care Med.* 2005;172:1556–1562.

48. Mascaux C, Laes JF, Anthoine G, Haller A, et al. Evolution of microRNA expression during human bronchial squamous carcinogenesis. *Eur Respir J.* 2009;33:352–359.

49. Sozzi G, Oggionni M, Alasio L, et al. Molecular changes track recurrence and progression of bronchial precancerous lesions. *Lung Cancer.* 2002;37:267–270.

50. Salaün M, Sesboüé R, Moreno-Swirc S, et al. Molecular predictive factors for progression of high-grade preinvasive bronchial lesions. *Am J Respir Crit Care Med.* 2008;177:880–886.

Atypical Adenomatous Hyperplasia

27

▶ Keith M. Kerr

This chapter considers the current theories of adenocarcinogenesis in the human lung and the place that atypical adenomatous hyperplasia (AAH) has in this process. AAH is a putative precursor of lung adenocarcinoma and recognized in the WHO classification of lung tumors as a preinvasive lesion.[1] It is now believed that at least a proportion of lung adenocarcinomas, most of which arise in the peripheral parenchymal compartment of the lung, develop through what has been referred to as an adenoma-carcinoma sequence. In making this comparison with adenocarcinogenesis in the colon, AAH is the equivalent of the adenoma. Indeed, when the late Dr. Roberta Miller of Vancouver made this comparison between the colon and the lung, she referred to AAH lesions as bronchioloalveolar adenomas.[2,3] The term AAH has, however, emerged from a number of different synonyms as the preferred term.

With the benefit of hindsight there are descriptions of lesions we would now consider AAH in work published in the 1950s and 1960s, but the first clear description of AAH with a suggestion of the importance of this lesion in adenocarcinogenesis was made by Shimosato et al.[4] in 1982. The lesions were referred to as "atypical alveolar cuboidal cell hyperplasia" and Shimosato speculated that "one can assume that some peripheral adenocarcinomas arise without any association with preexisting scar tissue as an in-situ carcinoma from almost normal appearing bronchioloalveoli. However, it is not certain whether or not cancer develops through a stage of atypical hyperplasia." Several years elapsed before a few more publications appeared on this subject, including Roberta Miller's two seminal papers in 1988 and 1990[2,3]: the vast majority of the literature on AAH, however, emanates from Japan. Shimosato et al.[4] and Noguchi et al.[5] deserve credit for formulating the hypothesis of a step-wise progression of disease in the lung periphery whereby AAH lesions transform into a lesion currently known as localized nonmucinous bronchioloalveolar carcinoma (LNMBAC), a lesion that could better be referred to as adenocarcinoma in situ. LNMBAC lesions tend to undergo alveolar collapse and fibroelastosis. At some point invasion supervenes, usually in the center of the lesion, and invasive adenocarcinoma is defined.

The epithelial compartment of the peripheral lung is functionally diverse and is regarded quite separately from central bronchial epithelium. Peripheral epithelium has a different population of stem cells from those in the bronchus. There are a number of stem cell candidates, most of which reside in the peripheral bronchiolar epithelium which, with alveolar epithelium, makes up the peripheral bronchioloalveolar epithelial compartment. Some differentiated cells appear to have stem-like properties.[6,7] A variant of the Clara cell which shares an immunophenotype with alveolar pneumocytes and is found at the bronchioloalveolar duct junction is one such putative stem cell. Cells with neuroendocrine characteristics, found in bronchiolar neuroendocrine bodies, also appear to behave like stem cells. Not much is known about the biology of these particular cells but it seems likely that they, perhaps especially the variant Clara cells, are the population that gives rise to AAH. This concept fits neatly with the terminology, proposed by Yatabe et al.,[8,9] of terminal respiratory unit (TRU) carcinogenesis and TRU-type adenocarcinomas.

Adenocarcinoma has replaced squamous cell carcinoma as the most prevalent form of lung cancer worldwide. For many years this was the case in many East Asian countries but it is a more recent development in North America and at least some European countries. In central and eastern Europe, squamous cell carcinoma still appears to dominate. Although the association between tobacco smoking and adenocarcinoma is less strong than it is with squamous or small cell carcinoma, there is a dose-response relationship between smoking and risk of developing adenocarcinoma. While it is true that most lung cancers encountered in nonsmokers are adenocarcinomas, most adenocarcinomas, at least in European and North American populations, are found in smokers. The reasons for this rise in adenocarcinoma are not clear but a number of factors may be relevant. Changes in cigarette manufacture have led to lower nicotine and tar levels in smoke but also a change in many other carcinogens, including a rise in N-nitrosamines such as the potent carcinogen NNK (see also Chapter 26). There is some evidence that NNK and other nitrosamines may be more carcinogenic to the TRU and give rise to more adenocarcinomas.[10,11] Smoking habits have changed. Lower nicotine and tar levels and other alterations to the "smoking experience" such as filters mean that smokers of the "modern cigarette" inhale more deeply than earlier consumers. This, it has been suggested, exposes the peripheral lung to more carcinogens. In many countries the proportion of women who smoke has risen. This accounts for the observed rise in female lung cancer. Women seem more prone to develop adenocarcinoma but whether this is because the female smoking generation is consuming a more "adenocarcinogenic" cigarette than their male predecessors is not clear. Adenocarcinoma has also risen in males, suggesting the cigarette may be the culprit. As is discussed below, however, women seem more prone to develop AAH. The relationship between AAH and smoking is not known; are AAH more likely to develop in female rather than male smokers or are females more likely than males to develop AAH for some other reason, and AAH then becomes transformed into LNMBAC and adenocarcinoma?

There have been no studies of the biochemical influences that smoking may have on AAH. A small number of studies have shown altered gene expression in morphologically normal peripheral lung epithelium in smokers. As with similar studies on bronchial epithelium (see Chapter 26), among the differentially expressed genes in the smokers studied were those coding for xenobiotic metabolizing enzymes involved in the detoxification but also activation of tobacco carcinogens, and genes involved in cell cycle regulation.[12]

Although the combined literature addressing the molecular biology of AAH is less than that concerning central bronchial carcinogenesis, some interesting facts are emerging which give insight into the probable molecular events driving peripheral lung adenocarcinogenesis. These are reviewed below. There is good evidence, however, that the stepwise morphological progression of disease from AAH to LNMBAC to invasive adenocarcinoma is accompanied by progressive accumulation of genetic changes. It has been suggested that between 3 and 12 critical genetic events must occur, in the correct order, during lung carcinogenesis.[13] This issue and how it relates to field carcinogenesis in the central airway's epithelial compartment is discussed in a little more detail in Chapter 2 but many of the principles are also relevant to TRU carcinogenesis. While some of the genetic events in the AAH-LNMBAC sequence are common to those seen in bronchial squamous dysplasia and carcinoma in situ (SD/CIS), there are also differences. As with SD/CIS, it is likely that the observed morphological progression of disease is a reflection of accumulation of genetic changes. The morphology of these lesions is discussed in the next section.

PREINVASIVE LESIONS OF THE PERIPHERAL LUNG

AAH is defined as a preinvasive lesion in the WHO classification of lung tumors as follows: "a localised proliferation of mild to moderately atypical cells lining involved alveoli and, sometimes, respiratory bronchioles, resulting in focal lesions in peripheral alveolated lung, usually <5 mm in diameter and generally in the absence of underlying interstitial inflammation and fibrosis."[1] The last part of the definition is important as it emphasizes one of the factors which helps distinguish this lesion from the reactive proliferation of bronchioloalveolar epithelium seen in a number of inflammatory and fibrosing conditions in the lung. Some of these latter pathological diseases do appear to be associated with an increased risk of developing lung cancer, together with other lung lesions that also appear to have the potential to undergo malignant change. Reactive bronchioloalveolar cell hyperplasia is also an important differential diagnosis of AAH; this is considered below.

Two relevant issues are raised in this thread of discussion. The first is the recognition that, as in the central airways, cell proliferation seems to be an important early step in the development of neoplasia in the lung periphery. The second is rather more semantic and concerns the distinction between hyperplasia, a reactive phenomenon, and neoplasia, also a "reactive" proliferation of sorts but one that has, by definition, become, to some extent, autonomous and independent of the original stimulus that triggered the "new growth". Sometimes the distinction between these two processes is distinctly blurred; this is certainly the case with AAH.

AAH is the best recognized and most widely studied preinvasive lesion in the peripheral lung. Another lesion named bronchiolar columnar cell dysplasia (BCCD) has been proposed as an alternative preinvasive lesion arising in the TRU epithelial compartment. Descriptions of this lesion are few but seem to describe cytological atypia in bronchiolar epithelium. While this cannot be dismissed as a possible alternative precursor of lung cancer in the peripheral lung (one of the two papers describing this lesion considers BCCD, a potential precursor lesion, for peripheral squamous cell as well as adenocarcinoma), it is poorly recognized.[14] Until there are more published studies on BCCD, and experience of the lesion is more widespread, it is difficult to come to any conclusion regarding this lesion's place in the current discussion. The lesion will be more widely recognized only when clear criteria for diagnosis are established and accepted. One may occasionally identify what might be BCCD, but there is no data to relate it to the development of pulmonary carcinomas.

The evolution of cancer through a series of morphologically recognizable precursor stages has been referred to as the "sequential model" of carcinogenesis; examples would be SD/CIS as precursors of bronchial squamous cell carcinoma and AAH/LNMBAC (adenocarcinoma in situ) as precursors of adenocarcinoma. The "parallel model" of carcinogenesis considers the possibility that carcinoma may arise de novo from an epithelium without passing through a morphologically recognizable precursor stage.[15] This has been proposed as a mechanism through which small cell lung carcinoma (SCLC) may arise.[16] Although SCLC has been linked with SD/CIS, it is impossible to deny that SCLC may also arise in this rather more abrupt fashion, without a progenitor lesion; there is some molecular evidence to support this suggestion. Equally, it is possible that some lung adenocarcinomas may arise in this way, from the TRU epithelium or, indeed, from more central bronchial epithelium.

ATYPICAL ADENOMATOUS HYPERPLASIA, GROSS FEATURES

The identification of AAH is largely the preserve of pathologists. There is an emerging literature on the high resolution computed tomographic (HRCT) scanning appearances of AAH discovered in the course of lung cancer screening using this imaging modality. This work comes almost exclusively from Japanese and other East Asian centers.[17] Reference to this work will be made below. Most AAH lesions are incidental findings during microscopic examination of the alveolated lung. A proportion of AAH lesions may be identified macroscopically but success in this search is highly dependent upon the absence of concurrent pathology in the lung parenchyma under examination and upon how well prepared the lung tissue is before and during sectioning.

In well-prepared material, AAH lesions appear as poorly defined pale patches of a few millimeters in diameter on the cut surface of the lung parenchyma (Fig. 27-1). Their color ranges from gray through tan to cream or yellowish. The margins of the lesions are indistinct, blending into the surrounding lung. AAH lesions are rarely palpable on the lung cut surface. The surface of some lesions may be stippled by a few tiny pits that represent the alveolar spaces within the lesion. Occasional lesions may appear cystic; this is due to small foci of centriacinar emphysema arising in the same area as the AAH. These gross findings are not specific; the author finds that many lesions with this gross appearance are nonspecific inflammatory foci or tiny areas of fibrosis.

FIGURE 27-1 Gross image of AAH lesion. The small holes in the lesion represent individual alveolar spaces.

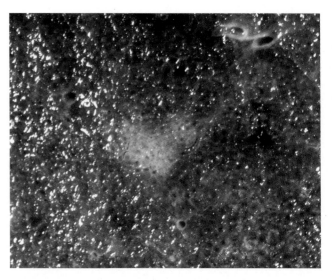

It should be clear from this description that the presence of other pathology such as pneumonia, extensive emphysema, or lung fibrosis will make the macroscopic identification of AAH more or less impossible.

Adequate preparation of the lung tissue before gross inspection is required to maximize the chances of identifying AAH lesions, at gross inspection or during microscopy. Whenever possible, all lung resection specimens (lobectomy, pneumonectomy, wedge resections, etc.) received fresh from the operating room should be inflated with 10% neutral buffered formalin, either per-bronchially or by needle and syringe. After 24 hours suspended floating in fixative, the specimens are serially sectioned. Larger resection specimens are cut into 1-cm thick parasagittal slices using a specially designed cutting board. Lung slices are then laid out on the cutting bench and periodically flooded with clean water while being observed under a bright light. The water partially reexpands the lung parenchyma, making small lesions easier to identify. All possible AAH lesions are sampled; if none are seen, then three to six random parenchymal tissue blocks are taken. Methods of tissue preparation and sampling vary greatly and this may be one reason for the differences in reported prevalence of AAH.

ATYPICAL ADENOMATOUS HYPERPLASIA, HISTOLOGICAL FEATURES

The WHO definition of AAH is given above. It is relevant to note that, given the earlier discussion of the possible role of BADJ stem cells in the evolution of TRU adenocarcinogenesis, these lesions appear to arise in a centriacinar location, the alveolar walls within and surrounding the respiratory bronchioles and alveolar ducts forming the framework for lesion growth (Fig. 27-2). The alveolar walls of an AAH lesion are lined by a single intermittent layer of cells that may be flattened, cuboidal, or low columnar; some cells appear round or globular, and others have apical snouts, sometimes referred to as hobnail or "peg cells" (Fig. 27-3). The cell population typically is quite heterogeneous and gaps between the larger cells which protrude into the alveolar spaces give the cell lining its "intermittent" character (Figs. 27-4 and 27-5). The cell cytoplasm is generally fairly nondescript; occasionally, small vacuoles may be seen. Ultrastructural and immunohistochemical studies have shown that the cells in AAH can show alveolar pneumocyte or Clara cell differentiation. Both may be found in the same lesion. Ciliated cells or mucous cells are not found in AAH.

Nuclei are generally regular with little pleomorphism. Nuclear inclusions are not uncommon in AAH. Nuclei can appear quite hyperchromatic and occasional large and irregular nuclei can be found. Some cells may show double nuclei, often located in the apical cytoplasm of an enlarged cell (Fig. 27-6). Mitotic figures are extremely uncommon.

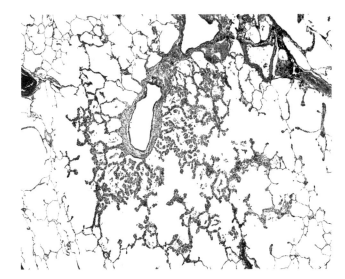

FIGURE 27-2 Low-power image of an AAH lesion in an obvious centriacinar location.

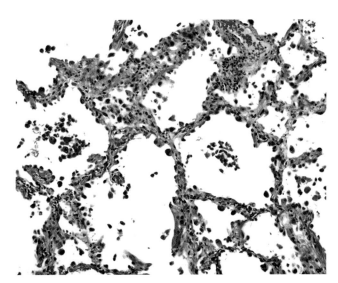

FIGURE 27-3 The cells lining the alveolar walls in AAH characteristically, in most lesions, form this interrupted lining with intercellular gaps. Some of the cells are quite large.

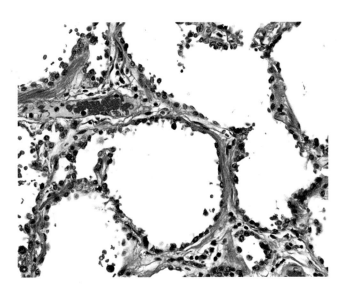

FIGURE 27-4 Higher power image of typical relatively low-grade AAH. The hobnail features of some of the cells can be seen. Some nuclei are apical as opposed to basally located.

FIGURE 27-5 High-power image of low-grade AAH in Figure 27-4 showing hobnail cells and occasional cells show intranuclear inclusions.

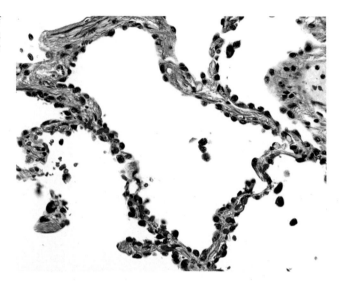

FIGURE 27-6 This high-power image of AAH shows cells with double nuclei.

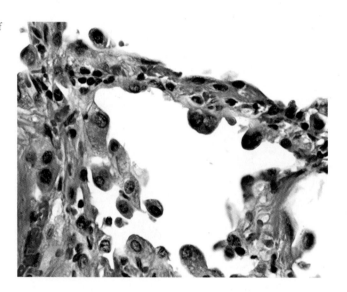

The alveolar walls within the AAH lesion are usually a little thickened due to an increase in collagen and also some elastosis. Occasional examples may be encountered where this process is more marked (Fig. 27-7). This may be associated with apparent shrinkage of the alveolar spaces or collapse of the alveolar architecture; this phenomenon is well described in LNMBAC but can also occur in AAH. The fibrotic interstitium may take on a rather hyalinized character. Chronic inflammatory cell infiltrates may be present. These are generally light in character but some lesions may be heavily infiltrated and lymphoid aggregates may be seen. This inflammatory process does not extend beyond the limits of the lesion as defined by the epithelial cell component, an important factor in distinguishing AAH from reactive hyperplasia in interstitial lung disease. Occasional lesions will be seen where only part of the lesion is fibrosed and the epithelial lining cells are lost. It is possible that this is a process that progressively leads to regression of the AAH lesion into a small hyalinized bronchioloalveolar scar.

AAH lesions are small localized foci of millimeter size, which usually stand out from the surrounding normal lung parenchyma due to the slight thickening of the alveolar walls and studding of the alveolar wall lining by enlarged epithelial cells. Lesions may also be highlighted by the

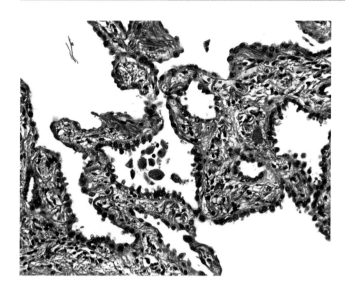

FIGURE 27-7 This example of AAH shows notably thickened alveolar walls with prominent elastic fibers. This is also a relatively cellular lesion with hobnail cells.

tendency for alveolar macrophages to accumulate within the alveolar spaces; this presumably, at least in part, is a result of the centriacinar location of AAH. Occasionally, in cases where there are very large numbers of AAH identified, larger AAH-like zones may be encountered where margins are difficult to discern, perhaps the result of merging of adjacent lesions.

AAH lesions vary in their cellularity. Some lesions may be encountered where there are few or no intercellular gaps, where more of the cells have a columnar or hobnail morphology and pleomorphism is a little more notable (Fig. 27-8). Occasional tiny tufts of cells may be seen but widespread stratification or papillary structures suggest LNMBAC. Such lesions tend to be slightly larger and show more interstitial fibrosis. The WHO classification recommends against separating AAH lesions into low or high grade, largely because there are no agreed, robust criteria for making the distinction. Nonetheless, some authors do make reference to low- and high-grade AAH. It is inevitable that there are "lower" and "higher" grade lesions, as poorly defined as these might be, if we accept that at least a proportion of AAH lesions progress to become what is recognized as LNMBAC, that is adenocarcinoma in situ. This is an arbitrary division of what is a biological continuum of disease. Criteria have been suggested for distinguishing AAH from LNMBAC and

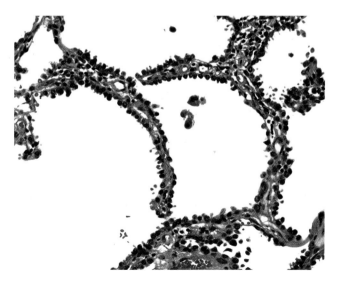

FIGURE 27-8 A more cellular AAH lesion with hobnail cells. This and the lesion in Figure 27-7 are higher grade AAH lesions but still falling short of features of localized nonmucinous bronchioloalveolar carcinoma (adenocarcinoma in situ).

these are discussed in the later section on differential diagnosis of AAH. There will be lesions that just fall short of being classifiable as LNMBAC, yet another "gray area" in this subjective discipline of surgical histopathology.

When AAH was first included in the WHO classification of lung tumors in 1999, it was stated that AAH always measured <5 mm in diameter. This was based upon Roberta Miller's assertion, as discussed above, that any lesion over 5 mm in diameter should be regarded as LNMBAC.[3] Not infrequently lesions are encountered which show the pathological features of AAH described above, which do not fulfill the suggested criteria for a diagnosis of LNMBAC, as discussed below, and which measure over 5 mm. This is the reason for the change in the definition of AAH published in 2004. It is true that AAH usually measures <5 mm across, around 65% to 75% of lesions measure 3 mm or less. Between 10% and 20% of lesions measure over 5 mm. About 10% of AAH lesions the authors measured were over 10 mm in diameter.[18] AAH lesions measuring up to 24 mm have been described.[19] As mentioned above, larger lesions also tend to be of "higher" grade, although this is not always the case.

The importance of properly prepared material cannot be overemphasized; some of the early skepticism around the existence of AAH stemmed from inadequate sampling of poorly inflated lung tissues. The presence of concurrent inflammation, fibrosis, or emphysema makes lesion identification very difficult. One must have a relatively high threshold for making the diagnosis of AAH; many possible lesions may be dismissed due to uncertainty. As is described below, the vast majority of AAH lesions described by pathologists have been found in the lung resected for carcinoma, especially adenocarcinoma. AAH may be found in any alveolated lung sample, provided there is sufficient expanded tissue present to allow tissue identification. AAH would be a very difficult diagnosis in a small transbronchial lung biopsy sample. It is unlikely that sufficient alveolated lung would be present to demonstrate the lesion and surrounding alveoli. At best, AAH-like areas could be described. AAH cannot be diagnosed by cytology. Various cytological samples may contain populations of atypical bronchioloalveolar cells but given the importance of architecture in the diagnosis of AAH and LNMBAC, a diagnosis of "atypical bronchioloalveolar cell proliferation" is all that should be offered.

ATYPICAL ADENOMATOUS HYPERPLASIA, DIFFERENTIAL DIAGNOSIS

The most important differential diagnosis of AAH is LNMBAC. Both these lesions consist of an abnormal cell population lining groups of adjacent alveoli. LNMBAC is considered adenocarcinoma in situ. The distinction between these two "grades" of lesions in what is regarded as an evolution of disease is arbitrary, but Minami et al.[20] have proposed a set of five criteria that may be sought in these lesions. LNMBAC will usually show at least three of these features; AAH lesions will rarely show more than one (Figs. 27-9 and 27-10). These five features are (1) prominent nucleoli and course chromatin; (2) high cell density, with notable nuclear overlapping and no intercellular gaps; (3) prominent cell stratification; (4) increased cell height, generally exceeding the height of normal columnar cells lining adjacent bronchioles; and (5) "picket fence" pattern of cell growth, which may be complex and may form papillae.

LNMBAC lesions often have a high proportion of hobnail cells. The cell population in LNMBAC tends to be rather more homogeneous than AAH, and this, together with the increase in cell size, tends to make the limits of the lesion more distinct from the surrounding lung than in AAH, the latter tending, at a microscopic level, to blend into the surrounding alveolar lining. Of course, as would be predicted from the proposed progression of AAH to LNMBAC, lesions will be encountered that show both areas fulfilling criteria for LNMBAC and parts that remain like AAH. In such circumstances the author diagnoses LNMBAC. Interstitial thickening and mild to moderate interstitial infiltration of lymphoid cells are frequent in LNMBAC; occasionally, the lymphoid infiltrate may be very heavy. LNMBAC lesions often measure more than 10 mm in diameter and lesions over 20 mm are not unusual.

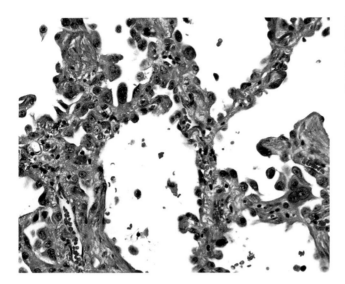

FIGURE 27-9 While this lesion shows intercellular gaps and cytological variability, which are features of AAH, the degree of atypia warrants a diagnosis of LNMBAC. Nonetheless, this is a difficult lesion to classify.

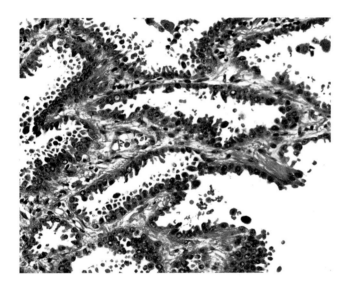

FIGURE 27-10 A clear example of LNMBAC with atypia, overlapping and stratification.

A number of benign lesions or processes enter the differential diagnosis of AAH.[21] There are very rare benign tumors which occur in the lung and which may show cells lining either native alveolar walls or alveolus-like spaces formed by the lesion.[22] In most circumstances, the distinction between these lesions and AAH is relatively straightforward if attention is paid to the cytology and architecture of individual lesions. Most clinically encountered examples of these benign tumors are considerably larger than AAH lesions. Papillary adenomas show alveoli lined by a homogeneous population of plump cuboidal or columnar cells but this lining is also thrown into papillary folds with fibrovascular cores. Ciliated cells may be seen. Alveolar adenoma is a benign tumor which shows microcystic alveolus-like spaces lined by cells which may resemble some of those found in AAH. However, the lesion architecture is nothing like that of native alveoli and the spaces are embedded in a fibrous and spindle cell stroma. Sclerosing hemangioma (pneumocytoma) is included here for completeness, as a lesion showing alveolar cell–type differentiation and which expresses thyroid transcription factor 1 (TTF1), a lineage marker for the TRU epithelium. AHH and LNMBAC both also express TTF1 but sclerosing hemangioma does not have an alveolar architecture.

Micronodular pneumocyte hyperplasia (MNPH) is a benign proliferation of alveolar pneumocytes. Lesions are usually only a few millimeters across and have a passing resemblance to

AAH.[23] However, the cells in MNPH tend to be rather homogeneous and plump and the alveolar spaces are small, distorted, rather fibrotic and frequently filled by macrophages giving the lesion a solid appearance. MNPH is extremely rare and is found in patients with tuberous sclerosis and lymphangioleiomyomatosis. Minute meningothelial nodules are tiny incidental findings in peripheral lung samples but there the resemblance with AAH ends. These lesions have a paravenular location and comprise plump pericyte-like cells aggregated in interstitial clusters. There is no proliferation of alveolar lining cells and these lesions are more likely to be confused with DIPNECH, a lesion discussed in Chapter 28.

An obvious and potentially difficult differential diagnosis concerns the separation of AAH from reactive proliferation of alveolar lining cells. In virtually any situation where there is alveolar interstitial inflammation and fibrosis, there may be proliferation of alveolar lining cells. When this fibro-inflammatory process is diffuse such as in idiopathic pulmonary fibrosis, nonspecific interstitial pneumonitis, organizing diffuse alveolar damage, etc., there should be no problem in differentiating associated epithelial proliferation from AAH. This is the reason why the statement regarding the lack of inflammation and fibrosis in the surrounding lung is included in the WHO definition of AAH. In AAH, any inflammation or fibrosis in the alveolar walls is confined to the lesion; the surrounding alveolar walls should lack these changes. The author would never make a diagnosis of AAH in the lung showing interstitial pneumonia.

If the fibro-inflammatory lesions are more localized it may be a little more difficult. Reactive lesions may be very irregular in shape and the alveoli may show signs of organizing pneumonia or even acute inflammation (Fig. 27-11). Generally speaking, the only cells found in the alveoli of AAH are macrophages. The cells in reactive hyperplasia associated with fibrosis and inflammation tend to be rather homogeneous populations of small regular cuboidal cells with round nuclei forming a continuous lining of affected alveoli. These lesions may be located in a centriacinar position, if the inflammation causing them began in small airways, but this is not always the case. Reactive proliferations of alveolar lining cells may also be seen covering alveolar walls abutting septa, bronchovascular bundles, large blood vessels, or the visceral pleura.

Peribronchiolar metaplasia (PBM), also known as Lambertosis or "bronchiolization of the alveoli," is a centriacinar lesion that should be distinguished from AAH. PBM probably results from small airway injury and consists of lesions, often multiple, in an affected area of lung where terminal bronchioles are distorted and bronchiolar-type epithelium lines what were the respiratory bronchioles and adjacent alveoli (Figs. 27-12 and 27-13). There may be quite marked fibrosis and some inflammation associated with this process. Florid examples may be mistaken for small "adenomas" or even well-differentiated adenocarcinoma. Important features of PBM are that the

FIGURE 27-11 Medium-power image of reactive pneumocyte hyperplasia. Hobnail cells are present. The context is that of alveolar interstitial inflammation and organizing pneumonia (Masson bodies).

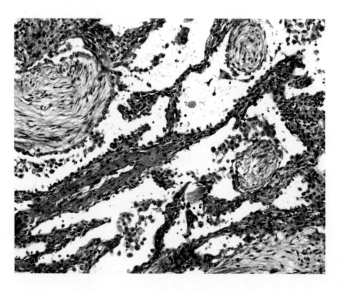

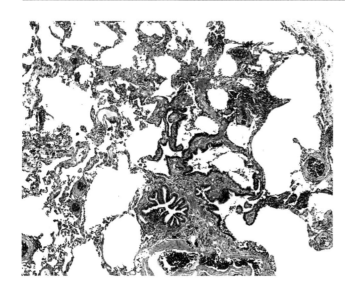

FIGURE 27-12 Medium-power image of PBM. This is, like AAH, a centriacinar proliferation lining alveolar walls.

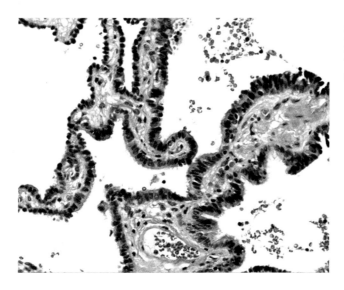

FIGURE 27-13 Note that the cell population in the specimen shown in Figure 27-12 is mixed and includes ciliated cells. These lesions may show marked scarring and chronic inflammation.

epithelial cell population is bronchiolar in type so shows not only Clara cells but also ciliated cells. Very occasionally mucinous cells may be present and cytokeratin 5/6 positive, p63 positive basal cells may also be identified.

The prevalence of AAH in the general population is unknown. Given that these lesions are asymptomatic, are almost impossible to identify in vivo, and are far from easy to find in pathological specimens, estimates of prevalence are prone to error. Even the most careful and assiduous search for lesions will underestimate the number present, and the extent to which specimens are sampled in the search for AAH will be tempered by practical realities in individual laboratories. Nonetheless, studies have been carried out with the aim of finding AAH lesions. There are four reported autopsy studies on AAH.[24–27] In one study, it is not clear if a prospective study was carried out; AAH was found in 3.6% of Japanese subjects. Three prospective studies have been published. One from the USA found AAH in 2% of 100 consecutive autopsies,[25] while two Japanese studies found that between 2.8% and 10.2% of subjects had AAH.[26,27] The higher figures were for older patients with a history of malignancy, both factors that may influence prevalence rates. Given what has already been said about the problems in finding AAH lesions, their discovery in autopsy lungs must be particularly challenging.

Almost all the reported cases of AAH lesions have been found in lungs resected for other reasons; the AAH lesions were incidental findings. AAH lesions are most often found in lungs resected for primary carcinoma.[2,19,28–32] This could be because this is the commonest reason for substantial lung resection in clinical practice, but our limited experience of finding AAH in lungs resected for other reasons suggests this is not the case. A number of studies have been published on the prevalence of AAH in lung cancer resection specimens. Most of these studies concern Japanese patients and some are retrospective series rather than prospective studies aimed at finding AAH lesions. Five prospective studies have been published, three from Japan,[28,30,31] one from Canada,[2] and one from the United Kingdom.[32] The overall prevalence of AAH in the Japanese studies is higher (16.4%, 23.2%, and 49%, respectively) than in the Canadian (9.3%) and UK (12.1%) studies. There were, however, differences between the studies, in the way the lung specimens were sectioned and sampled. The Japanese study that reported the highest prevalence of AAH also appeared to involve the finest sectioning of the lung and considerable tissue sampling.[31] These five studies, together with many other publications, report a higher prevalence of AAH in lungs resected for adenocarcinoma, when compared with resections for other tumor types.[33] In the three prospective Japanese studies, the prevalence of AAH in adenocarcinoma resections were, respectively, 17%, 29.3%, and 57%, as opposed to 11.6%, 9.8%, and 30% in squamous cell carcinoma resections. In the Canadian and UK studies, the findings showed AAH in 15.6% and 23.2% of adenocarcinoma resections and in 3% and 3.3%, respectively, of squamous cell carcinoma resections. These data suggest a number of things. The harder one looks for AAH the more is found. AAH is most prevalent in adenocarcinoma-bearing lungs, consistently across studies in all continents. It is tempting to speculate that the prevalence of AAH in lungs bearing squamous cell carcinoma approximates to a "background" prevalence; in which case, Japanese subjects may be more prone than Western individuals to develop AAH. The higher prevalence of AAH in those with adenocarcinoma implies a greater risk in this group of patients. It is not known whether this is the result of more AAH lesions per se or whether lesions in these patients are biologically different and more likely to progress to adenocarcinoma. Some of these studies reported AAH in association with large cell carcinoma and noted a prevalence intermediate between those of squamous and adenocarcinoma-bearing subjects.

While many of the reported cases concerned single AAH lesions, there is an inevitable underestimation of lesion numbers. It is likely that AAH lesions occur in multiple foci in affected lungs but that some patients seem to have more lesions than others.[33,34] Some patients have very large numbers of lesions, exclusively individuals with adenocarcinoma, their resection specimens often showing concurrent LNMBAC lesions and multiple synchronous primary invasive tumors. At the time of writing, the author has just reported a lobectomy specimen for primary T1N0M0 mixed-type adenocarcinoma, predominantly papillary pattern, which also shows a second mixed pattern adenocarcinoma (predominantly bronchioloalveolar/lepidic pattern with central scar and acinar invasive disease—see below and Chapters 3–5), ten further LNMBAC lesions, and around 130 AAH lesions. About 40 tissue blocks were taken from this left upper lobe. This is an unusual case but reflects well the issues around field carcinogenesis discussed earlier and in Chapter 26. In published Japanese studies, there is no clear gender difference in AAH prevalence. Chapman and Kerr,[32] however, noted that females had more AAH than males; this was true for all patients and for those with adenocarcinoma. The nature of the material in which AAH is found makes it difficult to comment of the association of AAH with age. There are case reports of AAH being found in 17-year-old patients, but the autopsy studies mentioned above suggest that more AAH are found in elderly subjects.[35,36]

ATYPICAL ADENOMATOUS HYPERPLASIA, ETIOLOGY

There are no clear etiological factors for AAH. Several Japanese studies have attempted to relate AAH to smoking but have been rather inconclusive.[30,34,37] One study did find smoking more common in patients with multiple AAH and adenocarcinoma.[37] Almost all of the AAH patients in the Chapman and Kerr[32] study were current or former smokers. Animal models of lung adenocarcinogenesis describe pulmonary lesions not unlike AAH as possible precursors of invasive disease. In the sheep disease ovine pulmonary adenomatosis (jaagsiekte), a retrovirus, is responsible for a disease rather like multifocal bronchioloalveolar adenocarcinoma; efforts to detect retroviral DNA in human disease have so far proved fruitless.[38] Rats exposed to asbestos develop AAH-like lesions as well as adenocarcinomas. AAH patients do not, as a group, show any greater tendency to have had occupations associated with asbestos exposure, when compared to similar patients without AAH.[39] A few studies have suggested that AAH may be commoner either in patients who have a history of previous nonpulmonary malignancy or in those who have a stronger family history of cancer.[30,32] There is little consistency between these studies and they are too few in number to allow proper conclusions to be drawn. There are single reports of a patient with Li-Fraumeni cancer syndrome[40] and another with familial adenomatous polyposis who had AAH.[41] All these studies suggest the possibility of a genetic predisposition to developing AAH, but without much more evidence, any such association remains purely speculative. There does seem to be circumstantial evidence at least that ethnicity may influence AAH prevalence.

ATYPICAL ADENOMATOUS HYPERPLASIA, CLINICAL IMPORTANCE

The importance of AAH and LNMBAC lies in the assumed risk that these lesions may progress to invasive adenocarcinoma. The degree of risk that either of these lesions poses to the individual is, however, unknown. There are no longitudinal studies of AAH lesions, mainly because they are more or less impossible to detect in vivo. Emerging HRCT-based lung cancer screening studies can identify very small so-called pure ground-glass opacities (GGOs). The GGO pattern corresponds to lesions in the peripheral lung parenchyma which still contain alveolar air but is a very nonspecific feature. Studies have been published describing HRCT software–based methods to distinguish AAH from LNMBAC but a reliable distinction has, so far, been elusive.[17] AAH cannot be distinguished radiologically from nonspecific fibro-inflammatory lesions or other artifacts. Both AAH and LNMBAC lesions can only be confidently diagnosed by pathologists after the lesions are removed. Longitudinal study of individual lesions will have to await more reliable radiological diagnosis. This may be possible for some LNMBAC lesions but seems an unlikely prospect for AAH.

There have been several studies comparing the prognosis (postoperative survival) of lung cancer patients with and without AAH.[33] One hypothesis is that patients with AAH in their resected lung are also likely to have AAH in their remaining lung tissue and that this poses an excess risk for future lung cancer development. All of these studies have failed to demonstrate a poorer prognosis for AAH patients. In the only case controlled study, of the largest cohort of AAH patients to be followed up, the author found a trend toward poorer survival in patients with larger numbers of AAH patients.[33,42] A review of the case records of patients in this study, however, demonstrated that the AAH-bearing cohort subsequently developed twice the number of second primary lung cancers and that most of these were second adenocarcinomas. Relatively few of the non-AAH patients developed a second adenocarcinoma.

ATYPICAL ADENOMATOUS HYPERPLASIA, MOLECULAR BIOLOGY

There is a growing body of data that exists regarding the molecular events that accompany and possibly drive the progression of AAH to LNMBAC and subsequently invasive disease, although this remains a smaller body of data than that exists for SD/CIS.[33,43] Generic comments were made in the introductory part of the equivalent section of the chapter on bronchial SD/CIS (Chapter 26) relating to the techniques used to study tumor molecular biology and the types of genomic alteration which appear important (see also Chapter 20). These comments are also relevant to studies of AAH and LNMBAC.

Numerous studies using morphometry, cytofluorimetry, and other measures of cell ploidy have demonstrated the "intermediate" position of AAH between normal brochioloalveolar epithelium and LNMBAC, with respect to cell size and shape, mean nuclear area, and nuclear DNA content. Interestingly, many of these studies show a proportion of cases with transitional features, shared between AAH and LNMBAC, more evidence that the former may progress into the latter.[18,33] Immunohistochemical studies demonstrating cell cycle activity have consistently shown AAH has a greater proliferative activity than normal alveolar epithelium but less than LNMBAC. Nonetheless, for a lesion considered hyperplastic, the growth fraction of AAH is remarkably low at around 1% to 4%.

p53 is an important tumor suppressor gene (TSG) which controls cell proliferation and promotes cell death pathways. Published values for *p53* positivity range widely, anywhere from 3% to 35% of AAH lesions.[33,44] In part, this will be a function of different anti-*p53* antibodies being used but also differing definitions of a "positive" case. Several studies report that *p53* positivity is higher in more cellular and atypical AAH lesions when compared to those of apparently lower grade. In contrast to LNMBAC, where *p53* mutation is reported in 16% to 33% of lesions, *p53* mutation is very rare in AAH. *p53* loss of heterozygosity (LOH—17p13) is also uncommon; one study reported this loss in 6% of AAH, 11% of LNMBAC, and 36% of early invasive adenocarcinomas.[45] p63 protein may be found in some AAH and LNMBAC lesions; data on bcl2 in these lesions seem to be very variable, while some studies report surviving levels low in low-grade AAH but markedly higher in high-grade lesions. There is very little work on the proteins and genes for factors upstream and downstream of p53: of p53 itself, its role in this disease progression is not entirely clear. The upregulation of the protein and gradual emergence of mutation suggest a potential role for loss of function of this TSG. Most of the mutational work has been done in Japan where the proportion of smokers in case series is likely to be relatively low; p53 mutation is associated with tobacco carcinogenesis.

With respect to the *P16ink4-cyclinD1-CDK4-RB* pathway, there are few studies in AAH. This is an important pathway, partially controlled by p53, which serves to promote G1-S arrest and limit cell cycle activity. Cyclin D1 has been found upregulated in AAH with less expression in LNMBAC and adenocarcinoma. *p16* gene promoter hypermethylation has been described in AAH, more so in higher grade lesions. *p16* function may also be lost through LOH at 9p21. This is described in 5% to 33% of AAH lesions and some studies found more loss in higher grade lesions.[46] All this suggests that, as with SD/CIS, cell cycle progression in AAH may be promoted through upregulation of cyclin D1 and loss of p16 function.

The HER cell membrane receptors, when activated by ligand binding or by activating mutation, stimulate a number of intracellular signalling pathways promoting cell cycle activity, proliferation, and angiogenesis and inhibit apoptosis. EGFR (HER1) is probably the most important of these in adenocarcinogenesis; HER2 may also have a role. The *KRAS* pathway is one of the downstream targets of activated *EGFR*. *EGFR* mutation appears to be an important driver of adenocarcinogenesis in nonsmokers, who are often also female and of East Asian ethnicity. *KRAS* mutation is more associated with smoking. Studies of EGFR protein expression and gene copy number are few. Neither has been shown increased in AAH; increased protein but not gene copy number are described in LNMBAC but both are more often seen in adenocarcinomas. Several studies have sought *EGFR* mutations at various stages in this proposed pathway of adenocarcinogenesis. The results show enormous variation, probably the result of technical differences and the evolution of more sensitive methods for detecting mutation in what are often very small DNA samples. *EGFR* mutation has been described in 3% to 44% of AAHs, 10.8% to 100% of LNMBACs, and 8% to 90% of adenocarcinomas. All but one of these studies concerns Japanese patients and these show a consistent rise in *EGFR* mutation prevalence as disease grade increases.[47,48]

KRAS mutation is an important genetic abnormality in many adenocarcinomas, especially those occurring in smokers. *KRAS* mutations tend to be commoner in adenocarcinomas in

Caucasians, when compared to East Asian subjects. *KRAS* mutation has been described in anything up to 39% of AAHs examined.[33,48,49] There is a sense that while *KRAS* mutation may fall in frequency from AAH to LNMBAC to adenocarcinoma in Japanese patients, the reverse is true in Western populations. This may be because EGFR is more important in nonsmoking Japanese patients and *KRAS* and *EGFR* mutations are mutually exclusive in the same lesion. Indeed some Japanese workers have asserted that *KRAS* mutant AAH lesions are much less likely than *EGFR* mutant AAH lesions to progress to LNMBAC and invasive disease. More data are needed on this topic, especially in non-Japanese subjects.

HER2 protein is occasionally overexpressed in higher grade AAH; more is found in LNM-BAC and adenocarcinoma. *HER2* mutation is rare in adenocarcinoma and has not been described in AAH. Progressive telomere shortening during cell division is an important mechanism in cell ageing and promoting cell death. Reversal of this process leads to cell immortalization and this is a common finding in cancer cells, mediated by the upregulation of various components of the telomerase complex. Several telomerase related molecules have been shown to be progressively upregulated in the progression through low to higher grade AAH, LNMBAC, and adenocarcinoma.

A number of other potentially important molecules such as eIF4E, LAT1, and NF-kappaB show progressive upregulation with disease progression. Occasional studies have shown evidence of loss of other TSGs such as *FHIT, P27, and LKB1* during adenocarcinogenesis. Data on all these factors are too few to draw any conclusions. Many other factors, such as cell adhesion molecules, matrix metalloproteinases, differentiation markers, and cytochrome P450s, have been immuno-histochemically evaluated in AAH, LNMBAC, and adenocarcinomas. It is difficult to draw many conclusions from these studies, but there is a tendency for expression to reflect the gradual progression in phenotype toward malignancy through grades of AAH to LNMBAC.

Several studies have shown that AAH lesions demonstrate clonality. LOH in various 3p loci has been described in 10% to 43% of AAH lesions. Findings are very variable between studies, depending on the particular loci studied and there are inconsistencies. Other losses in AAH at 9q,13q, 16p, and 17q hint at potentially important TSGs in these regions but, with the exception of 9q34 (*TSC1* or a nearby gene), none of these data concern more than one of two AAH lesions in single studies.[33,45] LOH is more frequent and widespread in LNMBAC.

EGFR and *KRAS* mutation analyses of multiple AAH, LMBAC, and/or adenocarcinomas in the same patient support the belief that these lesions are independently arising synchronous lesions. This is also the conclusion of studies of *HUMARA* polymorphisms, patterns of mutation in mitochondrial DNA D-loop regions and LOH studies. All this is in keeping with the theory of field carcinogenesis. Apart from the data on *p16* mentioned above, there is emerging evidence that other genes in AAH lesions may be silenced by promoter hypermethylation and that there may be progressive accumulation of more methylated genes during disease progression.

It is clear from the above synopsis that much is known about changes in the molecular characteristics of various lesions in this proposed pathway of adenocarcinogenesis. It is not at all clear, however, which are the key changes. More work is needed on the potentially interesting issue of *EGFR* and *KRAS* mutation and their respective importance according to the patient's ethnicity and smoking habit. Emerging evidence suggests gene hypermethylation may play an important role in this process. It is likely that further improvements in molecular investigative techniques will allow better analysis of the small nucleic acid samples derived from AAH in particular. With luck, new data will clarify rather than confuse our understanding of the molecular biology of pulmonary adenocarcinogenesis.

CONCLUSION

This chapter has reviewed many issues relating to the morphology, prevalence, association, and molecular biology of AAH and discussed the place of this lesion as a progenitor lesion in a step-wise progression of disease leading to invasive adenocarcinoma. Probably only very few AAH lesions progress into LNMBAC, which is now regarded as adenocarcinoma in situ. Although the histopathological distinction between AAH and LNMBAC may, in some cases, be difficult, and our knowledge of the risks and rate of progression of AAH to LNMBAC is essentially nil, this may be of limited clinical importance. Currently, with the exception of occasional larger LNMBACs, these lesions cannot be reliably identified in vivo. When they are diagnosed by the pathologist, they pose no (further) threat to the patient, having been excised.

Assuming we could identify LNMBAC in vivo, a more important question is the identification of invasion. This process appears to follow on, after a process of collapse of the alveolar framework in the LNMBAC lesion, converting a so-called Noguchi type A lesion, without collapse, into a type B LNMBAC that shows focal collapse and fibroelastosis.[5] Each of these lesion types has a 100% 5-year survival consistent with adenocarcinoma in situ. Invasion in the centre of the collapsed LNMBAC is heralded by neofibroplasia, probably a stromal response to invasive carcinoma. Microscopic foci of invasion within alveolar septa or at the margin of the collapsed "fibrotic" lesion center similarly have no effect on patient prognosis. If the central focus of new fibroblastic growth or area of invasive carcinoma measures <5 mm in diameter, there still appears to be no metastatic risk; larger foci herald a fall in survival. These invasive adenocarcinomas with peripheral BAC-pattern disease are sometimes referred to as Noguchi type C lesions. These issues are of clinical importance since the pathological identification of invasion may be very difficult yet is an important determinant of patient management. There is also, therefore, an implied "minimally invasive" stage of disease, evidence of invasion without detriment to prognosis. This potentially important category has still to be clearly defined. More discussion of these issues can be found in Chapter 5.

References

1. Kerr KM, Fraire AE, Pugatch B, et al. Atypical adenomatous hyperplasia. In: Travis WD, Brambilla E, Muller-Hermelink HK, et al., eds. *World Health Organisation Classification of Tumours. Pathology and Genetics of Tumours of the Lung, Pleura, Thymus and Heart.* Lyon: IARC press; 2004:73–75.
2. Miller RR, Nelems B, Evans KG, et al. Glandular neoplasia of the lung. A proposed analogy to colonic tumours. *Cancer.* 1988;61:1009–1014.
3. Miller RR. Bronchioloalveolar cell adenomas. *Am J Surg Pathol.* 1990;14:904–912.
4. Shimosato Y, Kodama T, Kameya T. Morphogenesis of peripheral type adenocarcinoma of the lung. In: Shimosato Y, Melamed MR, Nettesheim P, eds. *Morphogenesis of Lung Cancer.* Vol 1. Boca Raton, FL: CRC Press; 1982:65–90.
5. Noguchi M, Morokawa A, Kawasaki M, et al. Small adenocarcinoma of the lung. Histologic characteristics and prognosis. *Cancer.* 1995;75:2844–2852.
6. Kotton DN, Fine A. Lung stem cells. *Cell Tissue Res.* 2008;331:145–156.
7. Giangreco A, Groot KR, Janes SM. Lung cancer and lung stem cells. Strange bedfellows? *Am J Respir Crit Care Med.* 2007;175:547–553.
8. Yatabe Y, Mitsudomi T, Takahashi T. TTF-1 expression in pulmonary adenocarcinoma. *Am J Surg Pathol.* 2002;26:767–773.
9. Tanaka H, Yanagisawa K, Shinjo K, et al. Lineage-specific dependency of lung adenocarcinomas on the lung development regulator TTF-1. *Cancer Res.* 2007;67:6007–6011.
10. Hecht SS. Tobacco smoke carcinogens and lung cancer. *J Natl Cancer Inst.* 1999;91:1194–1210.
11. Hecht SS. Cigarette smoking: cancer risks, carcinogens and mechanisms. *Langenbecks Arch Surg.* 2006;391:603–613.
12. Woenckhaus M, Klein-Hitpass L, Grepmeier U, et al. Smoking and cancer-related gene expression in bronchial epithelium and non-small-cell-lung cancers. *J Pathol.* 2006;210:192–204.
13. Mao L. Molecular abnormalities in lung carcinogenesis and their potential clinical implications. *Lung Cancer.* 2001;34:S27–S34.
14. Ullman R, Bongiovanni M, Halbwedl I, et al. Bronchiolar columnar cell dysplasia—genetic analysis of a novel preneoplastic lesion of peripheral lung. *Virchows Arch.* 2003;442:429–436.

15. Wistuba II, Behrens C, Milchgrub S, et al. Sequential molecular abnormalities are involved in the multistage development of squamous cell lung carcinomas. *Oncogene*. 1999;18:643–650.

16. Wistuba II, Berry J, Behrens C, et al. Molecular changes in the bronchial epithelium of patients with small cell lung cancer. *Clin Cancer Res*. 2000;6:2604–2610.

17. Travis WD, Garg K, Franklin WA, et al. Evolving concepts in the pathology and ct imaging of lung adenocarcinoma and bronchioloalveolar carcinoma. *J Clin Oncol*. 2005;23:3279–3287.

18. Kerr KM. Morphology and genetics of preinvasive pulmonary disease. *Curr Diag Pathol*. 2004;10: 259–268.

19. Nakanishi K. Alveolar epithelial hyperplasia and adenocarcinoma of the lung. *Arch Pathol Lab Med*. 1990;114:363–368.

20. Minami Y, Matsuno Y, Iijima T, et al. Prognostication of small-sized primary pulmonary adenocarcinomas by histopathological and karyometric analysis. *Lung Cancer*. 2005;48:339–348.

21. Kerr KM, Popper HH. The differential diagnosis of pulmonary pre-invasive lesions. *Eur Respir Mon*. 2007;39:37–62.

22. Travis WD, Brambilla E, Muller-Hermelink HK, et al., eds. *World Health Organisation Classification of Tumours. Pathology and Genetics of Tumours of the Lung, Pleura, Thymus and Heart*. Lyon: IARC press; 2004.

23. Kobashi Y, Sugiu T, Mouri K, et al. Multifocal micronodular pneumocyte hyperplasia associated with tuberous sclerosis: differentiation from multiple atypical adenomatous hyperplasia. *Jpn J Clin Oncol*. 2008; 38:451–454.

24. Yanagisawa M. A histopathoogical study of proliferative changes of the epithelial components of the lung. A contribution to the histogenesis of pulmonary carcinoma (in Japanese). *Jpn J Cancer Clin*. 1959;5:667–680.

25. Sterner DJ, Masuko M, Roggli VL, et al. Prevalence of pulmonary atypical alveolar cell hyperplasia in an autopsy population: a study of 100 cases. *Mod Pathol*. 1997;10:469–473.

26. Yokose T, Ito Y, Ochiai A. High prevalence of atypical adenomatous hyperplasia of the lung in autopsy specimens from elderly patients with malignant neoplasms. *Lung Cancer*. 2000;29:125–130.

27. Yokose T, Doi M, Tanno K, et al. Atypical adenomatous hyperplasia of the lung in autopsy cases. *Lung Cancer*. 2001;33:155–161.

28. Weng S-Y, Tsuchiya E, Kasuga T, et al. Incidence of atypical bronchioloalveolar cell hyperplasia of the lung: relation to histological subtypes of lung cancer. *Virchows Archiv A Pathol Anat*. 1992;420: 463–471.

29. Carey FA, Wallace WAH, Fergusson RJ, et al. Alveolar atypical hyperplasia in association with primary pulmonary adenocarcinoma: a clinicopathological study of 10 cases. *Thorax*. 1992;47:1041–1043.

30. Nakahara R, Yokose T, Nagai K, et al. Atypical adenomatous hyperplasia of the lung: a clinicopathological study of 118 cases including cases with multiple atypical adenomatous hyperplasia. *Thorax*. 2001;56:302–305.

31. Koga T, Hashimoto S, Sugio K, et al. Lung adenocarcinoma with bronchioloalveolar carcinoma component is frequently associated with foci of high-grade atypical adenomatous hyperplasia. *Am J Clin Pathol*. 2002;117:464–470.

32. Chapman AD, Kerr KM. The association between atypical adenomatous hyperplasia and primary lung cancer. *Br J Cancer*. 2000;83:632–636.

33. Kerr KM, Fraire AE. Pre-invasive disease. In: Tomashefski JF, Cagle PT, Farver CF, et al., eds. *Dail and Hammar's Pulmonary Pathology*. New York: Springer; 2008:II,158—215.

34. Kitagawa H, Goto A, Niki T, et al. Lung adenocarcinoma associated with atypical adenomatous hyperplasia. A clinicopathological study with special reference to smoking and cancer multiplicity. *Pathol Int*. 2003;53:823–827.

35. Shoji T, Isowa N, Hasegawa S, et al. Solitary atypical adenomatous hyperplasia in the lung of a 17-year-old man with spontaneous pneumothorax. *Respiration*. 2003;70:303–305.

36. Kodama K, Higashiyama M, Takami K, et al. Synchronous pulmonary atypical adenomatous hyperplasia and metastatic osteosarcoma in a young female. *Jpn J Thorac Cardiovasc Surg*. 2004;52:357–359.

37. Takigawa N, Segawa Y, Nakata M, et al. Clinical investigation of atypical adenomatous hyperplasia of the lung. *Lung Cancer*. 1999;25:115–121.

38. Yousem SA, Finkelstein SD, Swalsky PA, et al. Absence of jaagsiekte sheep retrovirus DNA and RNA in bronchioloalveolar and conventional human pulmonary adenocarcinoma by PCR and RT-PCR analysis. *Hum Pathol*. 2001;32:1039–1042.

39. Chapman AD, Thetford D, Kerr KM. Pathological and clinical investigation of pulmonary atypical adenomatous hyperplasia and its association with primary lung adenocarcinoma *Lung Cancer*. 2000;29(S1):215–216.

40. Nadav Y, Pastorino U, Nicholson AG. Multiple synchronous lung cancers and atypical adenomatous hyperplasia in Li-Fraumeni syndrome. *Histopathology*. 1998;33:52–54.

41. Goto A, Nakajima J, Hara K, et al. Lung adenocarcinoma associated with familial adenomatous polyposis. Clear cell carcinoma with beta-catenin accumulation accompanied by atypical adenomatous hyperplasia. *Virchows Arch*. 2005;446:73–77.

42. Kerr KM, Devereux G, Chapman AD, et al. Is survival after surgical resection of lung cancer influenced by the presence of atypical adenomatous hyperplasia (AAH)? *J Thorac Oncol*. 2007;2(suppl 4): S401–S402.

43. Wistuba II, Gazdar AF. Lung cancer preneoplasia. *Annu Rev Pathol*. 2006;1:331–348.

44. Kerr KM, Carey FA, King G, et al. Atypical alveolar hyperplasia: relationship with pulmonary adenocarcinoma, p53 and c-erbB-2 expression. *J Pathol*. 1994;174:249–256.

45. Yamasaki M, Takeshima Y, Fujii S, et al. Correlation between genetic alterations and histopathological subtypes in bronchiolo-alveolar carcinoma and atypical adenomatous hyperplasia of the lung. *Pathol Int*. 2000;50:778–785.

46. Licchesi JD, Westra WH, Hooker CM, et al. Promotor hypermethylation of hallmark cancer genes in atypical adenomatous hyperplasia of the lung. *Clin Cancer Res*. 2008;14:2570–2578.

47. Ikeda K, Nomori H, Ohba Y, et al. Epidermal growth factor receptor mutations in multicentric lung adenocarcinomas and atypical adenomatous hyperplasias. *J Thorac Oncol*. 2008;3:467–471.

48. Sartori G, Cavazza A, Bertolini F, et al. A subset of lung adenocarcinomas and atypical adenomatous hyperplasia-associated foci are genotypically related: an EGFR, HER2, and K-ras mutational analysis. *Am J Clin Pathol*. 2008;129:202–210.

49. Cooper CA, Carey FA, Bubb VJ, et al. The pattern of K-ras mutation in pulmonary adenocarcinoma defines a new pathway of tumour development in the human lung. *J Pathol*. 1997;181:401–404.

Diffuse Idiopathic Pulmonary Neuroendocrine Cell Hyperplasia

28

▶ Keith M. Kerr

Diffuse idiopathic pulmonary neuroendocrine cell hyperplasia (DIPNECH) is described in the WHO classification of lung tumors as a generalized proliferation of neuroendocrine cells (NECs), which may be associated with the development of carcinoid tumors, hence its inclusion in the classification as a preinvasive lung disease.[1] There is no clear statement regarding how much NEC proliferation there must be for a diagnosis of DIPNECH to be made.

This is an extremely rare condition. In a review of DIPNECH written by the author in 2004,[2] there were 17 cases published in the English literature including the original cases of Aguayo et al.[3] who coined the term DIPNECH in 1992. Reviewing older literature back to the 1950s reveals descriptions of cases variously referred to as multiple bronchial adenomas or carcinoid tumors, which are probably examples of DIPNECH.[4–6] A more recent study reported 19 cases of probable DIPNECH, collected from multiple institutions in the UK over a 15-year period.[7] These authors quite reasonably suggested that while their experience was in part a collection of cases referred for consultation, DIPNECH may be an under-recognized condition that will be encountered more often as high-resolution computed tomography scanning is used more frequently.

DIPNECH seems consistently to be found more frequently in females in the age range 30 to 70 years. All of the original cases of Aguayo et al.[3] and many of the examples subsequently reported have been symptomatic. The typical presentation is of a slow increase in breathlessness with cough. Chest pain and hemoptysis are uncommon. Not infrequently, the patient is diagnosed with bronchial asthma. There is no association with smoking; most patients are never smokers. There may be no radiological abnormality but a frequent finding is a mosaic attenuation pattern (mosaicism) on the HRCT. Small millimeter-sized pulmonary nodules may also be found throughout both lung fields and in some cases larger tumors are seen (Fig. 28-1).[8–10] It is apparent that cases of DIPNECH will also be encountered where pathology identical to that present in such symptomatic cases (see below) may be found incidentally in patients who have lung tissue resected for another reason, for example a solitary pulmonary nodule or a known primary lung cancer. There has been some doubt as to whether or not these asymptomatic cases should be diagnosed as DIPNECH, especially as such material does not allow the full pathological examination of the lungs for "generalized proliferation" of pulmonary NEC afforded by autopsy examination. The author is quite comfortable with the diagnosis of DIPNECH being given to asymptomatic cases but is still unsure regarding how much NEC hyperplasia is required for a diagnosis (see below).

By definition, there is evidence of generalized diffuse hyperplasia of pulmonary NEC in this condition. Pulmonary NECs are normally present as singleton cells scattered within bronchial and bronchiolar epithelium. Very occasional small clusters of cells (neuroendocrine bodies) may be found in normal lungs. In DIPNECH, there is an increase in the number of singleton NEC;

FIGURE 28-1 Gross image of wedge biopsy containing DIPNECH, showing focal small carcinoid tumorlets, predominantly within the central portion of the specimen.

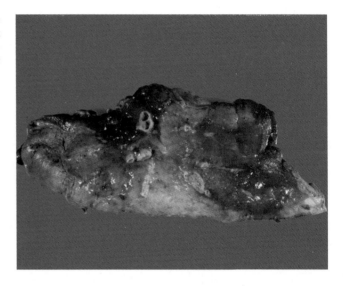

cells are found in rows of linear proliferation within the bronchial and especially bronchiolar epithelium and more nodules/neuroendocrine bodies are seen (Figs. 28-2–28-6). These nodules may be large enough to protrude into the bronchiolar lumen and may cause airway obstruction (Figs. 28-7–28-11). The proliferations of NEC may be associated with variable amounts of fibrosis (Figs. 28-12 and 28-13). Small airways remote from the NEC lesions may show fibrosis of the subepithelial connective tissue, sufficient to deserve classification as constrictive bronchiolitis (bronchiolitis obliterans), and these changes may be associated with a little chronic inflammation. This combination of changes seen in widespread distribution in pulmonary parenchyma would be a reasonable minimum requirement for a diagnosis of DIPNECH. The diagnosis of DIPNECH is normally made in the absence of significant background fibroinflammatory disease in the lung since the latter is associated with NEC hyperplasia (see below).

The obstruction of small airways is responsible for the asthma-like symptoms with which some patients with DIPNECH present seeking medical attention. The small airway pathology is also the cause of the signs of air trapping (mosaicism) on the HRCT scans. As a result of the small airways obstruction, there may be distal bronchiolectasis and mucous retention, as well as

FIGURE 28-2 Linear extensions of NEC in DIPNECH may be seen deep to bronchiolar columnar cells.

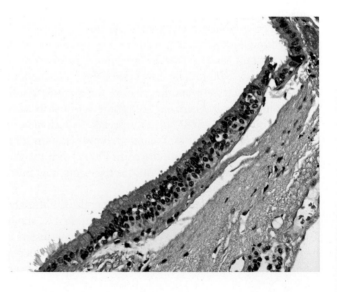

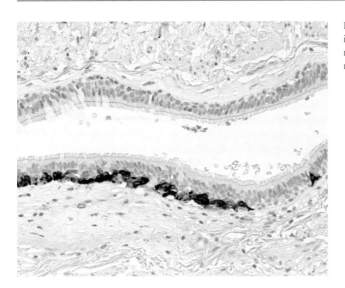

FIGURE 28-3 Linear extensions of NEC in DIPNECH can be highlighted using neuroendocrine markers such as chromogranin.

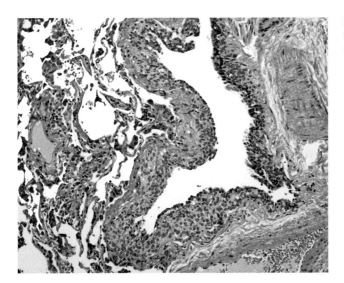

FIGURE 28-4 In some airways such as the one shown here, NEC hyperplasia is marked.

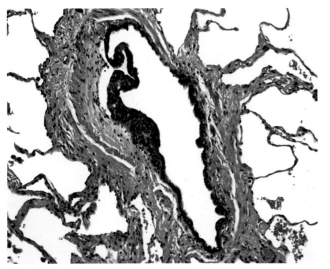

FIGURE 28-5 A prominent NEC nodule can be seen in this airway.

FIGURE 28-6 Chromogranin stain highlights the NEC nodule. Note the fine crescent of fibroblastic tissue between the bronchiolar muscle and the NEC nodule.

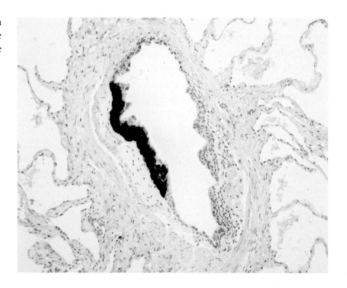

FIGURE 28-7 Nodule of NEC hyperplasia in DIPNECH obstructing a bronchiole, which is dilated distal to the obstruction with retained secretion.

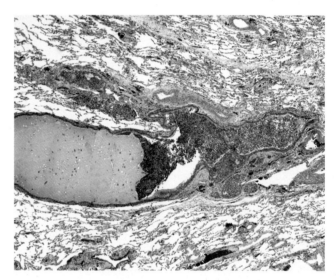

FIGURE 28-8 Medium power image of a carcinoid tumorlet in DIPNECH.

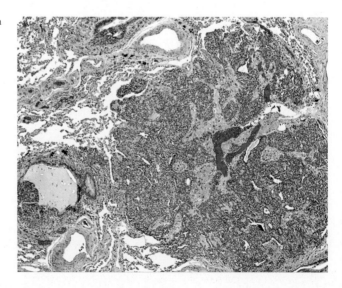

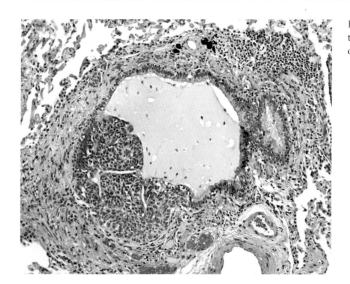

FIGURE 28-9 Adjacent to the carcinoid tumorlet shown in Figure 28-8, a bronchiole is partly occluded by a NEC nodule.

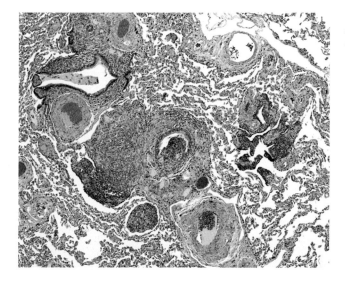

FIGURE 28-10 This DIPNECH tumorlet shows peribronchiolar fibrosis as well as extrabronchiolar NEC.

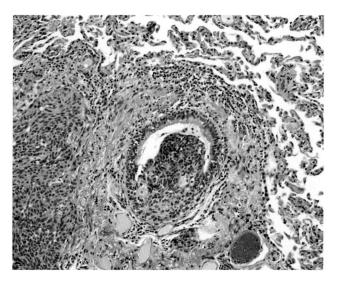

FIGURE 28-11 Adjacent to the DIPNECH tumorlet shown in Figure 28-10, a nodule is identified obstructing the constricted airway lumen.

FIGURE 28-12 This bronchiole shows NEC hyperplasia and striking fibroplasia between the epithelium and the smooth muscle.

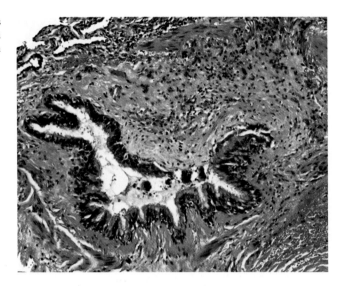

FIGURE 28-13 Chromogranin stain of the bronchiole in Figure 28-12 highlights the hyperplastic NEC.

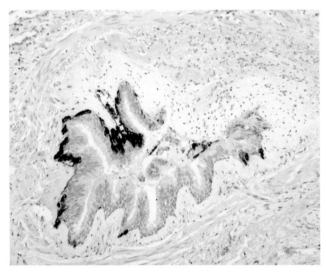

accumulation of alveolar macrophages. Clinically, this condition is either stable or very slowly progressive. Oral steroids may be used with occasional success; at least one patient is reported, having been treated by lung transplantation.

When these collections of hyperplastic NEC extend beyond the bronchiolar epithelial basement membrane, the term carcinoid tumorlet is used to describe the resulting lesion, which comprises small nodules of NEC set in an often quite dense fibrous stroma. These cells may give the impression of infiltration of the interstitium around the bronchiole. They may also protrude into and even partly line adjacent alveoli (Figs. 28-14–28-16). The cells are generally small, plump, fusiform, or spindle shaped. Cytoplasm is eosinophilic and cell borders are indistinct. The nuclei are often quite hyperchromatic and devoid of nuclear detail. Occasionally, the lesion may appear crushed. There is no atypia, nuclear molding is absent, and neither apoptosis nor mitoses are seen. Carcinoid tumorlets may cause complete obliteration of the associated bronchiole, the adjacent pulmonary arteriole being the only clue as to the site of the lesion. They are generally around 2 to 3 mm in diameter, may be visible on the cut surface of a well-prepared formalin-fixed specimen, and account for the micronodularity sometimes reported on HRCT scans (Fig. 28-17). By definition, carcinoid tumorlets never measure 5 mm or more in diameter. When a lesion reaches this size, it is classified as a carcinoid tumor.[1]

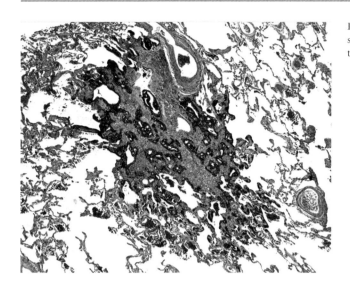

FIGURE 28-14 This carcinoid tumorlet shows less nodular expansion of NEC than in the lesion in Figure 28-7.

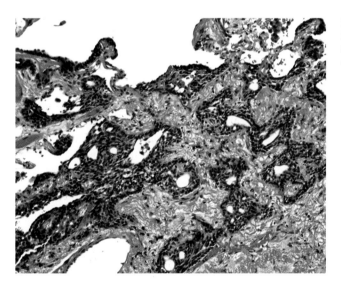

FIGURE 28-15 In the carcinoid tumorlet shown in Figure 28-14, there is more fibrosis, and NEC can be seen lining adjacent alveoli.

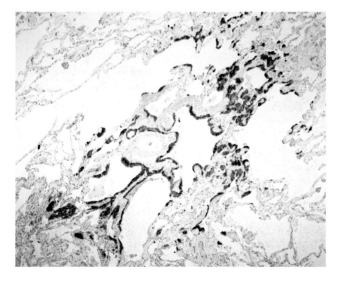

FIGURE 28-16 Chromogranin stain highlights the carcinoid tumorlet shown in Figure 28-14. (Chromogranin, 4×).

FIGURE 28-17 Low-power view of a wedge lung biopsy from a patient with DIPNECH showing multiple carcinoid tumorlets. This patient's case also is shown in Figures 28-2, 28-7 to 28-10, 28-20, and 28-21.

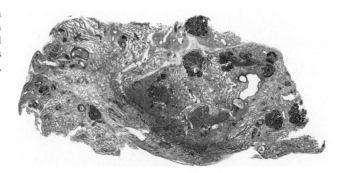

It is the finding of carcinoid tumors in some, though not all, cases of DIPNECH that merits the classification of DIPNECH as a preinvasive lung disease. It is a curious fact that the classification of these lesions regards an aggregate of NEC <5 mm across a hyperplastic lesion, yet over this size the lesion is regarded as neoplastic. This issue is discussed further in the section on molecular biology. The carcinoid tumors that occur in DIPNECH are usually of the peripheral, spindle cell type (Figs. 28-18 and 28-19). Central insular-trabecular pattern carcinoid tumors of the large cartilaginous airways are not found. The majority of carcinoid tumors reported in DIPNECH are of typical in morphology, lacking necrosis, and show <2 mitotic figures per 2 mm^2 (10 HPF). However, in the series of 19 DIPNECH cases reported by Davies et al.[7] while 9 patients had typical carcinoid tumors, three patients had atypical carcinoid tumors; the first time such tumors have been reported in DIPNECH. In one of these cases, the atypical carcinoid tumor has metastasized. One of the author's patients with DIPNECH also had an atypical carcinoid tumor (Figs. 28-20 and 28-21). Carcinoid tumors may be multiple in patients with DIPNECH.

The fibrosis that accompanies foci of NEC hyperplasia and even affects small airways lacking excess NEC has been attributed to the secretion of bombesin or other paracrine substances secreted by the NEC and capable of inducing fibrosis.[11] The NECs found in DIPNECH have also been shown to have high levels of neutral endopeptidase, probably due to the presence in these cells of bombesin-like peptides that are the substrate of this enzyme.[12,13]

FIGURE 28-18 Typical spindle cell carcinoid tumor in DIPNECH.

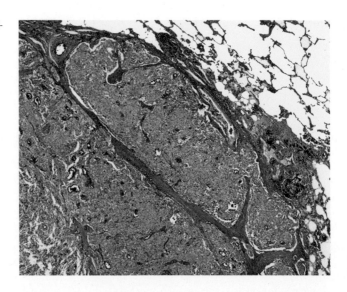

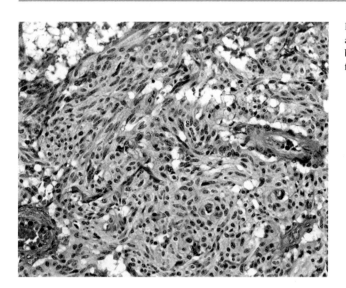

FIGURE 28-19 Many carcinoid tumors are of spindle cell type and closely resemble overgrown tumorlets with fewer fibrous bands between nodules of NEC.

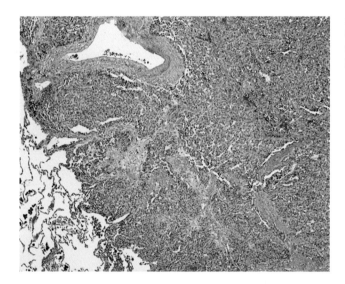

FIGURE 28-20 An atypical carcinoid tumor, diagnosed on the basis of more than 2 mitoses per 2 mm², identified in a patient with DIPNECH.

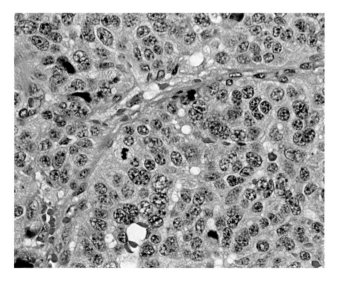

FIGURE 28-21 High-power view of the atypical carcinoid tumor shown in Figure 28-20, showing a central mitotic figure.

NEC HYPERPLASIA IN THE ABSENCE OF DIPNECH

Given the lack of a precise definition regarding the amount of NEC hyperplasia required for a diagnosis of DIPNECH, the occurrence of, relatively speaking, lesser amounts of NEC hyperplasia may raise some diagnostic questions. In one study of 25 peripheral-type spindle cell carcinoid tumors, around three quarters of the patients had evidence of concurrent NEC hyperplasia; one third had pathological evidence of small airways obliteration by NEC hyperplasia, tumorlets, and fibrosis, while two patients had measurable airflow limitation that could not be attributed to COPD.[14] This raises the possibility, indeed the likelihood, that NEC hyperplasia may occur in the lung to varying degrees, not all of which appear "generalized" enough to deserve the diagnostic label of DIPNECH; probably only a minority of cases are extensive enough for this classification.

NEC hyperplasia, including carcinoid tumorlets, is well described in association with a number of fibrotic and, especially, inflammatory conditions in the lung. Although tumorlets occurring in this setting have historically been considered neoplastic, even in situ or invasive carcinomas, they are almost certainly examples of reactive hyperplasia. The most common associated lung conditions in which carcinoid tumorlets are found are bronchiectasis and chronic lung abscess, but they have also been described in cystic fibrosis, COPD, Langerhans cell histiocytosis, diffuse panbronchiolitis, bronchopulmonary dysplasia, and intralobar sequestration.[11,12,15–18] There are rare reported cases of carcinoid tumorlets associated with lymph node "metastases." While some of these may be dismissed as probable cases of true carcinoid tumor, as currently defined, others cannot.[19,20] However, the finding of cells in a lymph node draining the location of a particular lesion is not proof of malignancy, as evidenced by the occasional finding of melanocytes in lymph nodes associated with benign melanocytic nevi.

Carcinoid tumorlets may also be encountered in small numbers, insufficient for a diagnosis of DIPNECH, in morphologically normal lung, in patients who do not have peripheral spindle cell carcinoid tumors. The significance of such a finding is not clear. They are of no consequence to the patient and possibly represent a reactive hyperplasia, the stimulus for which is not apparent in the sample examined or has disappeared, leaving behind carcinoid tumorlets.

Review of the literature on carcinoid tumorlets arising in the setting of fibroinflammatory lung disease has failed to identify a single case of carcinoid tumor arising in this setting. This suggests that there is some qualitative, possibly molecular, difference, as well as the apparent quantitative difference, between the NEC hyperplasia seen in fibroinflammatory disease and that which occurs in DIPNECH.

DIPNECH AND MOLECULAR BIOLOGY

Thyroid transcription factor 1 (TTF1) is a lineage marker for the peripheral bronchioloalveolar epithelium.[21] It is expressed in basal and some differentiated cells of the peripheral so-called terminal respiratory unit epithelium, and in NEC found in this location. It is therefore no surprise that the hyperplastic NEC lesions, including tumorlets, found in both DIPNECH and fibroinflammatory NEC hyperplasia express TTF1. Furthermore, and despite claims to the contrary, TTF1 expression, as demonstrated using immunohistochemistry, is frequent in peripheral spindle cell carcinoid tumors, with or without DIPNECH.[22] The regular absence of TTF1 staining in central bronchial insular-trabecular carcinoid tumors reflects the origin of this tumor from the biologically distinct bronchial or bronchial gland duct epithelium.

There are no other reports of molecular studies carried out on DIPNECH-associated lesions. One of the 19 cases of DIPNECH reported by Davies et al.[7] a case with a concurrent atypical carcinoid tumor, occurred in a patient with MEN1 syndrome. This is the only reported case of DIPNECH in this condition. Pulmonary carcinoid tumors are a rarely reported association in MEN1 syndrome, but the pathological detail of these tumors is not clear. It is of interest, however, that around one third of sporadic carcinoid tumors show *MEN1* gene mutation while between

22% and 47% of such tumors have shown loss of heterozygosity in chromosome 11, in particular in the region of 11q13, close to the *MEN1* gene locus. In one study that demonstrated 11q13 imbalance in almost three quarters of typical carcinoid tumors, a similar change was found in one carcinoid tumorlet found in the absence of a carcinoid tumor, representing 9% of those tumorlets examined.[23–26] Similar studies in the equivalent lesions occurring in DIPNECH patients are awaited.

DIPNECH is an interesting but very rare condition that may be under-recognized. It is not terribly clearly defined, always a problem in uncommon conditions, but provides interesting insights into the possible origins of some carcinoid tumors. It also creates a rather awkward juxtaposition of two supposedly different pathological processes, hyperplasia and neoplasia, in the same progression of disease. While this is not unknown in other pathways of pulmonary tumor development (see Chapters 26 and 27), in the case of DIPNECH, the discrimination is based purely on lesion size, with no differences in architectural features or cytological atypia.

References

1. Gosney JR, Travis WD. Diffuse idiopathic pulmonary neuroendocrine cell hyperplasia. In: Travis WD, Brambilla E, Muller-Hermelink HK et al., eds. *World Health Organisation Classification of Tumours. Pathology and Genetics of Tumours of the Lung, Pleura, Thymus and Heart.* Lyon: IARC press; 2004:76–77.
2. Kerr KM, Fraire AE. Pre-invasive diseases. In: Tomashefski J, Cagle P, Farver C, eds. *Dail & Hammar's Pulmonary Pathology.* 3rd ed. New York, NY: Springer; 2008.
3. Aguayo SM, Miller YE, Waldron JA, et al. Idiopathic diffuse hyperplasia of pulmonary neuroendocrine cells and airway disease. *N Engl J Med.* 1992;327:1285–1288.
4. Felton WL, Liebow AA, Lindskog GF. Peripheral and multiple bronchial adenomas. *Cancer.* 1953;6: 555–567.
5. Gmelich JT, Bensch KG, Liebow AA. Cells of Kulchitsky type in bronchioles and their relation to the origin of peripheral carcinoid tumours. *Lab Invest.* 1967;17:88–98.
6. Miller MA, Mark GJ, Kanarek D. Multiple peripheral pulmonary carcinoids and tumourlets of carcinoid type, with restrictive and obstructive lung disease. *Am J Med.* 1978;65:373–378.
7. Davies SJ, Gosney JR, Hansell DM, et al. Diffuse idiopathic pulmonary neuroendocrine cell hyperplasia: an under-recognised spectrum of disease. *Thorax.* 2007;62:248–252.
8. Jessurun J, Manivel JC, Simpson R. Idiopathic diffuse hyperplasia of pulmonary neuroendocrine cells (IDHPNC): a consequence of diffuse bronchiolitis. *Lab Invest.* 1994;70:151A.
9. Brown MJ, English J, Muller NL. Bronchiolitis obliterans due to neuroendocrine hyperplasia: high-resolution CT- pathologic correlation. *Am J Roentgenol.* 1997;168:1561–1562.
10. Lee JS, Brown KK, Cool C, et al. Diffuse pulmonary neuroendocrine cell hyperplasia: radiologic and clinical features. *J Comput Assit Tomogr.* 2002;26:180–184.
11. Johnson DE, Wobken JD, Landrum BG. Changes in bombesin, calcitonin, and serotonin immunoreactive pulmonary neuroendocrine cells in cystic fibrosis and after prolonged mechanical ventilation. *Am Rev Respir Dis.* 1988;137:123–131.
12. Aguayo SM, King TE Jr., Waldron JA Jr, et al. Increased pulmonary neuroendocrine cells with bombesin-like immunoreactivity in adult patients with eosinophilic granuloma. *J Clin Invest.* 1990;86: 838–844.
13. Cohen AJ, King TE, Gilman LB, et al. High expression of neutral endopeptidase in idiopathic diffuse hyperplasia of pulmonary neuroendocrine cells. *Am J Respir Crit Care Med.* 1998;158:1593–1599.
14. Miller RR, Muller NL. Neuroendocrine cell hyperplasia and obliterative bronchiolitis in patients with peripheral carcinoid tumours. *Am J Surg Pathol.* 1995;19:653–658.
15. Johnson DE, Lock JE, Elde RP, et al. Pulmonary neuroendocrine cells in hyaline membrane disease and bronchopulmonary dysplasia. *Pediatr Res.* 1982;16:446–454.
16. Churg A, Warnock ML. Pulmonary tumourlet. A form of peripheral carcinoid. *Cancer.* 1976;37: 1469–1477.

17. Watanabe H, Kobayashi H, Honma K, et al. Diffuse panbronchiolitis with multiple tumourlets. A quantitative study of the Kultschitzky cells and the clusters. *Acta Pathol Jpn*. 1985;35:1221–1231.
18. Gosney JR, Sissons MC, Allibone RO, et al. Pulmonary endocrine cells in chronic bronchitis and emphysema. *J Pathol*. 1989;157:127–133.
19. Hausman DH, Weimann RB. Pulmonary tumourlet with hilar lymph node metastases. *Cancer*. 1967;20:1515–1519.
20. D'Agati VD, Perzin KH. Carcinoid tumorlets of the lung with metastasis to a peribronchial lymph node. Report of a case and review of the literature. *Cancer*. 1985;55:2472–2476.
21. Yatabe Y, Mitsudomi T, Takahashi T. TTF-1 expression in pulmonary adenocarcinoma. *Am J Surg Pathol*. 2002;26:767–773.
22. Du EZ, Goldstraw P, Zacharias J, et al. TTF-1 expression is specific for lung primary in typical and atypical carcinoids: TTF-1-positive carcinoids are predominantly in peripheral location. *Hum Pathol*. 2004;35:825–831.
23. Debelenko LV, Brambilla E, Agarwal SK, et al. Identification of MEN1 gene mutations in sporadic carcinoid tumours of the lung. *Hum Mol Genet*. 1997;6:2285–2290.
24. Walch AK, Zitzelsberger HF, Aubele MM, et al. Typical and atypical carcinoid tumours of the lung are characterised by 11q deletions as detected by comparative genomic hybridisation. *Am J Pathol*. 1998;153:1089–1098.
25. Petzmann S, Ullmann R, Klemen H, et al. Loss of heterozygosity on chromosome arm 11q in lung carcinoids. *Hum Pathol*. 2001;32:333–338.
26. Finkelstein SD, Hasegawa T, Colby T, et al. 11q13 allelic imbalance discriminates pulmonary carcinoids from tumourlets. A microdissection-based genotyping approach useful in clinical practice. *Am J Pathol*. 1999;155:633–640.

Preexisting Lung Disease and Lung Cancer

29

▶ Keith M. Kerr

lsewhere in this book are reviews of the three preinvasive lung diseases that are recognized in the WHO classification of lung cancer as precursors of malignancy. This chapter considers the association between lung cancer and a number of different lung diseases that, apart from causing morbidity and sometimes mortality associated with the underlying pathology of the disease in question, are also associated with a risk of lung cancer development.

By far the most important of these is the association of lung cancer with a variety of forms of diffuse pulmonary fibrosis. Other conditions include a number of cystic conditions that occur in the lung and human papilloma virus (HPV)-induced papillomatosis. It is probable that most of these conditions owe their risk of carcinogenesis to the upregulation of epithelial proliferation that occurs in each case for a variety of reasons. The interaction between this background of cell proliferation and the "usual" lung carcinogens such as those found in tobacco smoke is variable but undoubtedly of importance in some cases.

It is very difficult to say how many lung cancers could be accounted for by transformation of a preexisting lung disease. Many of these conditions are rare. During routine examination of resected lung cancer specimens, the pathologist can sometimes find evidence of what appears to be intercurrent interstitial lung disease. The author has not made a formal study of this but would estimate that such cases account for very approximately 5% of resections. These are, of course, a very select group of lung cancers, due to the patients' suitability for operation and the resectability of the tumor. The presence of intercurrent disease such as diffuse pulmonary fibrosis is more likely to render the patient unfit for surgery, denying the pathologist the opportunity for full pathological assessment of such cases. On occasion, it may be difficult to distinguish between preexisting lung fibrosis, and that actually caused by the tumor through obstructive pneumonitis. In any such case where the patient smoked tobacco, it is probable that the tumor would be attributed to that particular cause, ignoring the contribution that any concurrent disease may have made.

LUNG CANCER AND PULMONARY FIBROSIS

Localized Pulmonary Fibrosis

As discussed in Chapter 3, fibrosis is a common occurrence in the center of peripheral pulmonary adenocarcinomas and the development of fibroelastosis, followed by neofibrogenesis are notable features of significance in the development of these tumors. A proposal was made by Rossle in 1943, in which localized scars in the lung could act as a nidus for the growth and development of peripheral forms of lung cancer; the so-called scar cancer or Narbenkrebs hypothesis.[1] Beyond the observed presence of central scars in lung adenocarcinomas, anthracotic pigment is often also seen and alveolar cell hyperplasia is recognized in association with lung scars, interpreted as evidence that the scar must predate the growth of the tumor and that fibrosis can stimulate epithelial change, which may lead to malignancy.[2–4] The proposal seemed plausible and was welcome, since the origin of pulmonary adenocarcinoma was otherwise quite unknown. Several reports followed, documenting cases of peripherally located lung cancer, with central scars.[5–7] Most of these tumors were adenocarcinomas, but squamous and undifferentiated tumors were also described (Fig. 29-1). A majority of these cases were located in the upper lobes. Favored etiology for the scars was tuberculosis and pulmonary infarction. In one large series of almost 1,200 resected lung cancers, 7% of cases were considered scar carcinomas.[5] These tumors were not associated with smoking, a finding that probably help acceptance that the scar was the cause of the tumor. A rise in incidence of scar cancer, mostly adenocarcinomas, was described during the 1960–1970s.

The scar cancer hypothesis is now considered incorrect. The above description would fit perfectly well with what we now know about the evolution of adenocarcinomas from atypical adenomatous hyperplasia and localized nonmucinous bronchioloalveolar adenocarcinoma (LNMBAC), effectively adenocarcinoma in situ, and the well-documented rise in the prevalence of adenocarcinoma in many countries. Much of the work in refuting the scar cancer hypothesis was carried out by Shimosato et al.[8–10] (see also Chapter 27), but others contributed to the following observations:

1. Adenocarcinoma is common in lungs without parenchymal scars.
2. Examination of patients' old chest radiographs, taken prior to presentation with cancer, rarely shows a preexisting scar.
3. Distant metastases from primary lung cancer and metastatic tumors in the lung often show a central scar.
4. Scars may contain psammoma bodies, suggesting there may have been viable tumor at that site, prior to the onset of fibrosis.
5. In most cases, the size of the scar and the tumor are in proportion, suggesting they develop in tandem.

Subsequent high-resolution computed tomography studies have shown that the scar indeed develops within the focus of adenocarcinoma in situ (LNMBAC), as a result of alveolar network collapse and fibroelastosis, followed by neofibrogenesis as invasion occurs and stimulates a stromal response.[11,12] Growth of the tumors also seems to be accompanied by growth of the "scar"; this is, after all, the invasive part of the lesion. As the scar is the harbinger of invasion, so its appearance is associated with metastatic risk and a poorer prognosis for the patient. Other studies have shown that the central scars in tumors show myofibroblasts and collagen type III, both typical of new fibroblastic growth.[13–15] This contrasts with findings in longstanding localized pulmonary scars that are not associated with cancer. Here, myofibroblasts are few and collagen types I and V are

FIGURE 29-1 This appearance of peripheral lung adenocarcinoma with a central anthracotic scar was the type of lesion formerly regarded as "scar cancer." It is now understood that the central fibrosis is the result of alveolar collapse and fibroplasia secondary to tumor growth.

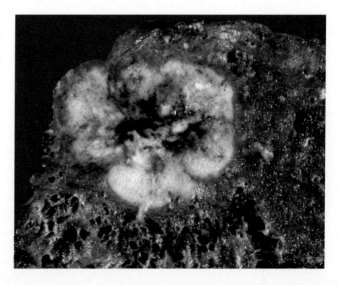

found. The term "scar cancer" may be retained as a descriptive label, but most evidence suggests the scar is not the cause of the cancer.

Diffuse Pulmonary Fibrosis

There are many different forms of diffuse pulmonary fibrosis. Among the most important associated with the development of lung cancer are idiopathic pulmonary fibrosis (IPF—Usual interstitial pneumonia), pulmonary fibrosis associated with autoimmune connective tissue diseases (CTDs), and the mineral pneumoconioses, principally asbestosis and silicosis. Why these patients should have a higher risk of developing lung cancer is not entirely clear. Tobacco smoking is probably an importance etiological cofactor. The reactive bronchioloalveolar epithelial hyperplasia, which is common in these conditions, may provide the "at risk" epithelial field within which malignant transformation can take place and asbestos, silica, or other minerals may have carcinogenic properties. Increasing interest has also been shown in the role that inflammation may play in the development of malignancy in the lung.[16] In a study of over 1,100 cases of sarcoidosis, however, no excess of lung cancer was found.[17]

Idiopathic Pulmonary Fibrosis and Lung Cancer

The presence of atypia in the reactive epithelium of IPF and lung honeycombing is commensurate with an association between IPF and malignancy (Figs. 29-2–29-6). There are, however, historical records of the atypical squamous metaplasia occurring in the proliferative and reparative stages of diffuse alveolar damage syndrome being overdiagnosed as squamous cell carcinoma. On the other hand, such squamous epithelium has been shown to bear some genetic changes that are consistent with early progression toward malignancy. Lung cancers have been described in a number of autopsy studies of patients with IPF. In Caucasian cohorts, prevalence of lung cancer reported in IPF autopsies varies from 4.8% to 21% of cases.[18–20] In Japanese studies, the reported prevalence of lung cancer in IPF autopsies appears to be higher at 42% to 48.2%, with 15% of these showing multiple synchronous primary tumors.[21–23] It has been estimated, in a study which controlled for age, gender, and smoking history, that IPF rendered a 14-fold increase in lung cancer risk in males and a sevenfold increase in women.[24]

Much of the evidence suggests that adenocarcinoma is especially likely to occur in IPF patients. While this is consistent with malignant transformation in the peripheral lung bronchioloalveolar epithelium (see Chapter 27), the data could be confounded by the fact that many studies are of Japanese patients, a population that seems more prone than Caucasians to develop adenocarcinoma.[20,23] An excess of adenocarcinoma has, however, been reported in non-Japanese

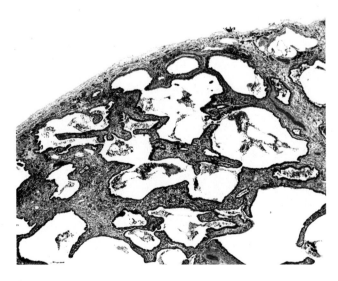

FIGURE 29-2 This patient had a history of IPF. Their lung biopsy showed remodeling of the lung architecture with honeycomb cysts.

FIGURE 29-3 In some areas, a transition from nonatypical ciliated bronchiolar epithelium to atypical alveolar lining epithelium is evident.

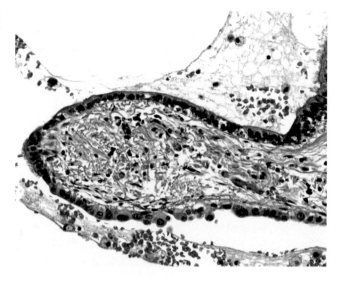

FIGURE 29-4 In other areas, there is atypical epithelium reminiscent of that seen in lepidic-pattern (bronchioloalveolar) adenocarcinoma.

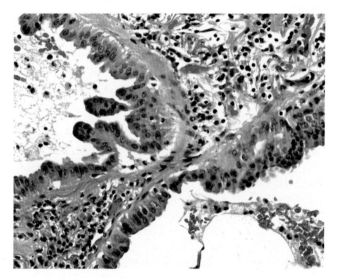

FIGURE 29-5 In some areas, small irregular glandular structures, lined by atypical epithelium, are present.

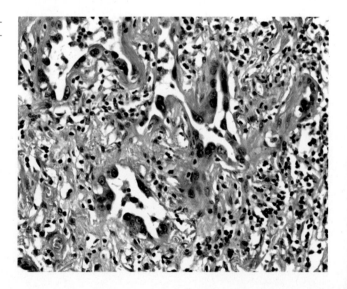

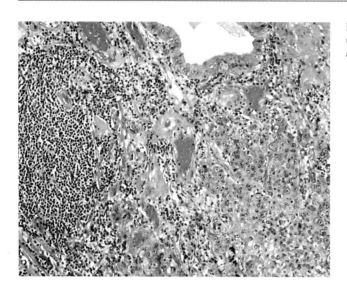

FIGURE 29-6 This patient also had unequivocal invasive poorly differentiated solid-pattern adenocarcinoma.

studies.[24,25] The finding of an adenocarcinoma predominance in IPF cancers is not universal; some studies have reported a similar distribution of cell types to that seen in a non-IPF smoking populations, over a time period when squamous cell and small cell carcinomas were more prevalent.[26,27]

IPF-associated cancers tend to occur within or at the margins of the zone of fibrosis and are consequently more often found in the lower lobes. It is possible that the IPF and the malignancy may share common etiology.[21,23,27,28] This has been mooted in patients with IPF who have a history of exposure to metal dust[20,29] (this does, however, question the diagnosis of IPF, rather than that of pneumoconiosis, but whatever the correct diagnosis, the cases are still relevant to this discussion). IPF is also associated with smoking, raising the possibility of confounding but several studies have controlled for smoking habit and still demonstrated an increased risk of lung cancer in IPF patients.[30,31]

It is suggested that the combination of an atypically proliferating epithelium in the lung plus the carcinogenic effects of tobacco, metal dust, and inflammatory cytokines may be responsible for this lung cancer excess in IPF.[16] Studies have also shown a number of molecular abnormalities in IPF, and especially in IPF associated with cancer, to support the hypothesis concerning malignant transformation in the proliferating bronchioloalveolar epithelium. Overexpression of p53 protein has been found, as well as *P53* and *KRAS* mutations.[32,33] In experimental animal models of IPF cancer, the P63-jag1 pathway is upregulated.[34] Loss of heterozygosity (LOH) for certain gene loci may indicate that loss of genetic material is a mechanism for silencing tumor suppressor genes. LOH at loci bearing the *MYCL1, FHIT, SPARC, P16 (INK4A)*, and *P53* genes has been reported in epithelium in IPF tissue from patients with IPF-associated lung cancer.[35] Many of these studies involve very small numbers of cases but nonetheless suggest that the same genetic alterations seen in lung cancers in general are found in IPF associated cases and in the "progenitor" reactive epithelium. This could, of course, be a reflection of a common etiological factor, tobacco smoke.

Connective Tissue Disease and Lung Cancer

Lung cancer is also a well-recognized complication of pulmonary fibrosis associated with CTDs. Once again much of this literature is from Japan and its relevance to Caucasian populations is uncertain.[36,37] One Japanese study reported a lung cancer prevalence of 12% in patients with CTD,[36] while a follow-up study of Serbian patients with IPF found lung cancer arising in 6.4% of patients over 10 years.[38] In a general literature review, which noted that most of the studies published were case reports, there was a slight preponderance of females (54%) in the reported

cases of CTD-associated lung cancer.[37] Over half the reported tumors (56%) were adenocarcinomas, and over half of these were described as bronchioloalveolar carcinoma (BAC). It seems
unlikely that these were true BACs, essentially adenocarcinoma in situ, as defined in the current
WHO classification of lung cancer. It is rather more likely that they were adenocarcinomas with a
prominent BAC component. Squamous cell and small cell carcinomas each accounted for around
18% of the reported cases.

Of all the CTDs, progressive systemic sclerosis (PSS) seems to have a particularly strong association with malignancy; a relative risk of 16.5 has been calculated.[37,39] Adenocarcinoma seems to
be the dominant cell type found in PSS, with reported prevalence of "BAC" ranging from 24%
to 77% of all tumors. This latter diagnosis, as discussed above, probably means adenocarcinoma
with a prominent BAC component. Most reported cases are female, have pulmonary fibrosis, and
just over half are smokers (Fig. 29-7).

Around 18% of CTD-associated lung cancers occur in patients with rheumatoid arthritis
(RA).[37,40] Most of these patients are male smokers and most have pulmonary fibrosis. In contrast
to PSS, between a fifth and a quarter of cases were, each, either squamous cell, small cell or adenocarcinoma. There is no apparent excess of "BAC"-type tumors. In patients with polymyositis/
dermatomyositis (PM/DM) and lung cancer, male smokers are the largest group; bronchogenic
carcinomas such as squamous cell and small cell are predominant. Around 16% of CTD-associated lung cancers fall in this group; around half the patients have fibrosis.[37,41] Lung cancer seems
to be rare in patients with systemic lupus erythematosis (SLE). In a study of 9,500 patients with
SLE the lung cancer prevalence was 0.3%; patients were mostly females and smokers.[42] Histological data are scarce but adenocarcinomas appear to be prominent. As is the case with IPF, there are
suggestions, at least in the case of PSS, that a background of atypical epithelial proliferation associated with the pulmonary fibrosis is related to the increased risk of developing adenocarcinoma.
A role for inflammatory mediators in the carcinogenic process has also been proposed; similarly
for tobacco smoking. A role for immunosuppressive therapy in tumor development is supported
by some studies, but not by others.[43]

It is difficult to come to an overall conclusion about these data, especially since lung cancer
in CTD is a relatively rare occurrence and data are few. The data on PSS are most compelling. It
is not clear if fibrosis is a prerequisite for lung cancer to arise "because of" the CTD. Obviously in
the case of IPF, fibrosis is present by definition. In CTD, there may not necessarily be pulmonary
fibrosis. In those cases that arise in the absence of lung fibrosis, how can we be sure that the CTD
had anything to do with the development of the tumor? Although the mean age of CTD-lung cancer patients is 58 years, at least 10 years younger than "average" lung cancer cohorts, the tumors

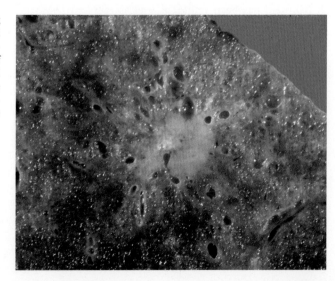

FIGURE 29-7 This patient was a life-long smoker with systemic sclerosis. A resected adenocarcinoma was located in associa-tion with a peripheral subpleural zone of fibrosis that had a nonspecific interstitial pneumonia pattern histologically. Note that the tumor has arisen at the bound-ary between the overtly fibrotic and the normal lung.

seen in RA and PM/DM seem to be fairly typical bronchogenic carcinomas in smoking males. The prevalence of lung cancer in SLE is only 3 per 100,000, well below the likely "background" lung cancer prevalence for the population under study. Of course, this could be confounded by a younger mean age in the SLE cohort. Careful epidemiological study of this issue is hampered by the relative rarity of cases.

Mineral Pneumoconiosis and Lung Cancer

Mention was made earlier of the possible role of metal dust exposure in conferring risk of lung cancer in IPF, notwithstanding the implications that such exposure may have for the diagnosis of IPF. More important, probably, in numerical terms are cases of lung cancer arising in patients exposed to asbestos. There also appears to be some risk of lung cancer in those exposed to silica.

The subject of asbestos exposure and lung cancer has some controversial aspects, due no doubt, in part at least, to the medicolegal implications of such disease attribution. It is accepted that significant asbestos exposure confers an excess risk of lung cancer, estimated to be around a fivefold increase (Fig. 29-8). Tobacco smoke exposure confounds many of the studies, but there seems to be a multiplicative effect when subjects are exposed to both asbestos and tobacco. This synergism may result in a 60-fold increased risk of lung cancer, compared to a fivefold risk for asbestos exposure alone, and a tenfold risk for non–asbestos-exposed smokers.[44]

Rather like the situation with CTD, however, there is controversy over the issue of whether fibrosis is required for lung cancer risk to be elevated in asbestos-exposed subjects.[45–48] Is asbestosis required for a patient to have an excess risk of lung cancer or is it simply a marker of a particularly heavy exposure to the mineral? There does appear to be an elevated risk of lung cancer in patients who have pleural plaques. These lesions are also markers of asbestos exposure but cannot in any way be considered an actual precursor lesion for lung cancer development. The same arguments regarding atypical epithelial proliferation associated with fibrosis in IPF and CTD, acting as an unstable progenitor epithelium for lung cancer development, may be applied in the case of asbestosis. Lung cancers do occur in the lower lobe fibrotic zones in asbestosis patients, and many of these tumors are adenocarcinomas. However, most evidence suggests that the tumors found in asbestos-exposed cohorts show the same cell type distribution to those found in non–asbestos-exposed smokers.[49,50] It has been questioned how pulmonary fibrosis could play a role in the development of bronchogenic squamous cell and small cell carcinomas. This seems a fair point although the possibility of inflammatory cytokines and other mediators being released in one part of the lung (the peripheral parenchyma), yet having an effect on more distant epithelium, for example that lining proximal airways, cannot be denied. These findings would rather

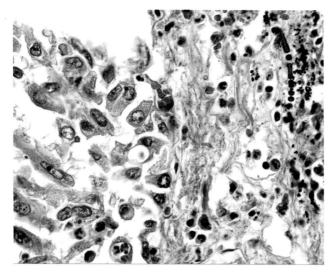

FIGURE 29-8 This is a case of poorly differentiated adenocarcinoma that arose in a lung affected by asbestosis in a smoker. Pleomorphic adenocarcinoma cells are seen spilling into an alveolar space on the left, while the fibrotic interstitium on the right shows both anthracotic pigment and a typical beaded ferruginous (asbestos) body.

FIGURE 29-9 This lung shows nodular silicosis with conglomerate nodules (the black lesions), but adenocarcinoma has also developed in a multifocal distribution, as seen in the white tissue infiltrates present in both lobes.

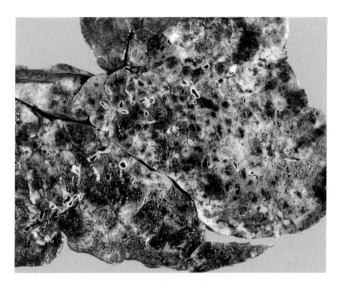

point to some synergism, at a cellular level, in either peripheral bronchioloalveolar or central bronchial epithelium, between asbestos and tobacco carcinogens.

If it is accepted that fibrosis (asbestosis) is not prerequisite for lung cancer in asbestos-exposed individuals, is there an association between degree of exposure and risk of lung cancer? Most evidence suggests that there is in effect a dose-response relationship; higher risk in those with heaviest exposure.[44,45] Thus, asbestos fiber counts amounting to those levels associated with asbestosis would be associated with a greater risk than lesser levels, which still pose some risk to the affected individual. Some authors point to the excess risk of lung cancer in those with pleural plaques but no asbestosis in support of this assertion. It is more difficult to define a lower limit, but there is probably a fiber count below which there is only a negligible risk of lung cancer due to that mineral burden.

The mechanism of asbestos-related carcinogenesis is not clear. Originally considered a promoter of tobacco carcinogen-initiated tumors, asbestos is now accepted as a complete carcinogen. Asbestos appears to be able to induce chromosomal damage; certain loci of chromosomes 2p, 19p, and 19q seem especially at risk.[51,52] Recent work has demonstrated that there may be a particular mRNA expression signature, characteristic of lung cancer in asbestos-exposed subjects.[53] If this proves to be a robust, repeatable finding, it could have important implications for attribution of cause in individual lung cancer cases. It has also been suggested that asbestos may induce malignancy by acting as a vector for carcinogens, by transporting into cells molecules adsorbed onto the fiber surface.[52] Immunological mediators and oxidative damage have been suggested as causes of disruption to intracellular signaling pathways, as a mechanism of carcinogenesis in those with asbestos in their lungs. Of course, this argument can equally well be applied to those who smoke tobacco.

Very similar arguments apply in the case of silica-induced lung cancer. There is controversy around whether or not fibrosis (silicosis) is required for the increased risk of lung cancer (Fig. 29-9).[54-56] Similar pathogenesis of disease is suggested, involving inflammatory and immune mediators with a questionable role for fibrosis-associated epithelial proliferation.[57] Certainly silica is a more cytotoxic mineral than asbestos; unlike asbestos, it appears to induce death in macrophages that phagocytose the mineral.

CONGENITAL CYSTIC ADENOMATOID MALFORMATIONS

In patients with type 1 congenital cystic adenomatoid malformation (CCAM), the surrounding lung tissue may show small groups of sometimes atypical mucous cells lining alveolar walls; cells similar to those found in the cyst lining. These cells in the alveoli are believed to be the progenitors of the mucinous adenocarcinomas showing a lepidic growth pattern (the so-called multifocal mucinous bronchioloalveolar carcinoma) that may be found in patients with CCAM.[58] The malignancy of these lesions has been questioned, but there are reports of cases that are slowly progressive; some patients have developed invasive mixed-type adenocarcinoma. Cases have been reported in patients as young as 11 years old but also in adults, in some cases many years after resection of the original CCAM. Excision of the cyst would not remove any foci of mucigenic cells in the surrounding lung parenchyma. Several studies have reported molecular changes in these mucigenic cell foci consistent with their putative role as a tumor precursor. Gains of genetic material in chromosomes 2 and 4 have been found using comparative genomic hybridization. *KRAS* mutations have been found in both intracystic and pericystic parenchymal foci of mucous cell hyperplasia, as well as in associated carcinomas. Some hyperplastic mucous cell foci have demonstrated LOH for the *P16, FHIT,* or *RB* genes, all potentially relevant to lung carcinogenesis.[59,60] CCAM may also, rarely, be associated with rhabdomyosarcoma. Type IV CCAM is also reported to carry a risk of transformation into pleuropulmonary blastoma.

JUVENILE TRACHEOBRONCHIAL SQUAMOUS PAPILLOMATOSIS

This condition is associated with HPV infection and malignant transformation to squamous cell carcinoma is an uncommon occurrence in this rare disease (Figs. 29-10 and 29-11). Malignant transformation appears to be variably associated with a history of tobacco smoking, previous radiation therapy for control of multifocal papillomatosis, or infection with HPV types 6a, 11, 16, and 18.[61,62] Papillomas may develop dysplastic prior to the onset of invasion, although in the limited literature on this subject this is not a universal finding. Some authors report overexpression of Rb and p53 protein and a decrease in expression of p21(waf1/cip1) with the onset of dysplasia.[63]

OTHER CYSTS, BRONCHIECTASIS, AND PULMONARY SEQUESTRATION

There are occasional reports in the literature of other lesions that were associated with a lung cancer. In reported cases of tumor in association with either a bronchogenic cyst or a "lung cyst," the carcinoma present was described as mucinous bronchioloalveolar in type.[64,65] This raises a question as to whether or not these cystic lesions were, in fact, CCAMs. The author has recently

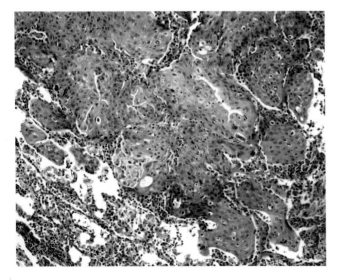

FIGURE 29-10 Medium-power image of squamous papillomatosis showing extension of nests of squamous papillomatosis epithelium within alveolar spaces.

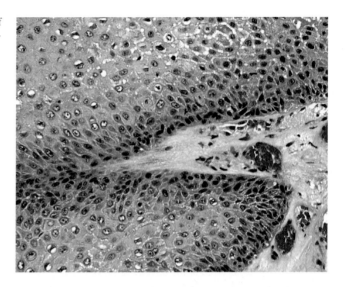

FIGURE 29-11 High-power image of squamous papillomatosis showing koilocytic cells and condylomatous atypia.

diagnosed a case of invasive acinar pattern adenocarcinoma arising in the wall of a chronic tuberculous cavity that was colonized by aspergillus fungi. Cases of squamous carcinoma have been reported, arising in the walls of chronic bronchiectatic airways or within a pulmonary sequestration.[66–68] In each of these circumstances, it is easy to speculate that squamous metaplasia, common in the chronically inflamed airways in both these conditions, may provide the "at risk" epithelium in each case. Several mentions have already been made of the possibility of inflammatory mediators, which would undoubtedly be present in these cases, being involved in the carcinogenic process. When dealing with any such case, the pathologist should be sure that bronchiectasis or any cystic change associated with a carcinoma has not actually been caused by the tumor through airway obstruction, before ascribing the origin of the carcinoma to preexisting chronic lung disease.

SUMMARY

This discussion has considered the risks and associations of primary lung carcinoma in a variety of different preexisting lung diseases. Although there are many differences between at least some of these conditions, a possible unifying factor is the presence of an abnormal epithelium, pathogenetically related to the underlying condition, which predisposes the individual to developing malignancy. In some cases, the etiological agents responsible for the underlying disease (asbestos, silica, etc.) may also be carcinogens capable of inducing tumors. In other circumstances, the preexisting disease may provide a background "field" of abnormal epithelium that is vulnerable to the transforming effects of regular carcinogenic agents such as tobacco smoke. A recurring theme in these conditions is the possible role that inflammation and immunological mediators may play in driving the carcinogenic process. This hypothesis also has its advocates in the context of chronic bronchitis as a factor in the development of lung cancer. Certainly, patients with COPD and a reduced FEV1 are included in cohorts considered at particularly high risk of developing lung cancer in some lung cancer screening studies.

References

1. Rossle R. Die Narbenkrebse der Lungen. *Schweiz Med Wochenschr*. 1943;73:1200–1203.
2. Raeburn C, Spencer H. A study of the origin and development of lung cancer. *Thorax*. 1953;8:1–10.
3. Carroll R. The influence of lung scars on primary lung cancer. *J Path Bact*. 1962;83:293–297.

4. Spencer H. Lung scar cancer. In: Shimosato Y, Melamed MD, Nettesheim P, eds. *Morphogenesis of Lung Cancer.* Vol 1. Boca Raton, FL: CRC Press; 1982:111–120.

5. Auerbach O, Garfinkel L, Parks VR. Scar cancer of the lung. Increase over a 21 year period. *Cancer.* 1979;43:636–642.

6. Bakris GL, Mulopulos GP, Korchik R, et al. Pulmonary scar carcinoma. A clinicopathological analysis. *Cancer.* 1983;52:493–497.

7. Edwards C, Carlile A. Scar adenocarcinoma of the lung: a light and electron microscopic study. *J Clin Pathol.* 1986;39:423–427.

8. Shimosato Y, Hashimoto T, Kodama T, et al. Prognostic implications of fibrotic focus (scar) in small peripheral lung cancers. *Am J Surg Pathol.* 1980;4:365–373.

9. Shimosato Y, Kodama T, Kameya T. Morphogenesis of peripheral type adenocarcinoma of the lung. In: Shimosato Y, Melamed MR, Nettesheim P, eds. *Morphogenesis of Lung Cancer.* Vol 1. Boca Raton, FL: CRC Press; 1982:65–90.

10. Suzuki A. Growth characteristics of peripheral type adenocarcinoma in terms of roentgenologic findings. In: Shimosato Y, Melamed MR, Nettesheim P, eds. *Morphogenesis of Lung Cancer.* Vol 1. Boca Raton, FL: CRC Press; 1982:91–110.

11. Kishi K, Homma S, Kurosaki A, et al. Small lung tumors with the size of 1cm or less in diameter: clinical, radiological, and histopathological characteristics. *Lung Cancer.* 2004;44:43–51.

12. Takashima S, Maruyama Y, Hasegawa M, et al. Prognostic significance of high-resolution CT findings in small peripheral adenocarcinoma of the lung: a retrospective study on 64 patients. *Lung Cancer.* 2002;36:289–295.

13. Madri JA, Carter D. Scar cancers of the lung: origin and significance. *Hum Pathol.* 1984;15:625–631.

14. El-Torkey M, Giltman LI, Dabbous M. Collagens in scar carcinoma of the lung. *Am J Pathol.* 1985;121:322–326.

15. Barsky SH, Huang SJ, Bhuta S. The extracellular matrix of pulmonary scar carcinomas is suggestive of a desmoplastic origin. *Am J Pathol.* 1986;124:412–419.

16. Daniels CE, Jett JR. Does interstitial lung disease predispose to lung cancer? *Curr Opin Pulm Med.* 2005;11:431–437.

17. Le Jeune I, Gribbin J, West J, et al. The incidence of cancer in patients with idiopathic pulmonary fibrosis and sarcoidosis in the UK. *Respir Med.* 2007;101:2534–2540.

18. Stack BH, Choo-Kang YF, Heard BE. The prognosis of cryptogenic fibrosing alveolitis. *Thorax.* 1972;27:535–542.

19. Fraire AE, Greenberg SD. Carcinoma and diffuse interstitial fibrosis of lung. *Cancer.* 1973;31:1078–1086.

20. Ma Y, Seneviratne CK, Koss M. Idiopathic pulmonary fibrosis and malignancy. *Curr Opin Pulm Med.* 2001;7:278–282.

21. Matsushita H, Tanaka S, Saiki Y, et al. Lung cancer associated with usual interstitial pneumonia. *Pathol Int.* 1995;45:925–932.

22. Qunn L, Takemura T, Ikushima S, et al. Hyperplastic epithelial foci in honeycomb lesions in idiopathic pulmonary fibrosis. *Virchows Arch.* 2002;441:271–278.

23. Mizushima Y, Kobayashi M. Clinical characteristics of synchronous multiple lung cancer associated with idiopathic pulmonary fibrosis. A review of Japanese cases. *Chest.* 1995;108:1271–1277.

24. Turner-Warwick M, Lebowitz M, Burrows B, et al. Cryptogenic fibrosing alveolitis and lung cancer. *Thorax.* 1980;35:496–499.

25. Meyer EC, Liebow AA. Relationship of interstitial pneumonia honeycombing and atypical epithelial proliferation to cancer of the lung. *Cancer.* 1965;18:322–351.

26. Aubry MC, Myers JL, Douglas WW, et al. Primary pulmonary carcinoma in patients with idiopathic pulmonary fibrosis. *Mayo Clin Proc.* 2002;77:763–770.

27. Sakai S, Ono M, Nishio T, et al. Lung cancer associated with diffuse pulmonary fibrosis: CT-pathologic correlation. *J Thorac Imaging.* 2003;18:67–71.

28. Hironaka M, Fukayama M. Pulmonary fibrosis and lung carcinoma: a comparative study of metaplastic epithelia in honeycombed areas of usual interstitial pneumonia with or without lung carcinoma. *Pathol Int.* 1999;49:1060–1066.

29. Samet JM. Does idiopathic pulmonary fibrosis increase lung cancer risk? *Am J Respir Crit Care Med.* 2000;161:1–2.

30. Hubbard R, Venn A, Lewis S, et al. Lung cancer and cryptogenic fibrosing alveolitis. A population-based cohort study. *Am J Respir Crit Care Med.* 2000;161:5–8.

31. Baumgartner KB, Samet JM, Stidley CA, et al. Cigarette smoking—a risk factor for idiopathic pulmonary fibrosis. *Am J Respir Crit Care Med.* 1997;155:242–248.

32. Kawasaki H, Ogura T, Yokose T, et al. p53 gene alteration in atypical epithelial lesions and carcinoma in patients with idiopathic pulmonary fibrosis. *Hum Pathol.* 2001;32:1043–1049.

33. Takahashi T, Munakata M, Ohtsuka Y, et al. Expression and alteration of ras and p53 proteins in patients with lung carcinoma accompanied by idiopathic pulmonary fibrosis. *Cancer.* 2002;95:624–633.

34. Murata K, Ota S, Niki T, et al. p63—key molecule in the early phase of epithelial abnormality in idiopathic pulmonary fibrosis. *Exp Mol Pathol.* 2007;83:367–376.

35. Demopoulos K, Arvanitis DA, Vassilakis DA, et al. MYCL1, FHIT, SPARC, p16(INK4) and TP53 genes associated to lung cancer in idiopathic pulmonary fibrosis. *J Cell Mol Med.* 2002;6:215–222.

36. Ohno S, Oshikawa K, Kitamura S, et al. Clinicopathological analysis of interstitial pneumonia associated with collagen vascular disease in patients with lung cancer. (In Japanese. English abstract). *Nihon Kyobu Shikkan Gakkai Zasshi.* 1997;35:1324–1329.

37. Yang Y, Fujita J, Tokuda M, et al. Lung cancer associated with several connective tissue diseases: with a review of literature. *Rheumatol Int.* 2001;21:106–111.

38. Adzi TN, Pesut DP, Nagorni-Obradovi LM, et al. Clinical features of lung cancer in patients with connective tissue diseases: a 10-year hospital based study. *Respir Med.* 2008;102:620–624.

39. Wooten M. Systemic sclerosis and malignancy: a review of the literature. *South Med J.* 2008;101: 59–62.

40. Matteson EL, Hickey AR, Maguire L, et al. Occurrence of neoplasia in patients with rheumatoid arthritis enrolled on DMARD Registry. Rheumatoid Arthritis Azathioprine Registry Steering Committee. *J Rheumatol.* 1991;18:809–814.

41. Fujita J, Tokuda M, Bandoh S, et al. Primary lung cancer associated with polymyositis/dermatomyositis, with a review of the literature. *Rheumatol Int.* 2001;20:81–84.

42. Bin J, Bernatsky S, Gordon C, et al. Lung cancer in systemic lupus erythematosus. *Lung Cancer.* 2007;56:303–306.

43. Bernatsky S, Clarke A, Suissa S. Lung cancer after exposure to disease modifying anti-rheumatic drugs. *Lung Cancer.* 2008;59:266–269.

44. Selikoff EJ, Hammond EC, Churg J. Asbestos exposure, smoking and neoplasia. *JAMA.* 1968;204: 104–110.

45. Henderson DW, de Klerk NH, Hammar SP, et al. Asbestos and lung cancer: is it attributable to asbestosis or asbestos fibre burden? In: Corrin B, eds. *Pathology of Lung Tumours.* Edinburgh: Churchill Livingstone; 1997:83–118.

46. Henderson DW, Rödelsperger K, Woitowitz HJ, et al. After Helsinki: a multidisciplinary review of the relationship between asbestos exposure and lung cancer, with emphasis on studies published during 1997–2004. *Pathology.* 2004;36:517–550.

47. Helsinki Consensus Report, Asbestos, asbestosis and cancer: the Helsinki criteria for diagnosis and attribution. *Scand J Work Environ Health.* 1997;23:311–316.

48. Gibbs A, Attanoos RL, Churg A, et al. The "Helsinki criteria" for attribution of lung cancer to asbestos exposure: how robust are the criteria? *Arch Pathol Lab Med.* 2007 Feb;131(2):181–183.

49. Auerbach O, Garfinkel L, Parks VR, et al. Histological type of lung cancer and asbestos exposure. *Cancer.* 1984;54:3017–3021.

50. Churg A. Lung cancer cell type and asbestos exposure. *JAMA.* 1985;253:2984–2985.

51. Nymark P, Wikman H, Hienonen-Kempas T, et al. Molecular and genetic changes in asbestos-related lung cancer. *Cancer Lett.* 2008;265:1–15.

52. Toyokuni S. Mechanisms of asbestos-induced carcinogenesis. *Nagoya J Med Sci.* 2009;71:1–10.

53. Ruosaari S, Hienonen-Kempas T, Puustinen A, et al. Pathways affected by asbestos exposure in normal and tumour tissue of lung cancer patients. *BMC Med Genomics.* 2008;1:55.

54. Weill H, McDonald JC. Exposure to crystalline silica and risk of lung cancer: the epidemiological evidence. *Thorax.* 1995;51:97–102.

55. Brown T. Silica exposure, smoking, silicosis and lung cancer—complex interactions. *Occup Med (Lond).* 2009;59:89–95.

56. Lacasse Y, Martin S, Gagn? D, et al. Dose-response meta-analysis of silica and lung cancer. *Cancer Causes Control.* 2009;20:925–933.

57. Otsuki T, Maeda M, Murakami S, et al. Immunological effects of silica and asbestos. *Cell Mol Immunol.* 2007;4:261–268.

58. MacSweeney F, Papagiannopoulos K, Goldstraw P, et al. An assessment of the expanded classification of congenital cystic adenomatoid malformations and their relationship to malignant transformation. *Am J Surg Pathol.* 2003;27:1139–1146.

59. Stacher E, Ullmann R, Halbwedl I, et al. Atypical goblet cell hyperplasia in congenital cystic adenomatoid malformation as a possible preneoplasia for pulmonary adenocarcinoma in childhood: a genetic analysis. *Hum Pathol.* 2004;35:565–570.

60. Lantuejoul S, Nicholson AG, Sartori G, et al. Mucinous cells in type 1 pulmonary congenital cystic adenomatoid malformation as mucinous bronchioloalveolar carcinoma precursors. *Am J Surg Pathol.* 2007;31:961–969.

61. Popper HH, el-Shabrawi Y, Wockel W, et al. Prognostic importance of human papilloma virus typing in squamous cell papilloma of the bronchus: comparison of in situ hybridisation and the polymerase chain reaction. *Hum Pathol.* 1994;25:1191–1197.

62. Lele SM, Pou AM, Ventura K, et al. Molecular events in the progression of recurrent respiratory papillomatosis to carcinoma. *Arch Pathol Lab Med.* 2002;126:1184–1188.

63. Go C, Schwartz MR, Donovan DT. Molecular transformation of recurrent respiratory papillomatosis: viral typing and p53 overexpression. *Ann Otol Rhinol Laryngol.* 2003;112:298–302.

64. De Perrot M, Pache JC, Spiliopoulos A. Carcinoma arising in congenital lung cysts. *J Thorac Cardiovasc Surg.* 2001;49:184–185.

65. Prichard MG, Brown PJ, Sterrett GF. Bronchioloalveolar carcinoma arising in longstanding lung cysts. *Thorax.* 1984;39:545–549.

66. Bell-Thomson J, Missier P, Sommers SC. Lung carcinoma arising in bronchopulmonary sequestration. *Cancer.* 1979;44:334–339.

67. Konwaler BE, Reingold IM. Carcinoma arising in bronchiectatic cavities. *Cancer.* 1952;5:525–529.

68. Tonelli P. A morphological study of nodular lung carcinomas and their possible pathogenesis from a cluster of non-obstructive bronchiectasis. *Lung Cancer.* 1997;17:135–145.

30

Lung Cancer Stem Cells

▶ Timothy Craig Allen

Although lung stem cells and the hypothesis of lung cancer stem cells do not fit the typical paradigm of preneoplastic and preinvasive lesions, a brief review of lung cancer stem cells is warranted in this section, as the molecular changes and other characteristics of preneoplasia are associated with lung cancer stem cells. Human beings normally possess germ cells. Populations of germinal stem cells produce eggs and sperm. Embryonic stem cells are undifferentiated totipotent cells derived from blastocysts that have the capacity to propagate indefinitely, and develop into more differentiated cell lineages both in vivo and in vitro.[1–7] Originally, embryonic stem cells appeared to have the greatest potential to provide future therapeutic benefits; however, legal, ethical, and policy considerations, as well as medical and technical issues such as tumorigenicity of the embryonic stem cells, contamination with animal material, and genetic compatibility have prevented the potential benefits of embryonic stem cells from being fully explored.[8–10] Nonetheless, cultures of human embryonic stem cells have reportedly been differentiated into lung epithelial-like tissue.[11]

ADULT STEM CELLS

Somatic, or adult, stem cells are another population of stem cells identified in human beings. Somatic stem cells have a limited capacity for self renewal and play a role in tissue self-renewal. Important for tissue repair and regeneration, somatic stem cells have been identified in a variety of tissues, including hematopoietic, neural, epidermal mammary, hepatic, mesenchymal, gastrointestinal, and pulmonary tissues. Telomeres, attached to the inner nuclear surface, are required for stability of individual chromosomes and the appropriate segregation of chromosomes during cell division. It is suspected that telomerase, important in maintaining telomere activity, is limited in somatic stem cells, thus limiting the self-renewal capacity of somatic stem cells. Adult stem cells include hematopoietic stem cells, typically found in the bone marrow, mesenchymal stem cells, and stem cells residing in specific organs, termed progenitor cells. Organ-specific progenitor cells are generally believed to aggregate in special tissue microenvironments, termed the stem cell niche.[12–40] These stem cell niches are thought to be located in areas of an organ with abundant vasculature and with growth factors from surrounding cells promoting the survival and self-renewal of the stem cells, allowing for the proper balance of self-renewal and differentiation.[41] Besides for promoting survival, the stem cell niche microenvironment also appears to promote drug resistance.[41–43] While still controversial, it is thought that these progenitor cell populations in the lung may arise from differentiation of embryonic stem cells; however, these cells have also been considered to possibly arise from hematopoietic stem cells or mesenchymal stem cells.[44–46]

CANCER STEM CELLS, LUNG STEM CELLS, AND LUNG CANCER STEM CELLS

Currently, there is evidence suggesting that both hematopoietic tumors and solid tumors are derived from organ-specific cancer stem cells, or related progenitor cells.[47–49] The cancer stem cell hypothesis is generally accepted as relevant to the development of solid malignancies.[50,51] Stem cell transformation into malignant cells is the origin of tumor cell populations and has only relatively recently become the subject of much attention with the emergence of supportive evidence from the study of hematologic malignancies.[52] It is thought that these antigenically distinct cancer stem cells make up a population of expanding progenitor cells that sustain the tumor mass as variably differentiated, possibly heterogeneous tumor cells; as well as a population of renewing cancer stem cells. Stem cells, self-renewing and long-lived, are the cells most likely to live long enough to accumulate sufficient molecular changes necessary for malignant transformation.[41,53] As such, characterization and destruction of the terminally differentiated cells may be less important therapeutically than the identification, characterization, regulation, and destruction of the cancer stem cells.

Cancer stem cells, supposedly rare cells that have the self-renewal properties, have the pluripotentiality, and result in the production of a hierarchy of progenitor and differentiated cells as normal stem cells, have been relatively well examined in hematopoietic malignancies. Leukemia stem cells have been found to be necessary and sufficient for leukemia maintenance. Cancer stem cells have been identified in a variety of leukemias, including acute myeloid leukemia and chronic myeloid leukemia.[54–57] Initial genetic hits have been identified in stem cells associated with hematopoietic tumors.[41] Once stem cells in the lung become malignant, these cells then proliferate, dividing to form one differentiated daughter cell and one daughter stem cell, maintaining the lung cancer stem cell population. Similar findings have been shown with some solid malignancies, including brain and breast tumors.[50,51,56,58] Disseminated or migrating cancer stem cells probably play a causative role in the development of metastatic disease.[59] Studies also show these cancer stem cells to exhibit resistance to chemotherapy and radiotherapy.[51] Lung cancers are often heterogeneous; but it is currently uncertain whether different cancer stem cell clones cause tumor heterogeneity or whether cancer stem cells have the pluripotentiality of normal stem cells.[60]

Rather than the existence of a single, pleuripotential stem cell population in the lung, studies have provided evidence of several stem cell populations in normal lung that are relatively specific to certain areas of the lung.[29,61–66] Strongly CK5-immunopositive basal cells within submucosal gland ducts in the mouse trachea have been identified and are considered possible stem cells or progenitor cells involved in regeneration or repair of tracheal epithelium.[61] Clara cell secretory protein expressing cells, also termed CE cells, and basal cells that line mouse bronchi may be stem cells or progenitor cells.[65,67,68] The bronchioles in the mouse lung, CE cells, associated with pulmonary neuroendocrine cells, are arranged in small bodies of cells termed neuroepithelial bodies. The CE cells in the bronchioles are pollution resistant, most likely due to cellular deficiency of the drug-metabolizing enzyme CYP450 2F2.[66] The bronchioloalveolar duct junction in mice has been shown to contain pollution-resistant CE cells, not associated with neuroepithelial bodies, exhibiting both alveolar epithelia type II cell marker, surfactant protein C, and Clara cell secretory protein. These cells probably play a reparative role for the terminal bronchioles, alveolar ducts, and alveoli.[64] These cells were identified as stem cells due to their expression of stem cell surface markers Sca-1 and CD34. Another stem cell niche of "variant" Clara cells has been identified arising in the same location.[63,64,69] A third possible stem cell population has been identified, differing from the bronchioloalveolar stem cell population noted above by their CD34 immunonegativity, and their immunopositivity with Oct-4 and SSEA-1, both embryonic stem cell markers related to self-renewal and puripotency.[70,71] Oct-4 positivity suggests the possibility that bronchioloalveolar stem cells arise from Oct-4 positive neonatal lung cells.[69,72] Homeostatic regulation of bronchioloalveolar stem cell niches has been associated with expression of several tumor suppressor genes.[69] In mouse lung studies, stem cell niches have been identified that maintain epithelial differentiation within the airways. These niches are likely targets for lung cancer initiation and promotion.[26,64,65] It is thought that there may be as many as 40 different epithelial, mesenchymal, vascular, and lymphatic endothelial and immune cell lineages in the lung.[24,73] It is important to remember that "lung cancer" is actually a variety of malignant pulmonary neoplasms that arise from cells that are phenotypically different.[24,26,33]

LUNG CANCER STEM CELL REGULATION, GENE EXPRESSION, AND CELL SURFACE MARKERS

There have been some common molecular pathways identified that are important in the development of cancer stem cells. Three embryonic patterning pathways, Notch, Hedgehog, and Wnt, are involved in early events leading to expansion and malignant transformation of normal stem cells in the lung.[69,74] The Notch pathway is important for development and homeostasis in stem cells, and helps stem cells maintain viability by asymmetric cell division. Notch signaling is required for lung development, and elevated Notch ligand and receptor levels have been shown in non–small cell lung cancer cell lines.[69,75] The Hedgehog pathway is also important in early lung formation, and studies have shown it to be involved in epithelial-mesenchymal interactions controlling the branching of developing lung buds. In adult lungs, Hedgehog signaling is normally identified only at low levels in rare cells located in bronchial epithelium basal layers.[69,76–78] Persistent activation of the Hedgehog pathway has been shown in small cell lung cancers, but uncommonly in non–small cell lung cancer cell lines.[26,79] Wnt pathway signaling is also important in early lung development and lung disease.[26,80,81] Wnt pathway disruption has been found to be a factor in the development of non–small cell lung cancers.[26,82,83] These three pathways offer opportunities for future therapeutic intervention.

There are other genes involved with cancer stem cells, including Oct-4 (also termed "Oct-3" and "POU5F1"), a gene regulated by the Wnt pathway that is involved in the maintenance of stem cell pluripotency. Interestingly, Oct-4 has been shown to be capable of reprogramming committed somatic cells and induce those cells to dedifferentiate and revert to an earlier, more developmentally potent state. Keratinocytes that overexpress Oct-4 have been shown to differentiate into other cell types.[26,84,85]

There are various cell surface markers that may help identify cancer stem cells.[26,86] These and future markers are important in helping to identify these stem cell niches and to identify mechanisms that transform normal stem cells into cancer stem cells. CD44, a transmembrane cell surface adhesion glycoprotein involved in cell-cell interactions and cell-matrix interactions, linked to chemoresistance and poor prognosis in various malignant neoplasms, is increased in, and correlates with survival in, both non–small cell lung cancer and small cell lung cancer.[26,86–88] CD133, also termed Prominin-1, is a glycoprotein found in endothelial cells that has been identified in cancer-initiating stem cells of the brain, pancreas, and colon. As with CD44, CD133 is associated with chemoresistance.[89] Non–small cell lung cancers and small cell lung cancers have been found to have CD133 positive tumor cell subpopulations, showing similarities to a rare CD133 positive population of normal mouse lung cells that undergo significant expansion after naphthalene-induced lung injury.[26, 86, 90] Phosphatase and tensin homologue deleted on chromosome ten (*Pten*) inactivation in side population cells have been shown to result in spontaneous lung tumors; and studies have shown that activation of Mammalian Target of Rapamycin (mTOR), involved in expression of CD133 in cancer cells, is related to upregulation of stem cells and progenitor cells in *Pten* conditional deletion models, suggesting that mTOR may be a potential therapeutic target.[91–93]

CD117, also termed c-Kit, is a stem cell factor in neuroendocrine lung tumors that is related to poor prognosis in early stage non–small cell lung cancers; however, less than one third of patients exhibit CD117 tumor cell positivity.[26,86,94] While other solid organ cancers, such as brain and breast cancers, have demonstrated a variety of putative cancer stem cell markers, few other potential cancer stem cell markers have to date been identified in lung cancers. Unfortunately, two cell surface markers found in mouse bronchioloalveolar stem cells have given disappointing results in human studies. Sca1 does not have a human counterpart, and CD34 does not correlate with putative human non–small cell lung cancer stem cells. Additional studies are necessary to identify and confirm whether each type of lung cancer arises from a single, normal lung stem cell, or whether there are multiple stem cell origins responsible for each cancer's cellularity.[86,95] The cell surface markers urokinase plasminogen activator (uPA) and its receptor uPAR, also termed

CD87, have been identified in small cell lung cancer cells that coexpress CD44; however, their contribution to the development and maintenance of a lung cancer stem cell population is not currently known.[26,96]

LUNG CANCER STEM CELLS AND CHEMO- AND RADIORESISTANCE

Importantly, both normal stem cells and cancer stem cells have demonstrated resistance to toxic compounds, allowing these cells to generally survive frequent airborne damage. These stem cells often exhibit a so-called side population phenotype, based on the cells' expression of ATP Binding Cassette (ABC) Transporter proteins. These side population cells are detected by efflux of Hoechst and other dyes by ABC transporters that allows for efficient drug efflux. These cells show enhanced efflux of doxorubicin, cisplatinum, and mitoxantrone, and are associated with chemoresistance. While it is currently unknown whether this "side population" are true stem cells, these cells have been shown to exhibit characteristics of stem cells, including tumor formation *in vivo* and enhanced clonogenicity.[26,55,66,97–101] Aldehyde dehydrogenase, a drug-resistance gene identified in normal hematopoietic stem cells, has been identified in a variety of cancers, including non–small cell lung cancer. It is important in the oxidation of retinal to all-*trans* retinoic acid, conferring drug resistance to various chemotherapeutic agents, including cyclophosphamide.[26,102–104]

PRENEOPLASIA

Epithelial metaplasia, an initially adaptive reaction to persisting tissue injury, is the beginning of the metaplasia-dysplasia-carcinoma continuum. Whether the causes of tissue injury that lead to metaplasia also play a causative role in dysplasia and neoplasia, and whether the inflammatory response accompanying metaplastic changes has an effect cellular, including stem cell, gene expression, remain unknown. Studies have associated metaplastic epithelium with deregulated production of receptors, cell adhesion molecules, and soluble mediators of the inflammatory response, including cytokines, prostaglandins, free radicals, and chemokines, all of which could result in genetic changes.[105] Therefore, not surprisingly research suggests that injurious agents that lead to metaplasia may have a direct injurious effect on bronchial epithelium, as well as an indirect effect via soluble inflammatory mediators from metaplastic and immune cells. Indeed, antioxidative and chemopreventative therapies have decreased the incidence of the transformation of Barrett esophagus to esophageal cancer. Much needs to be determined about lung stem cells and their relationship to metaplasia and dysplasia, including whether characteristics of stem cells that produce metaplastic cells; whether there are stem cell niches within metaplastic epithelium, and if so, where they are located; how inflammatory mediators within the metaplastic microenvironment affect stem cell niches; and what signaling pathways are involved or altered in stem cells that produce metaplastic epithelium.[105–108]

FUTURE OUTLOOK

The study of lung cancer stem cells is, if not in its infancy, an emerging field that has great potential to increase understanding of lung cancer origin, development, and potential improved therapies. A main goal is to identify lung cancer stem cell surface markers that are robust enough to help identify lung cancer stem cell niches. Once these stem cells and their niches are identified, the intricate pathways that allow for the development of cancer stem cells from normal lung stem cells, including their roles in the development and advancement of the continuum of dysplasias, can be better understood, with the hope of more specific, molecular-based, lung cancer therapies.

Future lung cancer stem cell research may focus on signaling pathways that could be therapeutic targets, such as the ABC transporter activity identified in lung cancer side population cells, in an attempt to reduce or eliminate chemoresistance. Among many possible research avenues, future stem cell research geared toward improved lung cancer treatment may include further studies of Oct-4 in lung cancer; studies involving therapeutically targeting CD133 overexpression; further examination of the Wnt, Hedgehog, and Notch signaling pathways in an attempt to find therapeutic targets; targeting of stem cells or stem cell niches with nanoparticles; further study of stem cell niches, including the vascular and other properties involved in maintaining the niche; and further studies of gene therapy as it relates to stem cells. Future research will undoubtedly also attempt to provide a better understanding of the relationship between stem cells and preneoplasia.

References

1. Baylis F, Robert JS. Human embryonic stem cell research: an argument for national research review. *Account Res.* 2006;13:207–224.
2. Bhattacharya B, Puri S, Puri RK. A review of gene expression profiling of human embryonic stem cell lines and their differentiated progeny. *Curr Stem Cell Res Ther.* 2009;4:98–106.
3. Pera MF, Reubinoff B, Trounson A. Human embryonic stem cells. *J Cell Sci.* 2000;113(Pt 1):5–10.
4. Pittenger MF, Mackay AM, Beck SC, et al. Multilineage potential of adult human mesenchymal stem cells. *Science.* 1999;284:143–147.
5. Reubinoff BE, Pera MF, Fong CY, et al. Embryonic stem cell lines from human blastocysts: somatic differentiation in vitro. *Nat Biotechnol.* 2000;18:399–404.
6. Shamblott MJ, Axelman J, Wang S, et al. Derivation of pluripotent stem cells from cultured human primordial germ cells. *Proc Natl Acad Sci USA.* 1998;95:13726–13731.
7. Thomson JA, Itskovitz-Eldor J, Shapiro SS, et al. Embryonic stem cell lines derived from human blastocysts. *Science.* 1998;282:1145–1147.
8. Gruen L, Grabel L. Concise review: scientific and ethical roadblocks to human embryonic stem cell therapy. *Stem Cells.* 2006;24:2162–2169.
9. Cohen CB. Ethical and policy issues surrounding the donation of cryopreserved and fresh embryos for human embryonic stem cell research. *Stem Cell Rev Rep.* 2009;5:116–122.
10. Mertes H, Pennings G. Cross-border research on human embryonic stem cells: legal and ethical considerations. *Stem Cell Rev Rep.* 2009;5:10–17.
11. Van Haute L, De Block G, Liebaers I, et al. Generation of lung epithelial-like tissue from human embryonic stem cells. *Respir Res.* 2009;10:105.
12. Delorme B, Nivet E, Gaillard S, et al. The human nose harbours a niche of olfactory ecto-mesenchymal stem cells displaying neurogenic and osteogenic properties. *Stem Cells Dev.* 2010;19:853–866.
13. Kuhn NZ, Tuan RS. Regulation of stemness and stem cell niche of mesenchymal stem cells: Implications in tumorigenesis and metastasis. *J Cell Physiol.* 2010;222:268–277.
14. Robin C, Bollerot K, Mendes S, et al. Human placenta is a potent hematopoietic niche containing hematopoietic stem and progenitor cells throughout development. *Cell Stem Cell.* 2009;5:385–395.
15. Nishikawa SI, Osawa M, Yonetani S, et al. Niche required for inducing quiescent stem cells. *Cold Spring Harb Symp Quant Biol.* 2008;73:67–71.
16. Coura GS, Garcez RC, de Aguiar CB, et al. Human periodontal ligament: a niche of neural crest stem cells. *J Periodontal Res.* 2008;43:531–536.
17. Raaijmakers MH, Scadden DT. Evolving concepts on the microenvironmental niche for hematopoietic stem cells. *Curr Opin Hematol.* 2008;15:301–306.
18. Takao T, Tsujimura A. Prostate stem cells: the niche and cell markers. *Int J Urol.* 2008;15:289–294.
19. Shiozawa Y, Havens AM, Pienta KJ, et al. The bone marrow niche: habitat to hematopoietic and mesenchymal stem cells, and unwitting host to molecular parasites. *Leukemia.* 2008;22:941–950.
20. Xie T, Li L. Stem cells and their niche: an inseparable relationship. *Development.* 2007;134:2001–2006.
21. Quinones-Hinojosa A, Sanai N, Gonzalez-Perez O, et al. The human brain subventricular zone: stem cells in this niche and its organization. *Neurosurg Clin N Am.* 2007;18:15–20,vii.
22. Walker MR, Patel KK, Stappenbeck TS. The stem cell niche. *J Pathol.* 2009;217:169–180.
23. Alison MR, Lebrenne AC, Islam S. Stem cells and lung cancer: future therapeutic targets? *Expert Opin Biol Ther.* 2009;9:1127–1141.

24. Warburton D, Perin L, Defilippo R, et al. Stem/progenitor cells in lung development, injury repair, and regeneration. *Proc Am Thorac Soc.* 2008;5:703–706.

25. Bellusci S. Lung stem cells in the balance. *Nat Genet.* 2008;40:822–824.

26. Pine SR, Marshall B, Varticovski L. Lung cancer stem cells. *Dis Markers.* 2008;24:257–266.

27. Kotton DN, Fine A. Lung stem cells. *Cell Tissue Res.* 2008;331:145–156.

28. Loebinger MR, Janes SM. Stem cells for lung disease. *Chest.* 2007;132:279–285.

29. Giangreco A, Groot KR, Janes SM. Lung cancer and lung stem cells: strange bedfellows? *Am J Respir Crit Care Med.* 2007;175:547–553.

30. Liu X, Driskell RR, Engelhardt JF. Stem cells in the lung. *Methods Enzymol.* 2006;419:285–321.

31. Yen CC, Yang SH, Lin CY, et al. Stem cells in the lung parenchyma and prospects for lung injury therapy. *Eur J Clin Invest.* 2006;36:310–319.

32. Stripp BR, Shapiro SD. Stem cells in lung disease, repair, and the potential for therapeutic interventions: State-of-the-art and future challenges. *Am J Respir Cell Mol Biol.* 2006;34:517–518.

33. Berns A. Stem cells for lung cancer? *Cell.* 2005;121:811–813.

34. Kotton DN, Summer R, Fine A. Lung stem cells: new paradigms. *Exp Hematol.* 2004;32:340–343.

35. Pitt BR, Ortiz LA. Stem cells in lung biology. *Am J Physiol Lung Cell Mol Physiol.* 2004;286: L621–L623.

36. Otto WR. Lung epithelial stem cells. *J Pathol.* 2002;197:527–535.

37. Otto WR. Lung stem cells. *Int J Exp Pathol.* 1997;78:291–310.

38. Mason RJ, Williams MC, Moses HL, et al. Stem cells in lung development, disease, and therapy. *Am J Respir Cell Mol Biol.* 1997;16:355–363.

39. Soltysova A, Altanerova V, Altaner C. Cancer stem cells. *Neoplasma.* 2005;52:435–440.

40. Artandi SE, Depinho RA. Telomeres and telomerase in cancer. *Carcinogenesis.* 2010;31:9–18.

41. Gangemi R, Paleari L, Orengo AM, et al. Cancer stem cells: a new paradigm for understanding tumor growth and progression and drug resistance. *Curr Med Chem.* 2009;16:1688–1703.

42. De Toni F, Racaud-Sultan C, Chicanne G, et al. A crosstalk between the Wnt and the adhesion-dependent signaling pathways governs the chemosensitivity of acute myeloid leukemia. *Oncogene.* 2006;25: 3113–3122.

43. Dick JE, Lapidot T. Biology of normal and acute myeloid leukemia stem cells. *Int J Hematol.* 2005;82: 389–396.

44. Kannan S, Wu M. Respiratory stem cells and progenitors: overview, derivation, differentiation, carcinogenesis, regeneration and therapeutic application. *Curr Stem Cell Res Ther.* 2006;1:37–46.

45. Nilsson SK, Simmons PJ. Transplantable stem cells: home to specific niches. *Curr Opin Hematol.* 2004;11:102–106.

46. Kotton DN, Ma BY, Cardoso WV, et al. Bone marrow-derived cells as progenitors of lung alveolar epithelium. *Development.* 2001;128:5181–5188.

47. Kitamura H, Okudela K, Yazawa T, et al. Cancer stem cell: implications in cancer biology and therapy with special reference to lung cancer. *Lung Cancer.* 2009;66:275–281.

48. Lobo NA, Shimono Y, Qian D, et al. The biology of cancer stem cells. *Annu Rev Cell Dev Biol.* 2007;23:675–699.

49. Rapp UR, Ceteci F, Schreck R. Oncogene-induced plasticity and cancer stem cells. *Cell Cycle.* 2008;7:45–51.

50. Er O. Cancer stem cells in solid tumors. *Onkologie.* 2009;32:605–609.

51. O'Brien CA, Kreso A, Dick JE. Cancer stem cells in solid tumors: an overview. *Semin Radiat Oncol.* 2009;19:71–77.

52. Trosko JE. Review paper: cancer stem cells and cancer nonstem cells: from adult stem cells or from reprogramming of differentiated somatic cells. *Vet Pathol.* 2009;46:176–193.

53. Hanahan D, Weinberg RA. The hallmarks of cancer. *Cell.* 2000;100:57–70.

54. Lapidot T, Sirard C, Vormoor J, et al. A cell initiating human acute myeloid leukaemia after transplantation into SCID mice. *Nature.* 1994;367:645–648.

55. Reya T, Morrison SJ, Clarke MF, et al. Stem cells, cancer, and cancer stem cells. *Nature.* 2001;414:105–111.

56. Galmozzi E, Facchetti F, La Porta CA. Cancer stem cells and therapeutic perspectives. *Curr Med Chem.* 2006;13:603–607.

57. Guan Y, Gerhard B, Hogge DE. Detection, isolation, and stimulation of quiescent primitive leukemic progenitor cells from patients with acute myeloid leukemia (AML). *Blood.* 2003;101:3142–3149.

58. McDonald SA, Graham TA, Schier S, et al. Stem cells and solid cancers. *Virchows Arch.* 2009;455:1–13.

59. Brabletz S, Schmalhofer O, Brabletz T. Gastrointestinal stem cells in development and cancer. *J Pathol.* 2009;217:307–317.

60. Tesei A, Zoli W, Arienti C, et al. Isolation of stem/progenitor cells from normal lung tissue of adult humans. *Cell Prolif.* 2009;42:298–308.

61. Borthwick DW, Shahbazian M, Krantz QT, et al. Evidence for stem-cell niches in the tracheal epithelium. *Am J Respir Cell Mol Biol.* 2001;24:662–670.

62. Daniely Y, Liao G, Dixon D, et al. Critical role of p63 in the development of a normal esophageal and tracheobronchial epithelium. *Am J Physiol Cell Physiol.* 2004;287:C171—C181.

63. Kim CF, Jackson EL, Woolfenden AE, et al. Identification of bronchioalveolar stem cells in normal lung and lung cancer. *Cell.* 2005;121:823–835.

64. Giangreco A, Reynolds SD, Stripp BR. Terminal bronchioles harbor a unique airway stem cell population that localizes to the bronchoalveolar duct junction. *Am J Pathol.* 2002;161:173–182.

65. Hong KU, Reynolds SD, Watkins S, et al. Basal cells are a multipotent progenitor capable of renewing the bronchial epithelium. *Am J Pathol.* 2004;164:577–588.

66. Reynolds SD, Giangreco A, Power JH, et al. Neuroepithelial bodies of pulmonary airways serve as a reservoir of progenitor cells capable of epithelial regeneration. *Am J Pathol.* 2000;156:269–278.

67. Reynolds SD, Malkinson AM. Clara cell: progenitor for the bronchiolar epithelium. *Int J Biochem Cell Biol.* 2010;42:1–4.

68. Wong AP, Keating A, Waddell TK. Airway regeneration: the role of the Clara cell secretory protein and the cells that express it. *Cytotherapy.* 2009;11:676–687.

69. Peacock CD, Watkins DN. Cancer stem cells and the ontogeny of lung cancer. *J Clin Oncol.* 2008;26:2883–2889.

70. Saito S, Liu B, Yokoyama K. Animal embryonic stem (ES) cells: self-renewal, pluripotency, transgenesis and nuclear transfer. *Hum Cell.* 2004;17:107–115.

71. Ling TY, Kuo MD, Li CL, et al. Identification of pulmonary Oct-4+ stem/progenitor cells and demonstration of their susceptibility to SARS coronavirus (SARS-CoV) infection in vitro. *Proc Natl Acad Sci USA.* 2006;103:9530–9535.

72. Kim CB. Advancing the field of lung stem cell biology. *Front Biosci.* 2007;12:3117–3124.

73. Warburton D. Developmental biology: order in the lung. *Nature.* 2008;453:733–735.

74. Wicha MS, Liu S, Dontu G. Cancer stem cells: an old idea–a paradigm shift. *Cancer Res.* 2006;66:1883–1890 [discussion 1895–6].

75. Lowry WE, Richter L. Signaling in adult stem cells. *Front Biosci.* 2007;12:3911–3927.

76. Watkins DN, Berman DM, Baylin SB. Hedgehog signaling: progenitor phenotype in small-cell lung cancer. *Cell Cycle.* 2003;2:196–198.

77. Watkins DN, Berman DM, Burkholder SG, et al. Hedgehog signalling within airway epithelial progenitors and in small-cell lung cancer. *Nature.* 2003;422:313–317.

78. van Tuyl M, Post M. From fruitflies to mammals: mechanisms of signalling via the Sonic hedgehog pathway in lung development. *Respir Res.* 2000;1:30–35.

79. Vestergaard J, Pedersen MW, Pedersen N, et al. Hedgehog signaling in small-cell lung cancer: frequent in vivo but a rare event in vitro. *Lung Cancer.* 2006;52:281–290.

80. Pongracz JE, Stockley RA. Wnt signalling in lung development and diseases. *Respir Res.* 2006;7:15.

81. Warburton D, Bellusci S, De Langhe S, et al. Molecular mechanisms of early lung specification and branching morphogenesis. *Pediatr Res.* 2005;57:26R–37R.

82. Mazieres J, He B, You L, et al. Wnt inhibitory factor-1 is silenced by promoter hypermethylation in human lung cancer. *Cancer Res.* 2004;64:4717–4720.

83. You L, He B, Xu Z, et al. Inhibition of Wnt-2-mediated signaling induces programmed cell death in non-small-cell lung cancer cells. *Oncogene.* 2004;23:6170–6174.

84. Pesce M, Scholer HR. Oct-4: gatekeeper in the beginnings of mammalian development. *Stem Cells.* 2001;19:271–278.

85. Grinnell KL, Yang B, Eckert RL, et al. De-differentiation of mouse interfollicular keratinocytes by the embryonic transcription factor Oct-4. *J Invest Dermatol.* 2007;127:372–380.

86. Yagui-Beltran A, He B, Jablons DM. The role of cancer stem cells in neoplasia of the lung: past, present and future. *Clin Transl Oncol.* 2008;10:719–725.

87. Desai B, Rogers MJ, Chellaiah MA. Mechanisms of osteopontin and CD44 as metastatic principles in prostate cancer cells. *Mol Cancer.* 2007;6:18.

88. Liu J, Jiang G. CD44 and hematologic malignancies. *Cell Mol Immunol.* 2006;3:359–365.

89. Bertolini G, Roz L, Perego P, et al. Highly tumorigenic lung cancer CD133+ cells display stem-like features and are spared by cisplatin treatment. *Proc Natl Acad Sci USA*. 2009;106:16281–16286.

90. Eramo A, Lotti F, Sette G, et al. Identification and expansion of the tumorigenic lung cancer stem cell population. *Cell Death Differ*. 2008;15:504–514.

91. Hill R, Wu H. PTEN, stem cells, and cancer stem cells. *J Biol Chem*. 2009;284:11755–11759.

92. Matsumoto K, Arao T, Tanaka K, et al. mTOR signal and hypoxia-inducible factor-1 alpha regulate CD133 expression in cancer cells. *Cancer Res*. 2009;69:7160–7164.

93. Yanagi S, Kishimoto H, Kawahara K, et al. Pten controls lung morphogenesis, bronchioalveolar stem cells, and onset of lung adenocarcinomas in mice. *J Clin Invest*. 2007;117:2929–2940.

94. Pelosi G, Barisella M, Pasini F, et al. CD117 immunoreactivity in stage I adenocarcinoma and squamous cell carcinoma of the lung: relevance to prognosis in a subset of adenocarcinoma patients. *Mod Pathol*. 2004;17:711–721.

95. Ho MM, Ng AV, Lam S, et al. Side population in human lung cancer cell lines and tumors is enriched with stem-like cancer cells. *Cancer Res*. 2007;67:4827–4833.

96. Gutova M, Najbauer J, Gevorgyan A, et al. Identification of uPAR-positive chemoresistant cells in small cell lung cancer. *PLoS ONE*. 2007;2:e243.

97. Summer R, Kotton DN, Sun X, et al. Side population cells and Bcrp1 expression in lung. *Am J Physiol Lung Cell Mol Physiol*. 2003;285:L97–L104.

98. Majka SM, Beutz MA, Hagen M, et al. Identification of novel resident pulmonary stem cells: form and function of the lung side population. *Stem Cells*. 2005;23:1073–1081.

99. Reynolds SD, Shen H, Reynolds PR, et al. Molecular and functional properties of lung SP cells. *Am J Physiol Lung Cell Mol Physiol*. 2007;292:L972—L983.

100. Mitsutake N, Iwao A, Nagai K, et al. Characterization of side population in thyroid cancer cell lines: cancer stem-like cells are enriched partly but not exclusively. *Endocrinology*. 2007;148:1797–1803.

101. Sabisz M, Skladanowski A. Cancer stem cells and escape from drug-induced premature senescence in human lung tumor cells: implications for drug resistance and in vitro drug screening models. *Cell Cycle*. 2009;8:3208–3217.

102. Pearce DJ, Taussig D, Simpson C, et al. Characterization of cells with a high aldehyde dehydrogenase activity from cord blood and acute myeloid leukemia samples. *Stem Cells*. 2005;23:752–760.

103. Russo J, Barnes A, Berger K, et al. 4-(*N*,*N*-dipropylamino)benzaldehyde inhibits the oxidation of all-trans retinal to all-trans retinoic acid by ALDH1A1, but not the differentiation of HL-60 promyelocytic leukemia cells exposed to all-trans retinal. *BMC Pharmacol*. 2002;2:4.

104. Baum C, Fairbairn LJ, Hildinger M, et al. New perspectives for cancer chemotherapy by genetic protection of haematopoietic cells. *Expert Rev Mol Med*. 1999;1999:1–28.

105. Herfs M, Hubert P, Delvenne P. Epithelial metaplasia: adult stem cell reprogramming and (pre)neoplastic transformation mediated by inflammation? *Trends Mol Med*. 2009;15:245–253.

106. Zhou H, Calaf GM, Hei TK. Malignant transformation of human bronchial epithelial cells with the tobacco-specific nitrosamine, 4-(methylnitrosamino)-1-(3-pyridyl)-1-butanone. *Int J Cancer*. 2003;106:821–826.

107. Limburg PJ, Wei W, Ahnen DJ, et al. Randomized, placebo-controlled, esophageal squamous cell cancer chemoprevention trial of selenomethionine and celecoxib. *Gastroenterology*. 2005;129:863–873.

108. Martin RC, Liu Q, Wo JM, et al. Chemoprevention of carcinogenic progression to esophageal adenocarcinoma by the manganese superoxide dismutase supplementation. *Clin Cancer Res*. 2007;13:5176–5182.

Index

Note: Page numbers followed by t indicate table. Page numbers in italics indicate figure.